COCHLEAR IMPLANTS

COCHLEAR IMPLANTS

Edited by ROGER F. GRAY

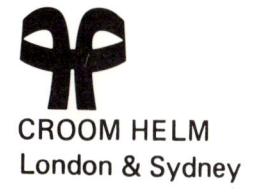

CROOM HELM
London & Sydney

COLLEGE-HILL PRESS, INC.
San Diego, CA 92105

© 1985 Roger F. Gray
Croom Helm Ltd, Provident House, Burrell Row,
Beckenham, Kent BR3 1AT
Croom Helm Australia Pty Ltd, First Floor, 139 King Street,
Sydney, NSW 2001, Australia

British Library Cataloguing in Publication Data

Cochlear implants.
  1. Cochlear implants
  I. Gray, Roger F.
  617.8'82   RF305

  ISBN 0-7099-1163-7

College-Hill Press, Inc.
4284 41st Street
San Diego, CA 92105

Library of Congress Cataloging in Publication Data
Main entry under title:

Cochlear implants.

  Includes bibliographies and index.
  1. Cochlear implants. I. Gray, Roger F.,
1946—   . [DNLM: 1. Auditory Prosthesis.
WV 274 C6614]
RF305.C629 1985   617.8'82   85-13320
ISBN 0-933014-70-8

Printed and bound in Great Britain

CONTENTS

Preface		vii
List of Contributors		ix
1.	The History of Cochlear Implants *William M. Luxford and Derald E. Brackmann*	1
2.	The Physiology of the Cochlea *James O. Pickles*	27
3.	Cochlear Anatomy and Histopathology *Lars-Goran Johnsson*	50
4.	Cochlear Implant Design and Construction *Stephen J. Rebscher*	74
5.	Selection of Patients *J. Graham Fraser*	124
6.	Surgical Implantation *Robert A. Schindler and Roger F. Gray*	141
7.	Complications and Failures of Cochlear Implants *Roger F. Gray and Robert A. Schindler*	152
8.	Speech Coding for Cochlear Implants *Brian C.J. Moore*	163
9.	The Results from Various Viewpoints *John Ballantyne*	180
10.	Rehabilitation of the Cochlear-Implant Patient *Brigitte Eisenwort, Karin Brauneis and Kurt Burian*	194
11.	The Engineering of Future Cochlear Implants *Graeme M. Clark and Yit C. Tong*	211
Glossary		229
Index		233

*To
Pat Jobson and David Wright for the opportunity,
and
Michael Merzenich and Robert Schindler for the inspiration*

PREFACE

This work brings together in book form, worldwide attempts to relieve total deafness by electronic means. Microphones exist which will detect sounds outside the range of normal human hearing. Video cameras exist which will show detail of the earth's surface from a satellite in space. These brilliant artefacts extend man's sensory powers by many orders of magnitude. Why can't the same technology relieve deafness, blindness or other sensory failure in man?

The stumbling block is the point of contact with the nervous system through which this torrent of information must pour. The auditory nerve has some 32,000 separate fibres. Designing and installing so many access points is not readily achieved! The following chapters illustrate the achievements made so far with a single or small number of channels and also the uncertainty about the best way to code the signals to be delivered.

About 450 people (most of whom lost hearing after the crucial years for acquisition of speech and language) have been fitted with a cochlear implant and declare that they hear environmental sounds and the rhythms of speech. There is no doubt that they do, nor doubt that it dramatically aids their lip reading. A small number of 'Star' patients are able to hear much more. Their abilities to understand test sentences and words, without lip reading, is remarkable. Research projects can be found in many countries, enthusiastically funded by agencies impressed by the performance of 'Star' patients.

Where is the need for such devices? Meningitis, trauma, ear infections and ototoxic drugs still deprive people all over the world of their hearing. For example, it is estimated that in China up to 5 million people are totally deaf as a result of streptomycin, an ototoxic antibiotic developed in the late 1940s, freely used for three decades to treat life-threatening and trivial infections alike. More generally, one child or more in a thousand is born deaf in all countries. It is therefore to be fervently hoped that cochlear implants will play as fine a part in minimising the educational and social effects of congenital deafness as hearing aids have done in the West since they were introduced forty years ago.

The story of cochlear implants is one of excitement and enthusiasm from those who have seen them in action, but it is also one of obstacles and obstructions of all sorts. Contributors to this book have addressed both sides of this story in the pages which follow.

Roger F. Gray

LIST OF CONTRIBUTORS

John Ballantyne, FRCS, Consultant Otolaryngologist, 18 Upper Wimpole Street, London W1M 7TB, England

Derald E. Brackmann, MD, Otologic Medical Group Inc., 2122 West Third Street, Los Angeles, California 90057, USA

Karin Brauneis, ENT Department, University of Vienna, University Hospital, Alser Strasse 4 1090 Vienna, Austria

Kurt Burian, MD, Professor of Otolaryngology, ENT Department, University of Vienna, University Hospital, Alser Strasse 4 1090 Vienna, Austria

Graeme M. Clark, FRCS, Professor of Otolaryngology, University of Melbourne, Department of Otolaryngology, Royal Victorian Hospital, 32 Gisborne Street, East Melbourne, Vic. 3002, Australia

Brigitte Eisenwort, ENT Department, University of Vienna, University Hospital, Alser Strasse 4 1090 Vienna, Austria

J. Graham Fraser, FRCS, Consultant Otolaryngologist, Royal Ear Hospital, Huntley Street, London WC1E 6AU, England

Roger F. Gray, FRCS, Consultant Otolaryngologist, Addenbrooke's Hospital, Hills Road, Cambridge CB2 2QQ, England

Lars-Goran Johnsson, MD, Consultant Otolaryngologist, University of Helskini, University Ear Hospital, Haartmaninkatu 4E 00290, Helskini 29, Finland, and visiting Professor, Kresge Hearing Research Institute, University of Michigan Medical School, Ann Arbor, Michigan, USA

William M. Luxford, MD, Otologic Medical Group Inc., 2122 West Third Street, Los Angeles, California 90057, USA

Brian C.J. Moore, PhD, Lecturer, University of Cambridge, Department of Experimental Psychology, Downing Street, Cambridge CB2 3EB, England

James O. Pickles, PhD, Lecturer, Department of Physiology, University of Birmingham, The Medical School, Vincent Drive, Birmingham B15 2TJ, England

Stephen Rebscher, BSc, Design Engineer, School of Medicine, Department of Otolaryngology 863 HSE, University of California, San Francisco, California 94143, USA

Robert A. Schindler, MD, Professor of Otolaryngology, School of Medicine, Department of Otolaryngology HSE 863, University of California, San Francisco, California 94143, USA

Yit C. Tong, FRCS, ENT Department, University of Melbourne, Department of Otolaryngology, Royal Victorian Hospital, 32 Gisborne Street, East Melbourne, Vic. 3002, Australia

1 THE HISTORY OF COCHLEAR IMPLANTS

William M. Luxford and Derald E. Brackmann

Electrical stimulation for medical purposes is not a new idea. Roman physicians in the early years after the birth of Christ recommended the electrical discharge of the torpedo fish for the treatment of headache and gout (McNeal, 1977, pp. 3–35). Electrical stimulation of the intact auditory system was attempted almost 200 years ago. Simmons (1966, pp. 2–54) has reviewed extensively the early history of electrical stimulation of the auditory system. The following historical review to the 1960s is from his work.

Volta, in 1790, inserted metal rods into each ear and connected them to a circuit which produced approximately 50 volts. Upon closing the circuit, he experienced the sensation which he described as a blow to the head, followed by a sound like the boiling of a viscous liquid. Volta's unpleasant experience probably discouraged others and only a few reported on electrical stimulation of the auditory system over the next 50 years.

Interest in electrical stimulation was revived in the latter half of the nineteenth century. Prominent otologists, including Politzer and Gradenigo, advocated electrical stimulation for diagnosis and therapy of many ear diseases. A new field of 'electro-otiatrics' was founded. This field soon fell into disfavour as other physicians advocated electricity for diagnosis and treatment in many diseases in which it had no benefit. Therefore, by the start of the twentieth century most reputable physicians had abandoned its use.

Two separate events resurrected the interest in electrical stimulation of the auditory system. (1) In 1925 radio engineers discovered that auditory sensations could be produced by stimulating electrodes near the ear with a modulated alternating current. (2) In 1930 Weaver and Bray discovered the electrical potential (now known as the cochlear microphonic) which arises in the cochlea as a result of acoustic stimulation.

Stevens termed the first event 'electrophonic hearing' in 1937 and he, Jones, Lurie and Flottorp studied this over several years (Figure 1.1). Electrophonic hearing results when an alternating electrical current in the audible frequency range is passed from an electrode to the skin. The electrode and the skin surface act as two plates of a condenser microphone. The resulting auditory vibrations are transmitted to the cochlea by air and bone conduction and auditory sensations are produced. The electrode may be placed in the external or middle ear, as well as on the skin. The possible frequency range for electrophonic hearing is from 150 Hz to 12,000 Hz. The maximum loudness is approximately 40 dB sensation level; the limiting factor is the pain threshold of the skin. In all types of electrophonic hearing, a normal or near normal cochlea is a prerequisite. Therefore, electrophonic stimulation of hearing has no application in the hearing impaired.

The discovery of the cochlear microphonic gave rise to the concept that the

Figure 1.1: Electrophonic Hearing. This is lost if the ear is damaged.

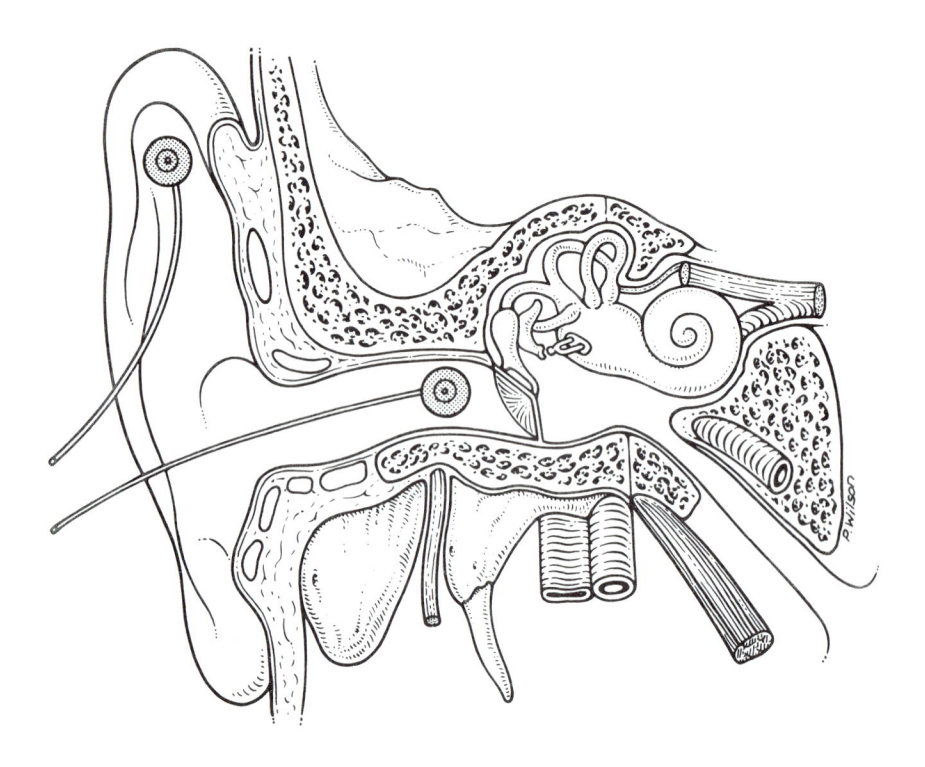

cochlea acted essentially as a transducer of acoustical to electrical energy, creating enthusiasm for the possibility of artificial hearing through direct electrical stimulation of the cochlear nerve.

The first report of stimulation of the acoustic nerve by direct application of an electrode in a totally deaf person was in 1957 by Djourno and Eyries (Figure 1.2). A 50-year-old man previously operated upon for cholesteatoma was being reoperated for repair of a facial nerve paralysis. During this surgery an induction coil and an indifferent electrode were permanently implanted in the temporalis muscle and an active lead was placed on a segment of the auditory nerve visible through an opening in the vestibule. The coil was later stimulated by induction currents from a second coil placed against the overlying skin. An electronic stimulator that generated pulse stimuli at a rate of 100 per second, interrupted 20 times per minute, was used. The subject reported sounds like 'crickets' or a 'roulette wheel'. When other signal generators were used, the subject perceived a change in stimulus up to but not above 1000 cycles per second. The patient was aware of background sound. He used his increased awareness of the speech rhythm to improve his speech reading ability and in time could apparently distinguish a few simple words. He was unable to develop any real speech discrimination.

Figure 1.2: Djourno and Eyries' Direct Stimulation of the Auditory Nerve in 1957. The induction coil is not shown.

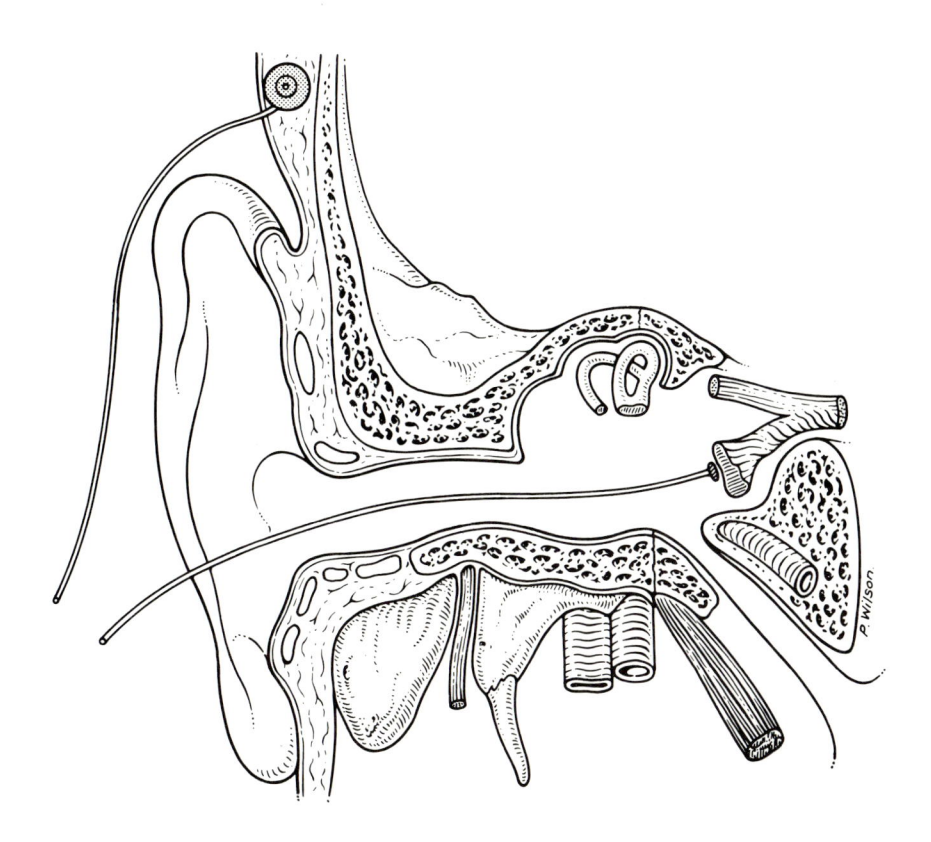

The optimistic view of the potential benefits of electrical stimulation of the inner ear, as detailed in newspaper accounts of the work of Djourno and Eyries, was dampened by the considerable doubt about the safety of inserting anything into the inner ear. However, the possibility of developing a safe cochlear implant accelerated in the late 1950s with the evolution and developments of microsurgical techniques, stapes surgery, and the mastoid facial recess approach to the middle ear and round window. Electrical stimulation as treatment for profound sensorineural hearing loss would become a reality in the following decades.

The Sixties

The Investigators — House, Simmons and Michelson

Stimulated by the reports of Djourno and Eyries, Dr William F. House (1976, pp. 3–6) began his investigation into the effect of electrical stimulation on the inner ear in 1960–1. He studied the responses to electrical stimulation of several patients undergoing stapes surgery. A square wave generator stimulated electrodes placed on the promontory and/or into the vestibule through the open oval window. Less current was needed when the electrode was in the vestibule than on the promontory, but the subjects reported the same sensation of hearing (electrophonic hearing) regardless of the electrode location. The important finding was that direct electrical stimulation of the perilymph did not seem to cause discomfort, dizziness, or facial nerve twitching for signals above 30 Hz. However, when frequencies at and below 20 Hz were used, the patient experienced a sensation of dizziness suggesting activation of the vestibular system. The sensation of sound was not reported at the frequencies the patient experienced dizziness. From this experience and that of others studying the electrode and tissue tolerance related to thermal, chemical and electrolytic factors in animals, it was felt that a profoundly hearing-impaired person could be implanted with reasonable safety.

In 1961 Dr House stimulated a postlingually deaf man. The aetiology of deafness was unknown. The patient reported a sensation of hearing with square wave stimulation through a promontory electrode within the range of 40–200 Hz. The patient was subsequently implanted with a single, hard-wire gold electrode placed in the scala tympani via the ear canal and round window.

A second patient, a woman deafened by congenital lues in her late twenties, also had a hard-wire gold electrode placed into her scala tympani. Gold was used at the time because it was felt a pure metal would cause less reaction by electrolysis. Both patients perceived a sensation of hearing with electrical stimulation. However, because of infection, the wire was soon removed from the second patient and in an attempt to obtain better loudness tolerance, the first patient was soon changed to a five-wire electrode induction coil system. Implantation was through the facial recess and round window into the scala tympani. The ground electrode was placed in the temporalis muscle. The electrodes were insulated with silicone rubber. The stimulus was a square wave frequency of 100 Hz, amplitude modulated with the electrical analogue of sound. The device was rejected two weeks after implantation.

Encouraged by the patients' reports of pleasant and useful hearing sensations with electrical stimulation, House worked with Jack Urban, an electrical engineer, in developing more sophisticated and reliable implant systems. Before completion of the first of these new systems in 1969, however, the work of other investigators added to the information available on electrical stimulation in man and animals.

Simmons (1966, pp. 2–54) reported extensively on the direct electrical stimulation of the auditory nerve in a 60-year-old man with a right profound and left severe sensorineural hearing loss. He was implanted with a hard-wire cluster of six stainless-steel electrodes into the auditory nerve through the modiolus on the right.

The electrodes were very well tolerated over a several-month period during which time the patient was studied intensively. Simmons found that electrical pulses through such electrodes could be used to excite relatively discrete groups of nerve fibres. The usual stimulus was a train of bisphasic pulses or a sinusoid. Both monopolar and bipolar stimulation was used. The dynamic range of stimulus amplitude from threshold to uncomfortable loudness was 15 to 25 dB. Loudness of the sensation increased with the amplitude and pulse duration of the stimulation current, and to a lesser extent, with repetition rate. Monopolar excitation at threshold required less current than bipolar stimuli. At threshold levels, excitation of two discrete groups of fibres did not summate or otherwise interact. At higher intensities, the fibres did interact. At times simultaneous stimulation in two electrodes produced sensations which retained their perceptual identity and sometimes they fused to form a different third sound. Subjective pitch sensation from 70 to 300 Hz was influenced by electrode selection, stimulus repetition rate, and current intensity.

From the study, Simmons felt both periodicity and place pitch were possible with modiolar electrodes. Speech and speech modulated waveforms were recognised by the patient primarily on the basis of their irregular envelopes and amplitudes. Separating the speech spectrum into frequency bands to channel the stimuli into the various electrodes failed to produce any speech discrimination. The electrodes were removed after the completion of the study.

Michelson (1968, pp. 626-44) working with cats found that intracochlear electrodes could function safely for long periods and were well tolerated in the experimental animals.

During the 1960s as in the 1950s there were other developments that aided the progress of cochlear implants. Advances in cardiac pacemakers increased the knowledge of biocompatible materials, insulation of electrodes, and effects of electrical stimulation. The developments in electronics as a spinoff of the space industry allowed for better and smaller circuit designs.

These initial efforts in electrically stimulating the acoustic nerve acted as a springboard for these three investigators and for several others into the 1970s.

Cochlear Implant Terminology

As the programmes developed, so did the cochlear implant terminology. For clarity it is best to describe the parts of the various systems. A glossary of technical terms can be found at the end of the book.

Though there are specific differences between implants, the main components are the microphone that sends an electrical equivalent of an acoustic stimulus to the signal processor. The processor transforms the electrical input into the desired electrical stimuli. From the processor the stimulus is transferred to the implanted system where the stimulus travels down one or more electrodes to excite the auditory nerve.

The stimulus is transferred from the processor to the implanted system in two ways: either directly by wires through the skin, or transcutaneously across intact skin. The transcutaneous system must be capable of transferring both the information of the signal processor and the power necessary to run the internal components. Transfer of the information and power is through electromagnetic induction, ultrasound, radiofrequency, or other methods. The stimulus signal may be the strict analogue of auditory input, sine or square wave pulses, an amplitude modulated high frequency carrier, or another scheme.

The implant can be a multichannel or single-channel system. A multichannel system delivers different processed information to each stimulating electrode. A single-channel system delivers the same information to each electrode. A multichannel system requires by definition multiple active electrodes while a single-channel system may have one or more active electrodes.

An indifferent or ground electrode creates three possible configurations. In the monopolar configuration, the indifferent or ground electrode is placed away from the active electrodes usually in the region of the temporalis muscle. This creates a fairly large electric field with a large amount of current shunting through the relatively low resistance of the perilymph resulting in stimulation of a large number of neurons. In a bipolar system, the active and ground electrodes are close together. The exciting current applied between the two electrodes creates a much smaller electric field than the monopolar configuration allowing for stimulation of a discrete population of neurons. The third configuration, termed 'pseudo-bipolar', is a compromise between the monopolar and bipolar configurations and is found in multichannel systems (Parkins and Houde, 1982, pp. 332–56). Each stimulus channel has a bipolar pair of electrodes with separate active electrodes but the ground electrodes are connected as one common return. Implant design and coding schemes will be discussed in much more detail in further chapters.

Within the normal cochlea the mechnical energy of sound causes a displacement of the basilar membrane which results in the shearing action of the cilia of the hair cells. The resulting electrical potential probably through release of a chemical mediator causes the eighth nerve action potential. The action potential produced in the auditory nerve is carried centrally through multiple synapses to the auditory cortex.

The frequency of sound arriving at the cochlea is coded in two ways: by its periodicity or by the place of maximum displacement of the basilar membrane. Low frequency stimuli below 500–600 Hz are thought to be perceived through periodicity pitch while high frequency information is coded by place pitch. This is the subject of Chapter 2.

The Seventies

The cochlear implant gained notoriety in the seventies with radio and television publicity. As a result of that exposure the implant provided access to improved hearing for many patients who had been told years before they had a loss that could not be helped. On seeking the new operation, most found that advanced hearing aids would probably help them more than the implant would.

A selected group of deaf patients with realistic expectations did consent to take part in cochlear implant projects. The hearing sensations noted by patients on electrical stimulation led both to enthusiastic reports and sceptical comments. Questions concerning the how and why of electrical stimulation of the auditory system in a deaf individual were not easily answered. Questions were also raised about who should be implanted, which device should be used, what were the criteria of success, when should an implant be used, and the safety of the electrical stimulation. The seventies was a decade of controversy for the implant.

American Otological Society — 1971 and 1973

Michelson (1971, pp. 914–19) presented his work on cochlear implants in humans at the meeting of the American Otological Society in 1971. Initially four patients with severe sensorineural hearing losses were tested with electrical stimulation under local anaesthesia. Two of them heard only noise. They were felt to have a neural loss and were dropped from the study. The other two could recognise changes in pitch and were later implanted with permanent devices. Michelson implanted one other deaf volunteer. He used a single-channel bipolar scala tympani system. The electrode pair was mounted in a SilasticTM carrier moulded to fill the first half turn of the scala tympani. The leads were routed via a subcutaneous channel in the external auditory channel to the mastoid. The electrode leads terminated in a tiny amplitude modulated radio receiver beneath the skin. The electrical stimulus transferred to the receiver was the analogue signal of the acoustic stimulus. The signal and power were transferred transcutaneously by radio-frequency. The transmitter antenna was positioned and held in place over the receiver by a headband.

The discussion following Michelson's presentation raised the possibility that discrimination exhibited in the presented cases was not the result of direct stimulation of the auditory nerve but the result of an electrophonic effect on the remaining neural tissue in his deaf patients.

These patients were analysed in detail over the next two years by Merzenich *et al*. (1973, pp. 486–503). During the same time they performed studies on cats implanted with an intracochlear device similar except in size to the human implant. They presented their findings from their animal and patient studies at the American Otological Society in 1973. They found that, while patients respond to electrical stimulation from approximately 25 Hz to 10 kHZ, the useful range of pitch discrimination is limited to frequencies below 600 Hz. The patients noted a subjective change in sensation from a low to a higher tone with an increasing frequency of stimulation. This pitch change was noted as the stimulus was increased from 50 HZ to 500 HZ. Above 500–600 Hz the pitch changed little with increasing frequency. Therefore, the low-tone sensations generated by electrical stimulation were probably a result of periodicity pitch coding. There was no place pitch coding with the single-channel electrode. A narrow dynamic range was noted with electrical stimulation. They concluded from their cat studies that the responses noted by the patients did arise from direct electrical stimulation of the acoustic nerve. It was not electrophonic hearing arising from electromechanical excitation of hair cells.

At that same meeting in 1973, House and Urban (1973, pp. 504–17) reported on three profoundly deaf patients implanted in 1969 and 1970. A multiple-electrode device was placed through the round window into the scala tympani. The five intracochlear electrodes and a sixth ground electrode were connected to a percutaneous button embedded in the mastoid cortex. One of the patients developed infection around the button a few months after implantation and it had to be removed. Studies were performed on the other two subjects.

House and Urban used multichannel electrodes in an attempt to achieve both periodicity and place pitch and a hard-wire system to have better control of signal input. A stimulator was constructed in which a complex incoming signal could be divided into bandwidths with progressive distribution of the higher to lower frequencies from the basal to more apical electrodes. They found that the patients experienced an increase in pitch with an increase in stimulus rate for lower frequencies (periodicity pitch) and an increase in pitch as electrodes were stimulated progressively closer to the basal turn (place pitch).

Many variations of the stimulating signal were tried especially with one patient. They found the patient was able to perceive a 1000 Hz frequency if a second high frequency signal at a voltage just below the threshold of response was applied, and that without this 'sensitising' signal he could not. Thus, the concept of a carrier wave was developed. After trying multiple stimulating signals, the patient empirically felt the best input signal for speech was a 16 kHz carrier wave amplitude modulated by the electric analogue of sound. This simple circuit gave the same information to each electrode. The incoming signal was not separated into bandwidths. Because the patient felt he received so much benefit from single-channel stimulation, a single-wire induction system was constructed and implanted in the patient's other ear. At the time of the 1973 meeting, the patient had used a wearable take-home stimulator for approximately one year. He felt the implant certainly did help him with environmental sounds and lip-reading, though he could not understand speech.

The patient maintained similar electrical thresholds over the year that he was stimulated. House felt the stable electrical threshold was evidence that gross electrolysis of the electrodes had not taken place and that presumably electrical stimulation within the cochlea had not caused further degeneration of the remaining neural elements.

Kiang began the discussion that followed these two presentations. He had previously published information concerning electrical stimulation of the auditory nerve as compared to auditory stimulation (Kiang and Moxon, 1972, pp. 714–30). The conclusions involved tuning, timing, and dynamic range. Tuning and timing of the auditory nerve discharge did not exist when the nerve was stimulated electrically. The dynamic range while typically 20 to 40 dB for acoustical stimulation of a normal cochlea was reduced to less than 10 dB for electrical stimulation. At this meeting he discussed the importance of making use of the basic auditory physiology known then and the need, if investigators chose to continue human implant studies, for parallel animal experiments.

Simmons followed. Though he had not implanted other patients since the mid-1960s, he had continued to evaluate the effects of electrical stimulation in cats showing that modiolar electrodes were well tolerated and that they were possibly more effective than scala tympani stimulation (Simmons and Glattke, 1972, pp. 731–8). He raised a question concerning nerve fibre degeneration and forms of sensorineural hearing loss. Which types of sensorineural hearing loss have enough neural elements remaining that can be electrically stimulated and which do not?

Merzenich then challenged Kiang, whose remarks suggested little or no discriminative hearing could be generated from a single-electrode pair, to explain in terms of auditory nerve physiology why implanted patients described 'hearing' tones.

First International Conference on Electrical Stimulation — San Francisco

In an attempt to answer some of the questions raised at earlier meetings, the First International Conference on Electrical Stimulation of the Acoustic Nerve As a Treatment for Profound Sensorineural Deafness in Man was held in San Francisco in 1973. The proceedings (Merzenich et al., 1974, pp. 1–213) contained reports on auditory physiology, pathology, and of electrical stimulation both in animals and man. A few will be discussed here.

Spoendlin (1974, pp. 7–24) studied the degeneration of neural tissue after the destruction of the organ of Corti in guinea pigs by ototoxic antibiotics and acoustic trauma. In all animals, even after survival times of one and one-half years, there were always 5–10 per cent surviving ganglion cells. Hawkins (1974, pp. 47–62) and Schuknecht (1974, pp. 37–46) reviewing human temporal bones noted that for certain aetiologies (ototoxic and acoustic trauma) ganglion cells do survive hair cell loss. Schindler (1974, pp. 93–104) examined temporal bones of cats chronically implanted for periods of 3 to 117 weeks. If the basilar partition was not disrupted, there appeared to be little evidence of loss of spiral ganglion cells or radial nerve fibres and these cells appeared responsive to electrical stimulation in studies performed prior to death. Apparently the neurons are metabolically and physiologically independent of the hair cells but they are somewhat dependent on the supporting cells of the organ of Corti; therefore, any cochlear prosthesis should as much as possible respect the integrity of the organ of Corti.

Carhart (1974, pp. 171–8) addressed the effect of the periodicity information presented by electrical stimulation with a single-channel implant. He stated that volley information alone could be used for speech detection and as a supplement to lipreading by providing recognition of the intonation, rhythm, and melody of ongoing speech. But volley information alone would not allow for full understanding of conversation. Simmons (1974, pp. 123–6) discussed the utilisation of mainly rate pitch information in three children who had essentially no functioning hearing bilaterally above 750 Hz and reasonably normal hearing at lower frequencies. Although the losses developed before two years of age, all three children were able to communicate effectively.

Even though it appeared from the Carhart presentation that the low frequency information presented by a single-channel cochlear implant might be theoretically beneficial, and from the clinical presentations that patients did subjectively receive benefit from their single-channel implants, several participants felt that implantation of single-channel cochlear devices should be curtailed. These participants felt, since single-channel information would never provide full speech discrimination, that only multichannel devices which could theoretically provide speech discrimination should be implanted. Others considered single-channel devices therapeutic and that the implantation of single-channel systems should continue. All felt that implants should be limited to carefully selected adults.

Pittsburgh Evaluation of Single-Channel Cochlear Implants

In 1976 an independent evaluation of patients then implanted with a single-channel cochlear prosthesis was conducted by the staff of the Eye and Ear Hospital of Pittsburgh, Pennsylvania. The investigation was sponsored by the National Institute of Health (Bilger *et al.*, 1977, pp. 1–176). Thirteen patients, eleven of Dr William House and two of Dr Robin Michelson, were evaluated extensively over five days undergoing audiologic, vestibular and psychological testing.

Evaluation Summary. The conclusions of the Pittsburgh group concerning single-channel stimulation in the 13 patients were: (1) Patients with a single-channel prosthesis could detect environmental sounds over the entire frequency range at a 50–60 dB level. (2) Patients fitted with the prosthesis had significantly improved identification of environmental sounds. (3) The dynamic range of the patients was improved with the prosthesis. (4) The patients had significantly improved lipreading with the prosthesis. (5) Implants assisted postlingually deaf adults in monitoring their speech. (6) None of the patients developed significant speech discrimination. (7) Many of the patients benefited psychologically from the procedure. (8) All of the subjects found noise bothersome. (9) Activation of the prosthesis disrupted the stability of the patients during postural testing, but few complained of unsteadiness.

Electrical Auditory Stimulation — Ballantyne, Evans, and Morrison

To determine the possible benefits for the profoundly hearing-impaired in Great Britain these English physicians and their staffs reviewed extensively the state of development of cochlear implant work in the United States (Ballantyne *et al.*, 1978, pp. 1–117). Their findings were an excellent summary of all aspects of cochlear implantation including patient selection, staffing, facilities, operative techniques, complications and systems failures, long-term safety factors, engineering and coding strategies. It is worthwhile to review briefly their findings of different implant programmes in 1977 and 1978.

Los Angeles, San Francisco, and Stanford. All programmes regarded cochlear implants as experimental. The Stanford group under Dr Blair Simmons and the San Francisco group under Drs Robin Michelson and Michael Merzenich were committed to an exploitation of multichannel stimulation, although the implants performed to that time were single-channel. Though the Los Angeles group under Dr William House had begun work with multichannel implants, it had concentrated its efforts on single-channel devices and rehabilitation strategies to exploit the limited gains of single-electrode systems.

Patient selection. All groups agreed that only profoundly deaf adults who received little, if any, benefit from appropriate hearing aids should be considered as implant candidates. At the time Dr House had implanted 22 patients, 18 postlingually deaf and four prelingually deaf. Of the seven patients implanted by Dr Michelson four were postlingual and three were prelingual. The two patients implanted by Dr Simmons in the mid-1970s were postlingual.

Aetiologies of deafness varied. Patients deafened by meningitis were regarded as less satisfactory subjects of implantation. Michelson believed young, ototoxically deafened adults to be the ideal candidates for multichannel implantation. Aetiology did not seem to have an effect on patient performance using the single-channel device.

None of the groups had yet developed a preoperative test that would map out surviving auditory nerve cells and determine patient suitability for either single- or multichannel stimulation. It is possible that there are patients in which neuronal survival is so sparse that single-channel stimulation is as effective as multichannel and because of the simplicity and reliability of the single-electrode system is the implant of choice in those patients.

Patients' selection differed. Patients' suitability was determined in Los Angeles by a positive auditory response to preoperative transtympanic promontory stimulation. The suitability in San Francisco and Stanford was determined by responses to acute stimulation of the implant under local anaesthesia at the beginning of surgery. Failure to elicit any auditory sensation by acute stimulation with an electrode on the round window would contraindicate permanent implantation.

All three felt that the greatest potential benefit of cochlear implant might ultimately be found in congenitally deaf children. Implantation of children, however, would be postponed until more was learned of the potential advantages and disadvantages of cochlear implantation.

Electrodes. Though gold and silver had been used initially, electrodes of the three groups were now made of platinum (alloyed with 10 per cent iridium or rhodium for greater malleability). Insulation of the electrodes, though better, was still not perfect. Pyre MLTM, epoxy overcoated with silicone rubber, or Teflon™ covered the electrodes.

Compared with monopolar stimulation, discrete polar paired electrodes situated in contact with the basilar membrane gave much more restricted patterns of excitation. The San Francisco group developed an eight-channel arrangement of eight pairs of wires (see Chapter 4). Simmons used four Teflon™-coated electrodes uninsulated at their tips placed directly into the modiolus with a monopolar ground. This site though technically more difficult required less stimulating current. The House single electrode placed into the scala tympani for approximately 18 mm was uninsulated along the entire intracochlear length and had a ball at its tip to reduce the chance of penetration of the basilar membrane.

Transmission link systems. The House-Urban single-channel system used a transcutaneous magnetic induction link. This passive system required neither a power source for the internal components nor demodulation of the audiofrequency signal. It was a simple and efficient system. A disadvantage of the audiofrequency inductive system was the critical alignment of transmitter and subcutaneous receiver needed for transfer of information.

The San Francisco group used a radiofrequency transmission system which is not as sensitive as the audiofrequency link to misalignment. However, transmission problems did occur because of difficulties in hermetically sealing the subcutaneous receiver package. Besides using the transcutaneous radiofrequency link, San Francisco also considered using a hard-wire connector of pyrolised carbon. The direct connection would allow for flexibility in the development of optimum coding schemes.

The Stanford group used a hard-wire system. The subcutaneous connector was designed to facilitate subsequent replacement of the percutaneous link system by a fully implanted integrated circuit package. The highly sophisticated package would accept stimulating power through a transcutaneous radiofrequency link. The data links for 'acoustic' information would be received as a digital code via an ultrasonic receiver. Each channel would be completely independent and could be individually programmed. The package would use a hybrid thick film technique.

Surgical considerations. Dr House approached the scala tympani through the mastoid, facial recess, and the round window allowing the single-electrode wire to be passed easily into the scala with minimal complications.

Dr Michelson used a postauricular incision and evaluation of the posterior external ear canal skin and annulus to enter the middle ear and visualise the round window. The wires from the subcutaneous receiver led down a gutter drilled in the posterior canal wall to the round window which was widely enlarged anteriorly to accept the moulded implant. Since the wires were laid close to the thin external canal skin there had been problems with wire breakage and development of external otitis with exposure of the wires. A concern was also raised regarding possible new bone formation at the site of drilling.

Dr Simmons used a modified endaural incision allowing exposure of the mastoid cortex. The antrum and attic were visualised through a mastoid opening and the middle ear visualised by elevating a tympanomeatal flap. After removal of the stapes arch the modiolus was approached by passing through a hole just anterior and inferior to the margin of the oval window into the scala vestibuli of the first turn of the cochlea, and then through its medial wall. Complications included temporary cerebrospinal fluid leak, external otitis, and vertigo.

Results. Responses to implant stimulation were similar to those noted in the Pittsburgh study. Also, the single-electrode single-channel system was as effective as multiple-electrode single-channel systems. Two patients had been chronically stimulated for six and seven years without changes in their electrical thresholds or their subjective responses to stimulation suggesting that long-term electrical stimulation did not cause further degeneration of auditory neural tissue and that chronic electrical stimulation close to the brain did not lead to psychological disturbance.

University of Utah and Ear Research Institute. This implant programme was the joint effort of Drs M. Mladyovsky, D. Eddington, and W. Dobelle of the University of Utah and Dr D. Brackmann of the Ear Research Institute (now known as the House Ear Institute). The programme involved four postlingually deaf patients (one patient had only a unilateral profound loss, the unimplanted ear was normal) implanted with a six-electrode multichannel monopolar array in the scala tympani. A seventh electrode was embedded in the bone of the promontory. Their purpose was to study stimulus and coding parameters necessary to provide speech discrimination through a multichannel stimulator. Patients were studied in the laboratory. No take-home device was constructed. The device consisted of platinum electrodes insulated with TeflonTM connected to a percutaneous pedestal made of pyrolised carbon anchored to the mastoid bone. The pyrolised carbon pedestal had been extremely well tolerated without infection or reaction in all patients. Following mastoidectomy, opening of the facial recess and round window, the wires with bell tips were easily passed individually into the scala tympani — the most apical being at 24–26 mm and the most basal at 3–4 mm from the round window. The seventh electrode was embedded in the promontory, the ground electrode under the temporalis muscle.

Extensive psychoacoustic data on frequency and intensity discrimination as well as the effects of different types of stimulation on threshold and electrode position was obtained. The patients reported both periodicity and place pitch with stimulation of the various intracochlear electrodes. The narrowed dynamic range from threshold to uncomfortable loudness was only 5 to 7 dB for pulse and 12 to 15 dB for sinusoidal waveform stimulation. The current levels required to reach threshold with the promontory electrode were higher than with the scala tympani electrode. At levels two to three times threshold, promontory threshold evoked pain in the distribution of the glossopharyngeal nerve probably by stimulating the tympanic branch (Jacobson's nerve). Otherwise there was no substantial difference between intracochlear and promontory stimulation.

University of Washington, Seattle. This group, led by Josef Miller, PhD, was investigating the behavioural responses and histological changes in monkeys and the physiological responses and histological changes in guinea pigs to short- and long-term electrode implantation and excitation in the scala tympani. The programme had just completed the first year of a five-year National Institute of Health grant. Histologically they found, in normal animals, that if the basilar membrane was ruptured by the electrodes or if the cochlear blood supply was compromised by a tight electrode carrier there was extensive damage to the organ of Corti with a loss of ganglion cells.

Recommendations for United Kingdom. Ballantyne *et al.* concluded that the efficacy of single-channel implants as compared to hearing aids or vibrotactile devices for profound, postlingually deafened adults should be established by using an extracochlear stimulator. If efficacy is proved, studies should be begun by multidisciplinary teams of the most reliable intracochlear systems, single- and multichannel, to determine the optimum stimulus and coding parameters.

Besides studying the programmes in the United States, the authors also reviewed the implant programme of Dr C. Chouard in France. A summary of that programme and of programmes begun in other countries during the 1970s will be presented next.

International Programmes

France. Mr A. Morrison visited Dr C. Chouard in the late 1970s. His thorough review and a paper presented by Chouard (1980, pp. 137–45) at the Fourteenth International Congress of Audiology in 1978 provide the information on the Paris implant programme.

Dr Chouard's studies began in the early 1970s. The exact nature of these early experiments and the number of patients studied is unclear. By 1975 he wrote that he had implanted 21 patients with multichannel devices having five to seven monopolar electrodes connected to a percutaneous TeflonTM plug. The electrodes were placed into the cochlea through the middle fossa and mastoid. Through the middle fossa Chouard approached the superior segment of the first coil, and following a radical mastoidectomy he had access to the remaining turns. He drilled a fenestra for each electrode, each separated by several millimetres. He placed sheets of SilasticTM into each hole in an attempt to isolate the electrodes and prevent shunting between them. Methylmethacrylate fixed the electrodes at the fenestra. The mastoid was obliterated with bone pate and the external auditory meatus sutured closed. Because of skin infection, the TeflonTM plugs in all 21 patients had to be removed after 6 to 18 months. The wires were left buried subcutaneously.

A new transcutaneous device was designed having 8 to 12 monopolar electrodes and by August 1978 Chouard had implanted 22 new patients; a few were children (younger than 18 years of age). The surgical technique remained the same. The platinum iridium, TeflonTM-insulated electrodes were attached to the subcutaneous receiver coil by SilasticTM connectors. The stimulus to each electrode was a pulse with frequency and amplitude fixed and duration of pulse variable. The information and power were transmitted from the external transmitter by radiofrequency to the implanted receiver coil. The signals were phased to stimulate the basal to the more apical electrodes in sequence within 1 ms. The signal processor was carried in a shoulder bag.

Chouard required that the patients be totally deaf and have a positive response to electrical stimulation of the round window (requires elevating a tympanomeatal flap). The response was assessed subjectively in patients having local anaesthesia and by auditory brainstem responses in patients stimulated while under general anaesthesia. Most of his totally deaf patients did have a positive response to round window stimulation. He felt that the positive response signified that viable auditory neurons were present though he also was unable to determine their number or their distribution along the basilar membrane.

All patients underwent intensive rehabilitation. Chouard felt his patients had intensity and frequency discrimination of several sounds having both periodicity and place pitch. The implant improved lipreading. Using only the implant, without lipreading, the discrimination of phonemes was improved with training. Speech discrimination was not present.

Australia. Dr Graham Clark (Clark *et al.*, 1977, pp. 127–40) who began studying the effects of electrical stimulation of the auditory nerve in animals in 1969 did extensive work in the 1970s developing a multichannel cochlear implant. The multichannel scala tympani electrode array with interweaving ground and active electrodes reduced the spread of electrical current in the scala tympani. This pseudo-bipolar system had, as did the bipolar system, a much more restricted pattern of excitation than the monopolar system. Therefore, Clark felt his device would be more useful for patients than the multichannel monopolar systems of Chouard and Eddington (Tong *et al.*, 1979, pp. 679–95).

In 1978 and 1979 three profoundly deaf adults had multichannel cochlear implant operations. The electrode array consisted of 20 individual platinum foil bands wrapped around a silicone rubber cylinder with the conductors to the rings carried within the centre of the cylinder. Every other ring was connected to form the common ground; therefore, of the 20 rings ten were active electrodes. The electrodes were connected to a subcutaneous receiver/stimulator.

The auditory stimulus was digitally coded by the computer in the single processor which sent the information to the transmitter. The transmitter formated the data and subsequently generated radiofrequency power and data signals which were inductively coupled to the receiver/stimulator. The data were decoded and the appropriate electrodes stimulated. The surgical approach to the round window and scala tympani was through a mastoidectomy with opening of the facial recess.

All three patients noted that the perceived pitch varied according to the rate and site of stimulation. A speech-processing strategy was developed from the results of extensive psychophysical tests with two of the three patients (the strategy will be discussed in detail in later chapters). A device failure within a few months of implantation prevented extensive testing of the third patient.

Austria. Drs Ingeborg J. Hochmair-Desoyer and Erwin S. Hochmair of the Department of Electrical Engineering at the Technical University of Vienna working with Dr Kurt Burian as their otologic surgeon implanted five patients during the 1970s (Hochmair-Desoyer *et al.*, 1981, pp. 107–19).

Their first two prostheses were multichannel electrode systems consisting of eight bipolar electrodes. The next two patients used a six-channel system and the fifth a four-channel. Initially the number of electrodes used in their implant design was based on the concept that possibly to attain speech understanding through electrical stimulation, 8 to 12 discrete points of stimulation would be necessary. Because the complex circuitry and speech coding strategies were not optimum, the Vienna group decided to change to a simpler device.

The four-channel system consisted of four bipolar pairs of electrodes placed 16 mm within the scala tympani. The electrode array was made of TeflonTM-insulated, 90 per cent platinum 10 per cent iridium wires embedded in a molded-silicone carrier. The array connected to a pair of two-channel receiver/stimulators. Analogue signals from the portable speech processor were passed transcutaneously from the external transmitter to the receiver/stimulator by radiofrequency. The array was placed through the mastoid–facial recess approach to the round window and scala tympani.

From their experiments the group felt that the role of periodicity pitch in speech understanding had been underestimated. Not only did their patients have the same benefits reported by previous single-channel users but the Vienna group found that stimulation of one single channel of a multichannel intracochlear electrode array using a simple correlate of the analogue speech signal did result in some useful speech understanding. Though a single-channel stimulator was used, it was important to implant several channels as stimulation of the different channels does not always produce the same speech results. The group felt this might be due to patchy nerve survival.

England. Mr Ellis Douek and his colleagues (1977, pp. 379–83) placed an extracochlear electrode in contact with the promontory near the round window membrane to avoid the difficulties and hazards of implanting an electrode into the scala tympani. The first tests of extracochlear stimulation were in patients with radical cavities. The initial observation that the information provided by extracochlear and single-channel intracochlear stimulation appeared similar was confirmed later (Fourcin *et al.*, 1979, pp. 85–107). Their electrical stimulation was based on the use of auditory speech pattern components stressing voicing. In order to use voice information in clinical testing and in speech training during rehabilitation they used the laryngograph which transduces voice frequencies at the larynx into an electrical signal.

Switzerland. Dr Ugo Fisch (Dillier *et al.*, 1980, p. 146–63) implanted a hard wired two-channel bipolar modiolar implant in 1977. Because of problems with the hardwire system, the group decided to develop a transcutaneous system. They began studying electrical stimulation of an electrode temporarily placed at the round window in five patients obtaining results showing (like Douek had) that extracochlear stimulation was similar to intracochlear.

The Eighties

Investigators in the seventies addressed a few of the questions raised concerning cochlear implants. Electrical stimulation of the auditory system with appropriate currents appeared safe. Most implant patients were postlingually deafened adults, some were prelingual adults, and a few were children. Investigators used both single- and multichannel devices. Though cochlear implant stimulation did not provide substantial speech discrimination, it did provide other benefits for the profoundly deaf.

Other aspects of cochlear implantations were not clear. Two important riddles unsolved were the following. First, there was not yet a preoperative test to determine how many surviving neurons were present and where along the basilar membrane these cells were. Second, investigators had not yet developed the appropriate stimulus code necessary for full speech understanding with electrical stimulation of the auditory system.

An international field of cochlear implant investigators met at two meetings held early in the eighties to address the issues of implantation. The first conference was held in April, 1982, by the New York Academy of Sciences (Parkins and Anderson, 1983, pp. 1–532). The second was held by the University of California, San Francisco, in June, 1983, as the Tenth Anniversary Conference on Cochlear Implant: An International Symposium (Schindler, 1984). The information concerning the recent and current activity of the international field of cochlear implant investigators has come from those two meetings and from a questionnaire we sent them.

Recent and Current Activity of Implant Programmes

Australia (G.N. Clark, Y.C. Tong, D. Dewhurst and associates). The group continues to study multichannel systems in a limited population. Because of the problems with the pseudo-bipolar multichannel device implanted in the late 1970s, design changes were made with the assistance of the Australian biomedical firm Nucleus Limited. The present device is described in Chapter 11.

Six patients implanted with the new system were assessed three months after surgery using the Minimal Auditory Capabilities (MAC) battery. There was marked improvement on almost every test as compared with preoperative hearing aid results. Lipreading was improved with implant and four patients have some open set speech discrimination. Patients reported an increased awareness of environmental sounds.

A great deal of research has been done on speech processing strategies and coding. Histopathological studies of the effects of insertion trauma, chronic electrical stimulation, secondary labyrinthine infection, and electrode electrolysis have been performed. The group felt from their study on new bone formation within the scala of implanted bones that the new bone formation may be a result of insertion trauma to the endosteal layer with resultant inflammation rather than of electrical stimulation.

Austria (I.J. Hochmair-Desoyer, E.S. Hochmair and K. Burian). This group, besides continuing to use single-channel stimulation of a multichannel intracochlear electrode array, has developed an extracochlear system for use in patients who have some limited residual hearing.

The intracochlear system consisting of a four-channel bipolar molded scala tympani electrode connected to a four-channel receiver/stimulator has been described. The extracochlear single-channel device consists of a pair of platinum iridium electrodes attached to an implanted receiver/stimulator. The active ball tip is placed in the round window niche — outside the scala. Fitting the speech processor is the subject of Chapter 8.

18 *The History of Cochlear Implants*

Up to 1 July 1983, 23 patients had received the intracochlear system and 22 patients the extracochlear. All patients were either pre- or postlingually hearing-impaired adults. Besides the benefits previously reported the group stated that approximately 70 per cent of the postlingually deafened patients reach some degree of understanding of untrained, unknown words or sentences (varying from 0 to 90 per cent correct) by electrical stimulation only, i.e. without additional lipreading.

The intracochlear implant has been designed to allow comparisons of a number of different single- and multichannel coding schemes in a laboratory setting. For both intra- and extracochlear systems the signal processor is individually fitted.

England. Ballantyne, Evans, and Morrison (1982, pp. 811–16), after receiving progress reports from different implant centres and revisiting a few, updated their recommendations to the Department of Health and Social Security. Encouraged by the reports they suggested that a limited number of implant centres be established. The following three groups are evaluating the cochlear implant.

The External Pattern Input (EPI) Group. The group, E.E. Douek, A.J. Fourcin, B.C.J. Moore and associates, has continued to study extracochlear stimulation developing coding techniques using speech pattern components and a rehabilitation programme to improve the patient's speaking ability as well as his/her hearing (see Chapter 8). The group has tested many individuals in the past and has implanted several patients only recently. The 'opened' ears (those having a radical cavity) received a ball-tipped electrode assembly that is held in a conventional earmold against the promontory. A tympanopexy (sealing of the intact tympanic membrane to the promontory) was performed in the patients without radical cavities.

The prosthesis consists of two boxes and the earmold assembly. The first box which is an acoustically driven fundamental frequency extractor with microphone receiver needs to be fairly close to the person speaking as it emits infrared light pulses corresponding to each vocal-fold closure. The second box is carried by the patient like a body aid. An infrared receiver inside this box triggers an electrical stimulus for each infrared pulse. The stimulus travels down the stainless-steel electrode to the promontory. The electrode is axially sprung; the spring assembly is embedded into the earmold. The mold itself is plastic and gold-plated so that it acts as the other electrode.

Project Ear Foundation. The implant of A.W. Morrison and E.F. Evans is in an early stage of development. The focus will be both rehabilitative and experimental. Selected patients will receive both intracochlear and extracochlear electrodes. Comparisons will be made between single- and multichannel stimulation strategies. Stimulus transfer will be by radiofrequency transcutaneous link using pulse or analogue waveforms. Implants will be limited initially to postlingually deaf adults.

University College Hospital, London. The implant team of J.G. Fraser, J.M. Graham, and R.F. Gray is working with the San Francisco group in evaluating the San Francisco multichannel implant. One or two patients have been implanted.

France (C.H. Chouard, C. Fugain, B. Meyer and associates). Through 1982 Dr Chouard continued to use the multichannel implant having twelve electrodes implanted one by one into the scala tympani through twelve fenestrations (see description under The Seventies). Of 48 patients who were implanted with this system between 1976 and 1982, eight were less than 18 years of age while the remaining adult patients were almost equally divided between pre- and postlingual deafness. For reasons not clear Chouard has switched to a twelve-channel multi-electrode bipolar scala tympani system. The array is carried by an electrode bearer through the round window into the scala. The older fenestration technique is now reserved for patients who have ossification of the labyrinth.

At least ten patients have been implanted with the new system. A positive response to round window electrical stimulation is still used by Chouard for selection of suitable implant candidates. The older implant system has been well tolerated in patients for up to six years without change in electrical thresholds. Chouard reports that all patients discriminate at least some words and sentences from a reference list without lip-reading. Discrimination of unknown words is more difficult. He has reported a significant effect of implant stimulation on an autistic child and two other patients, both deaf and blind. Chouard, like House, has noted that electrical stimulation through the implant has decreased tinnitus in several patients. Chouard's youngest patient was 9 years old at implantation. He plans progressively to lower the age limit. Chouard is extensively evaluating the patients implanted and is developing new techniques for multichannel stimulation.

Switzerland (U. Fisch, N. Dillier and T. Spillman). Encouraged by their results of round window stimulation with the temporary electrodes, the group developed a single-channel system. The single electrode is placed at the round window through a facial recess to round window approach. The wearable signal processor delivers biphasic pulses transcutaneously via radiofrequency to the receiver/stimulator. Four patients have been implanted and extensively tested. The group feels their results are similar to those of single-channel intracochlear devices.

West Germany (P. Banfai, G. Hortmann, A. Karczag and associates). Dr Banfai used a House single intracochlear electrode device for his first implant. Attempting to create a better device he has developed a multichannel system that is intracochlear but extrascalar. He drills individual fenestra for the eight electrodes; four in the second turn, three near the basal turn, one in the helicotrema. Each fenestra is drilled only to the endosteal layer — the scala tympani is not entered. A monopolar ground electrode is placed in the mastoid cavity. Percutaneous transmission is initially used to determine the electrical measurements and stimulation thresholds of each individual electrode. Once that is accomplished, the system is switched to transcutaneous radiofrequency transmission. The wearable signal processor divides the incoming signal into eight frequency bands by means of a band passer and delivers biphasic pulses to the receiver/stimulator.

As of June 1 1983, the group has implanted twelve postlingual adults, 24 prelingual adults and eight children. The results reported are similar to single-channel stimulation with respect to awareness of environmental sounds, lipreading, etc. However, 30 per cent of their patients are reported to recognise 75–80 per cent of the everyday sentences from an unfamiliar text.

House Ear Institute — Los Angeles (W.F. House, K.I. Berliner, B.J. Edgerton and associates). House and Berliner (1982, pp. 1–124) published a detailed review of the single-electrode programme at the House Ear Institute (HEI). The programme had not changed greatly from the late 1970s. Experience led to a few modifications and refinements. The current programme is basically the same except for changes in the engineering of the implant package which has been done by the Minnesota Manufacturing and Mining (3M) Company of St Paul, Minnesota. HEI and 3M have worked closely together since 1982 in all aspects of the programme including manufacturing and research.

The strategy of using a single-electrode system with emphasis on rehabilitation to assist selected profoundly hearing-impaired patients has not changed. The implant is undergoing clinical trials under the Food and Drug Administration (FDA) regulations governing investigational devices. Twenty-seven other otologists in the United States have implanted one or more patients as co-investigators with HEI in the clinical trials programme. The purpose of the programme is to gather safety and efficacy information on the single-electrode cochlear implant. The co-investigators and their implant teams are trained by HEI. As a result of the co-investigator programme more information on safety and efficacy is available from a variety of clinical settings. HEI has also recently trained implant teams from several countries. A few of these co-investigators have implanted the House/3M device in one or more patients.

There have been engineering changes in the device. A more energy-efficient coil system has allowed the creation of a smaller signal processor. Magnets in the external transmitter and internal receiver now keep the two coils more easily aligned. The active electrode placed in the scala tympani through the facial recess/round window approach has been shortened to 6 mm uninsulated length. The shortened electrode can be inserted with minimal risk of insertion trauma to the auditory system. Transmission of the amplitude modulated 16 kHz signal by electromagnetic induction is unchanged.

As of 1 September 1983, Dr William House and the co-investigators have implanted 288 deaf adults; the majority are postlingual. More than 85 per cent of all adult patients use their device on a regular basis. One patient has used the device daily for eleven years and 15 patients for five to seven years with no measurable or reported changes in auditory or psychological functioning. Prelinguals have a greater tendency than postlinguals to be non-users. Nine patients are now deceased (cause of death not related to implant use).

A wide variety of aetiologies have been found suitable for cochlear implantation including meningitis. Only seven of 288 patients have no perception of sound from the implant.

Research at both HEI and 3M is continuing to determine the optimum coding and processing techniques to increase single-channel benefits. Work is also being done, especially at 3M, in developing a preoperative evaluation of the surviving auditory neurons. The temporal bones of the deceased HEI patients are also being studied. The findings on the first set of temporal bones has been previously published (Johnsson et al., 1982, pp. 74–89). The extracochlear tissue of four other patients has been extensively examined. There was no evidence of inflammation. A fibrous tissue seal around the electrode at the round window effectively separated the middle ear from the scala tympani. The intracochlear tissues are in process and the findings of the HEI-3M histopathologists should be published soon. Two other present research projects are: to continue the investigation begun in the early 1970s of the effect of the cochlear implant on tinnitus, and to pursue hearing by cochlear nucleus stimulation in those patients who cannot benefit from a cochlear implant because the eighth nerve is not intact from the cochlea to the brain stem.

Experience gained from adults using the single-electrode cochlear implant showed that the device provided significant benefit with almost no measurable adverse effects (Berliner, 1982, pp. 90–8). As a result of this experience House decided to extend the benefits to children (Eisenberg et al., 1983, pp. 41–50).

Up to 1 September 1983, 78 children had been implanted with the single-electrode cochlear implant by House and three other selected co-investigators. Most of the children have acquired losses secondary to meningitis. Meningitis may lead to a labyrinthitis which causes the destruction of neural elements and in time the formation of fibrous tissue and often bone growth within the labyrinth. Though the degree of labyrinthine ossification ranged from mild to complete occlusion of the scala tympani in the meningitic children implanted, all patients except one stimulated with the cochlear implant. This is interesting because it implies that even in the presence of bone growth in the cochlea, stimulatable neural elements survive.

The great majority of children use their implants. Prelingual teenagers are more likely to be non-users. The test results are consistent with those of the adults. With the implant the children can differentiate changes of timing and intensity which could not be done with hearing aids. Electrical thresholds have not changed in several children who have used their device for more than two years. Several children have had episodes of acute otitis media that has responded to routine antibiotics. There have been no complications in these patients.

Stanford University (F.B. Simmons, R.L. White and associates). Initially Simmons selected the modiolus as the best site for electrode placement but after comparing data on scala tympani with modiolar stimulation he feels that there is no real difference. So, as a result of the size constraints of modiolar placement on the electrode bundle, Simmons has switched from modiolar to scala tympani placement. Research will continue to develop methods of obtaining speech discrimination with multichannel devices and a clinical programme will be started using a single-electrode device.

Two new systems are being developed. The first is a multichannel system.

Different engineering designs of the intracochlear array are being constructed. The implantable receiver/stimulator will be sealed in a titanium can. Transcutaneous power transmission will be by radiofrequency and data transmission by ultrasound. A variety of speech coding processes are being considered. Simmons feels this complex multichannel system is probably three to five years away from being ready. Therefore, he is working with Biostim Inc., developing a simple single-channel system. Though the single-electrode device will not provide speech discrimination, it will provide the benefits already described. The surgical approach to the scala tympani is through a routine tympanotomy flap with removal of the incus and exposure of the round window. A very high atticotomy is then done from the mastoid cortex to the fossa of the incus. The electrode(s) are passed via the atticotomy through the round window into the scala.

University of California, San Francisco (R.P. Michelson, M.M. Merzenich, R.A. Schindler, and associates). The group continues to research methods of obtaining speech discrimination. They have been using, in several subjects, an eight-bipolar electrode array with a single-channel stimulator. Recently in three other patients implanted with an eight-bipolar electrode array a four-channel stimulator has been used.

The electrode array has been redesigned for atraumatic insertion up to 24 to 26 mm into the scala tympani. This is discussed in detail in Chapter 4.

A few of the patients have initially reported that they have a strong preference for multichannel as compared to single-channel stimulation. The group states that highly significant levels of open speech recognition have been recorded with their multichannel device.

Auditory brainstem responses to electrical stimuli have recently been recorded intraoperatively and postoperatively in three implanted patients to explore the possibilities of using these measures as an objective index of implant performances. The group feels from their results that they could separate a device problem from a physiological or anatomical problem as the cause of a failure to stimulate. Also, they feel it is possible to determine position of surviving neural tissue, and therefore, the place of electrical stimulation.

Future histopathological studies in animals will attempt to determine long-term effects of chronic electrical stimulation on cochlear tissue at levels similar to those used by patients. Previous studies have shown high current levels do cause damage. Also being studied is the effect of middle ear infection in an implanted ear on cochlear structures.

University of Utah (D.K. Eddington, D.E. Brackmann and associates). The programme has remained essentially research oriented studying different coding strategies in the patients previously implanted. Only two of the four are presently being studied — one patient died and one patient was explanted. A take-home four-channel stimulator has been developed and is being used by a postlingual patient. The percutaneous pyrolised carbon plug has been well tolerated in each patient for approximately six years. These two patients, receiving analogue stimuli from a four-channel processor, were able to recognise approximately two-thirds (67 per cent and 64 per cent) of an open set unpractised list of two-syllable words. Though the results are better than the single-channel results reported (43 per cent and 35 per cent), Eddington cautions that not all patients might expect these results. However, it does suggest that a device can be developed that will provide speech discrimination for deaf patients. The University of Utah and Eddington have recently contracted with Kolff Medical to manufacture and distribute their cochlear implant.

University of Washington, Seattle (J.M. Miller, D. Sutton, B.E. Pfingst and associates). Work is continuing on the studies in guinea pigs and monkeys concerning the mechanisms of implant-induced damage and the histopathological changes secondary to stimulation. The group is also studying in monkeys through psychophysical tests the relation of an implant's function to the pattern and degree of nerve survival in the cochlea. Another project concerns the feasibility of evaluating experimental implant design in monkeys prior to implantation in man.

Summary

Cochlear implants are a significant benefit to the profoundly deaf. The work of implant investigators reviewed in this chapter (Table 1.1) and of others throughout the world over the last 25 years has shown that the implant provides, among other things, an awareness of environmental sounds, improved speechreading, and possibly some minimal speech discrimination. The various single- and multichannel devices, now available, provide similar benefits. Full speech discrimination is not yet possible. The 'perfect' device offering full speech discrimination is probably many years off. Increased interest in the implant by speech scientists and auditory physiologists will hopefully speed the development of the appropriate coding schemes necessary for electrical stimulation of the impaired auditory system within the cochlea to produce intelligible speech. The cooperation of private manufacturing companies with the investigators will improve the quality and reliability of the implant system.

The future implant system will probably be a combination of different devices, i.e. a simple single electrode device would be more effective for some patients while a multichannel device would be more effective for other profoundly deaf patients. The techniques necessary to map surviving auditory neurons and therefore determine which patient would benefit more from which device are being investigated.

Acknowledgements

We would like to thank Elaine M. Kalivoda for typing this chapter, and Karen I. Berliner, PhD, for her constructive remarks. Our study has been supported by

Table 1.1: Major Cochlear Implant Investigations

	Investigators	Location	Channels	Electrodes	Placement	Comment
EXTRACOCHLEAR	Douek	London, England	Single	Single	Promontory	
	Fisch	Zurich, Switzerland	Single	Single	Round window	
	Hochmairs	Vienna, Austria	Single	Single	Round window	
INTRACOCHLEAR/ EXTRASCALAR	Banfai	Cologne, West Germany	Multiple	Multiple	Fenestra of cochlear turns	8 channels
INTRACOCHLEAR	Chouard	Paris, France	Multiple	Multiple	Scala tympani	Fenestrates cochlear turns in cases of ossification — 12 channels
	Clark	Melbourne, Austrlia	Multiple	Multiple	Scala tympani	Working with Nucleus, Ltd.
	Eddington	Salt Lake City, UT	Multiple	Multiple	Scala tympani	Working with Kolff Medical. Hard wire system — 4 channels
	Hochmairs	Vienna, Austria	Multiple	Multiple	Scala tympani	Chooses best channel — then stimulates as single channel
	House	Los Angeles, CA	Single	Single	Scala tympani	Working with 3M
	Michelson	San Francisco, CA	Multiple	Multiple	Scala tympani	4-channel stimulator
	Simmons	Stanford, CA	Single	Single	Scala tympani	Working with Biostim Inc.

funds from the House Ear Institute, Los Angeles, an affiliate of the University of California School of Medicine.

References

Ballantyne, J.C., Evans, E.F. and Morrison, A.W. (1978) *J. Laryngol. Otol.* (Suppl. 1), 1–117
—— Evans, E.F. and Morrison, A.W. (1982) *J. Laryngol. Otol.*, 96, 811–16
Berliner, K.I. (1982) *Ann. Otol. Rhinol. Laryngol.*, 91 (Suppl. 91), 90–8
Bilger, R.C., Black, F.O., Hopkinson, N.T., Myers, E.N., Payne, J.L., Stenson, N.R., Vega, A. and Wolf, R.V. (1977) *Ann. Otol. Rhinol. Laryngol.*, 86 (Suppl. 38), 1–176
Carhart, R. (1974) in M.M. Merzenich, R.A. Schindler and F.A. Sooy (eds.), *Proceedings of the First International Conference on Electrical Stimulation of the Acoustic Nerve as a Treatment for Profound Sensorineural Deafness in Man*, University of California, San Francisco, pp. 171–8
Chouard, C.H. (1980) *Audiology*, 19, 137–45
Clark, G.M., Black, R., Dewhurst, D.J., Forster, I.C., Patrick, J.F. and Tong, Y.C. (1977) *Med. Prog. Technol.*, 5, 127–40
Dillier, N., Spillman, T., Fisch, U.P. and Leifer, L.J. (1980) *Audiology*, 19, 146–63
Douek, E.E., Fourcin, A.J., Moore, B.C.J. and Clarke, G.P. (1977) *Proc. R. Soc. Med.*, 70, 379–83
Eisenberg, L.S., Berliner, K.I., Thielemeir, M.A., Kirk, K.I. and Tiber, N. (1983) *Ear and Hearing*, 4, 41–50
Fourcin, A.J., Rosen, S.M., Moore, B.C.J., Douek, E.E., Clarke, G.P., Dodson, H. and Bannister, L.H. (1979) *Br. J. Audiol*, 13, 85–107
Hawkins, J. (1974) in M.M. Merzenich, R.A. Schindler and F.A. Sooy (eds.), *Proceedings of the First International Conference on Electrical Stimulation of the Acoustic Nerve as a Treatment for Profound Sensorineural Deafness in Man*, University of California, San Francisco, pp. 47–62
Hochmair-Desoyer, I.J., Hochmair, E.S., Burian, K. and Fischer, R.E. (1981) *Med. Prog. Technol.*, 8, 107–19
House, W.F. (1976) *Ann. Otol. Rhinol. Laryngol.*, 85 (Suppl. 27), 3–6
—— and Berliner, K.I. (eds.) (1982) *Ann. Otol. Rhinol. Laryngol.*, 91 (Suppl. 91), 1–124
—— and Urban, J. (1973) *Ann. Otol. Rhinol. Laryngol.*, 82, 504–17
Johnsson, L-G., House, W.F. and Linthicum, F.H., jr (1982) *Ann. Otol. Rhinol. Laryngol.*, 91 (Suppl. 91), 74–89
Kiang, N.Y.S. and Moxon, E.C. (1972) *Ann. Otol. Rhinol. Laryngol.*, 81, 714–30
McNeal, D.R. (1977) in F.T. Hambrecht and J.B. Reswick (eds.), *Functional Electrical Stimulation*, Marcel Dekker Inc., New York, pp. 3–35
Merzenich, M.M., Michelson, R.P., Schindler, R.A., Pettit, C.R. and Reid, M. (1973) *Ann. Otol. Rhinol. Laryngol.* 82, 486–503
——, Schindler, R.A. and Sooy, F.A. (eds.) (1974) in *Proc. First Int. Conf. Electrical Stimulation of the Acoustic Nerve as a Treatment for Profound Sensorineural Deafness in Man*. University of California, San Francisco, pp. 1–213
Michelson, R.P. (1968) *Trans. Am. Laryngol. Rhinol. Otol. Soc. Inc.*, pp. 626–44
—— (1971) *Ann. Otol. Rhinol. Laryngol.*, 80, 914–19
Parkins, C.W. and Anderson, S.W. (eds.) (1983) *Cochlear Prostheses: An International Symposium*, New York Academy of Sciences, New York, pp. 1–532
—— and Houde, R.A. (1982) in D.G. Sins, G.G. Walter and R.L. Whitehead (eds.), *Deafness and Communication: Assessment and Training*, Williams & Wilkins, Baltimore, pp. 332–56
Schindler, R.A. (1974) in M.M. Merzenich, R.A. Schindler and F.A. Sooy (eds.), *Proc. First Int. Conf. Electrical Stimulation of the Acoustic Nerve as a Treatment for Profound Sensorineural Deafness in Man*, University of California, San Francisco, pp. 93–104
—— (ed.) (1984) *Tenth Anniversary Conference on Cochlear Implants — An International Symposium*, Raven Press, New York
Schuknecht, H. (1974) in M.M. Merzenich, R.A. Schindler and F. A. Sooy (eds.), *Proc. First Int. Conf. Electrical Stimulation of the Acoustic Nerve as a Treatment for Profound Sensorineural Deafness in Man*, University of California, San Francisco, pp. 37–46
Simmons, F.B. (1966) *Arch. Otolaryngol.*, 84, 2–54
—— (1974) in M.M. Merzenich, R.A. Schindler and F.A. Sooy (eds.), *Proc. First Int. Conf. Electrical*

Stimulation of the Acoustic Nerve as a Treatment for Profound Sensorineural Deafness in Man, University of California, San Francisco, pp. 123-6
────── and Glattke, T.J. (1972) *Ann. Otol. Rhinol. Laryngol., 81*, 731-8
Spoendlin, H. (1974) in M.M. Merzenich, R.A. Schindler and F.A. Sooy (eds.), *Proc. First Int. Conf. Electrical Stimulation of the Acoustic Nerve as a Treatment for Profound Sensorineural Deafness in Man*, University of California, San Francisco, pp. 7-74
Tong, Y.C., Black, R.C., Clark, G.M., Forster, I.C., Millar, J.B., O'Loughlin, B.J. and Patrick, J.F. (1979) *J. Larnygol. Otol., 93*, 679-95

2 THE PHYSIOLOGY OF THE COCHLEA

James O. Pickles

Our knowledge of the physiology of the cochlea has been developing in a particularly rapid and exciting way in the last few years. Answers to many fundamental questions have recently been found. This has entailed a complete reassessment of some cherished concepts, and the proposing of some new and revolutionary principles. At the moment, the signs are that the pace of discovery will quicken rather than slacken in the near future.

Cochlear Mechanics

Recent measurements of the mechanical vibrations of the basilar membrane have shown the vibration to be much more sharply tuned, and much more non-linear, than previously demonstrated. In fact, the tuning of the cochlear vibration seems to be as sharp as the response of any neural stage in the auditory system, and it is therefore now recognised that the whole frequency resolving power of the auditory system is revealed at the mechanical stage.

Although the definitive accounts of basilar membrane vibration have appeared in the last year or so, understanding of the pattern of vibration is still best approached through the results of von Bekesy. It is a measure of von Bekesy's achievement that the definitive accounts only appeared, in 1982, 40 years after his original observations were published.

Von Bekesy, working with human cadavers, exposed a length of the cochlea. He scattered reflecting particles on Reissner's membrane (Figure 2.1A), so that he could observe its motion under a stroboscopic microscope. By stimulating with a fixed tone, he was able to plot out the pattern of vibration of the cochlear partition as a function of distance along the cochlea, and so show the now-classic travelling wave (Figure 2.2). For a sound of fixed frequency, the cochlear partition vibrated with a wave that grew in amplitude as it passed up the cochlea, came to a maximum, and then rapidly decreased in amplitude. Although the waves travelled continually up the cochlea, they did so within an envelope that, for a sinusoid of fixed frequency, was constant (von Bekesy, 1960). Von Bekesy also made plots in a second way. He opened the cochlea at certain fixed points, and plotted the amplitude of the travelling wave at those points as the stimulus frequency was varied, while the stimulus intensity was kept constant. This gives the frequency response of fixed points on the cochlea. When measurements were made in this way, each point on the cochlea was seen to vibrate with a constant amplitude of vibration up to a certain cut-off frequency, above which the response fell sharply. He therefore showed that the cochlear partition acted simply as a low-pass filter.

Hair cell and auditory nerve fibres have, however, a very sharply tuned bandpass

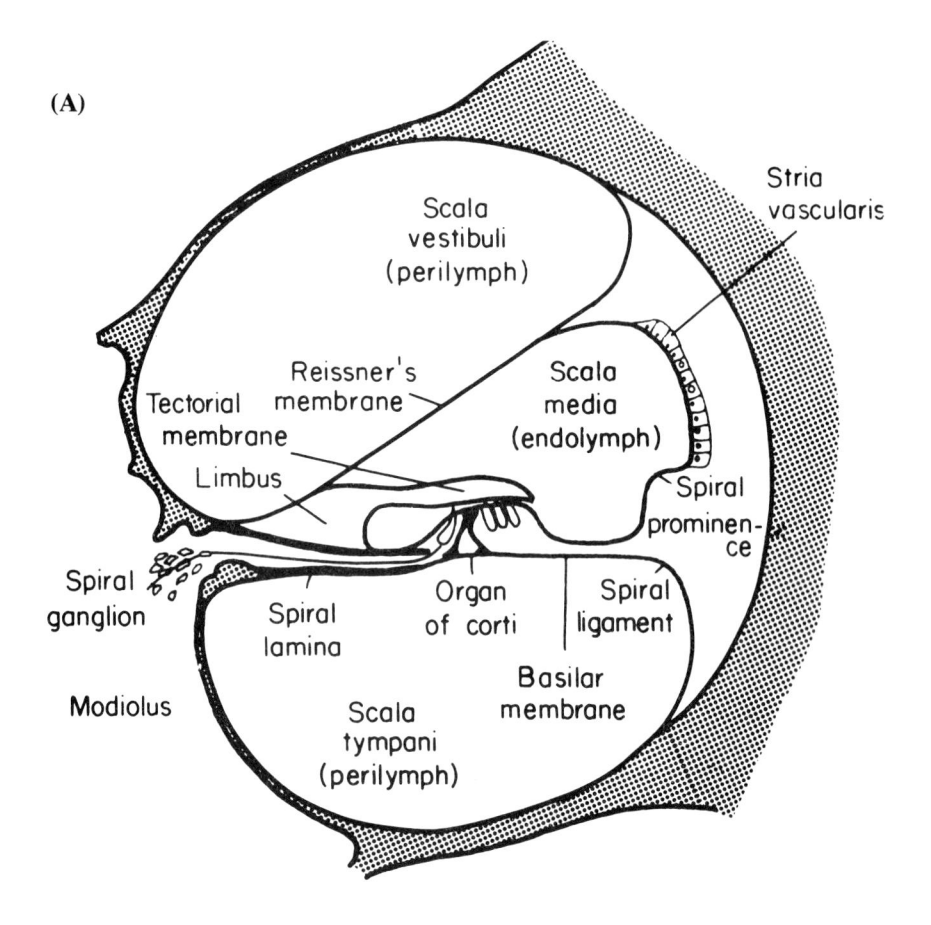

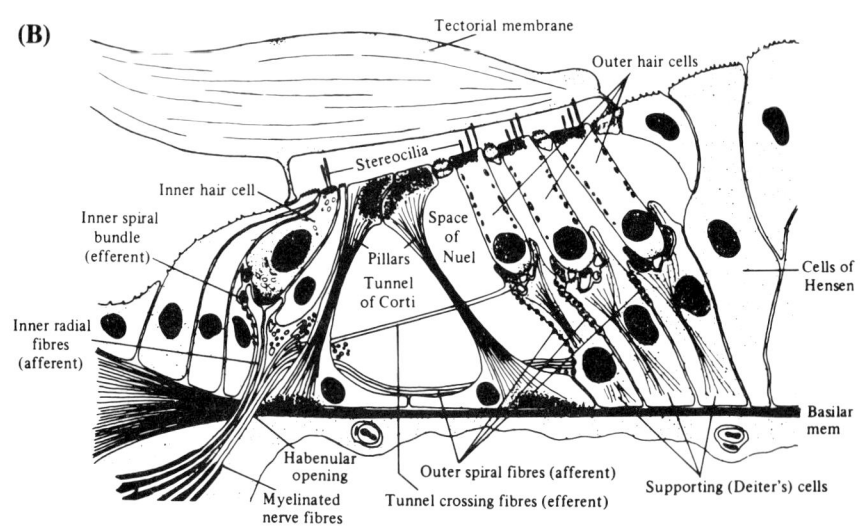

28   *The Physiology of the Cochlea*

The Physiology of the Cochlea 29

Figure 2.1: (opposite) (A) A Transverse Section of the Cochlear Duct, Showing its Division into Three Scalae by Reissner's Membrane and the Basilar Membrane. The nerve supply to the origin of Corti enters by way of the modiolus, on the left of the figure. (B) A transverse section through the organ of Corti. Note the position of the hair cells and the stereocilia, and their relation to the tectorial membrane.
Sources: (A) Pickles (1982). (B) Durrant, J.D. and Lovrinic, H.J. (1977), *Bases of Hearing Science*, Williams and Wilkins, Baltimore.

Figure 2.2: According to von Bekesy (1960), the Travelling Wave has a Broad Envelope (dotted lines). Here, the travelling wave is shown as a function of distance along the cochlear duct, for four successive instants (full lines). Points near the base of the cochlea are shown on the left, and those near the apex, on the right. Stimulus frequency, 200 Hz.

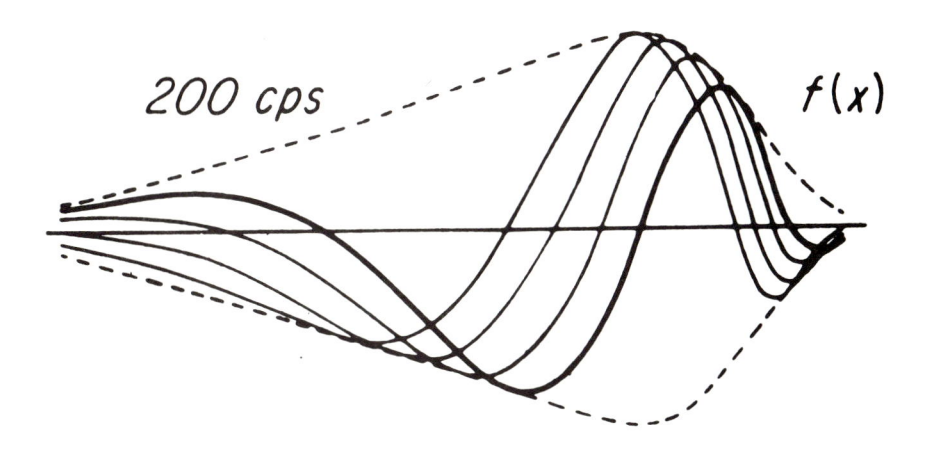

Source: von Bekesy (1960).

characteristic, rather than simply a low-pass characteristic. There has been an increasing suspicion over recent years that this sharp tuning arises in the mechanics, and that the cochlear partition is much more sharply tuned than von Bekesy showed. Although differing degrees of tuning have been found by the various investigators, the most recent, and probably definitive, results show the cochlear position to be as sharply tuned as the inner hair cells of the cochlea, or the auditory nerve fibres to which they are connected (e.g. Sellick *et al.*, 1982). Unlike von Bekesy, the recent investigators confined their measurements to single, isolated points on the cochlea, and so their measurements gave the frequency response at those points. Figure 2.3A shows the 'frequency threshold curve' or 'tuning curve' of a point on the basilar membrane of the guinea pig. In order to produce such a curve, the sound intensity (SPL) necessary to produce a certain, threshold, amplitude

30 *The Physiology of the Cochlea*

Figure 2.3

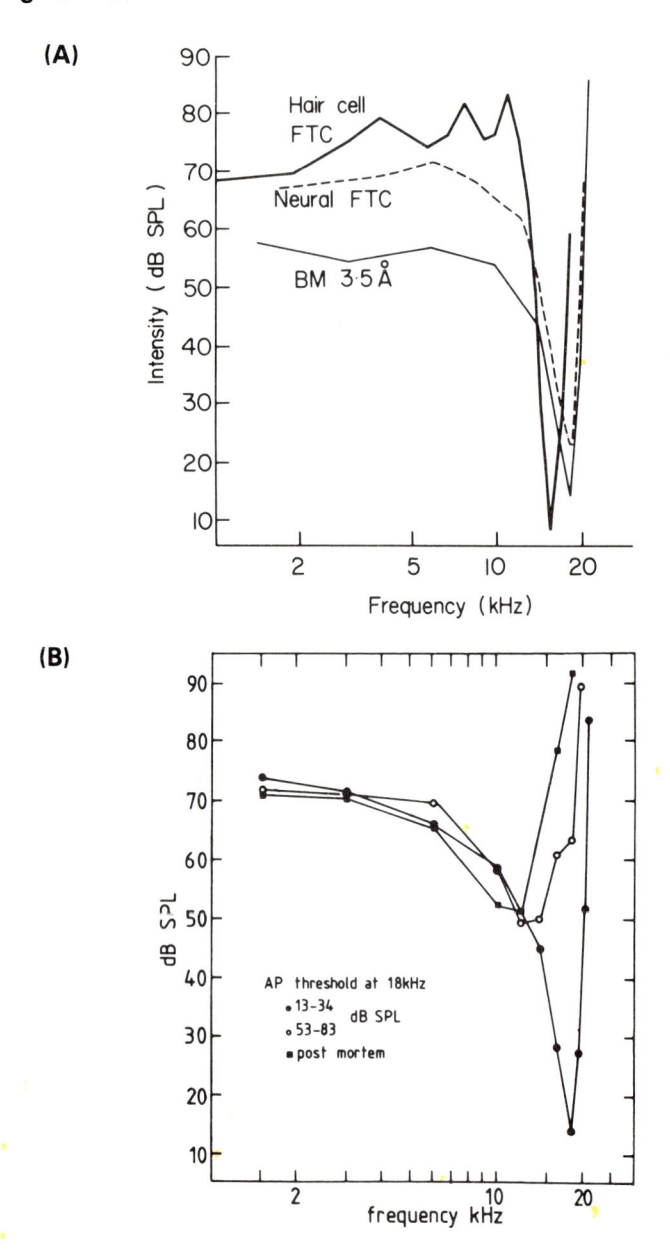

(A)

(B)

Source: Sellick *et al.* (1982).

The Physiology of the Cochlea   31

Figure 2.3: (opposite) (A) Tuning Curves for Basilar Membrane Vibration (BM 3.5 A), for an Inner Hair Cell Voltage Response (Hair Cell FTC), and for an Auditory Nerve Fibre (neural FTC; dotted). All curves show a similar sharply tuned frequency selectivity, except perhaps in the 'tail' of the tuning curve. The different measures were made at points nearly the same distance along the cochlea, and so the tip regions of the three curves lie at nearly the same frequency. (B) Basilar membrane tuning curves are shown for one animal while the cochlea was in good condition (filled circles), in poor condition in the living animal (open circles), and after death (filled squares). The tuning curve changes from a low-threshold, sharply-tuned bandpass characteristic, to a high-threshold, broadly-tuned, characteristic.

of movement, here 3.5 A peak to peak, was measured. In one frequency region, near 18 kHz, the basilar membrane had a very low threshold, so that at the tip of the tuning curve, the 3.5 A movement was produced by a sound stimulus of only 13 dB SPL. For frequencies on either side of this, the threshold sound intensity rose rapidly, with a slope of 400 dB/octave on the high frequency side, and a slope of 80 dB/octave on the low frequency side. On the high frequency side, the threshold sound intensity rose with a steep slope to the very highest sound pressures that were used. At low frequencies, however, the slope became shallow. Single points on the basilar membrane therefore have an asymmetric bandpass characteristic.

Why did von Bekesy not report this very sharp mechanical tuning? Three reasons can be suggested, in the light of recent results. First, and probably most importantly, the mechanical vibration is extremely sensitive to any small deterioration in the physiological state of the cochlea, as can be produced by for instance hypoxia, or bleeding into the perilymph. Von Bekesy's measurements, on the other hand, were performed after death. Figure 2.3B shows the changes in the tuning curve of a point on the basilar membrane, measured by Sellick *et al.* (1982), during the progressive deterioration of the cochlea, ending in death. The final tuning curve has very little of a bandpass characteristic, and looks rather like the low-pass tuning curves produced by von Bekesy. Secondly, techniques for measuring very low amplitudes of vibration were not available to von Bekesy, with the result that he had to use very high sound pressures (e.g. 130 dB SPL). Such high sound pressures will have produced rapid damage to the cochlea. In any case it is now recognised that the basilar membrane vibrates non-linearly, so that its sharpness of tuning deteriorates at high sound levels. He also made most of his measurements on Reissner's membrane, rather than the basilar membrane. While he had reason to believe that they vibrated together, this is now thought not necessarily to be the case.

What is unexplained in the recent measurements, is how the basilar membrane manages to resonate with such extraordinarily sharp tuning, and why the tuning is so vulnerable to any slight deterioration in the state of the cochlea. This has

The Physiology of the Cochlea

led investigators to suggest that a physiologically active process might be involved in producing the sharp tuning. This is a point to which we shall return, after considering details of cochlear transduction.

Cochlear Transduction

There have been advances in our knowledge of hair cell anatomy and physiology in recent years, and this had led to the hope that we may be on the threshold of understanding the transduction process itself. Our attention is focused on the stereocilia on the apical membrane of the hair cell, since it is these that are moved by the deflections of the cochlear partition resulting from the mechanical travelling wave. As pointed out by Davis (1958), vertical deflection of the basilar membrane will be translated into a shear, or relative movement, between the tectorial membrane and the reticular lamina (Figure 2.4). This will produce a deflection, in a radial direction, of the stereocilia of the hair cells. As shown by Figure 2.4, when the basilar membrane is moved upwards, the stereocilia are deflected in a direction which is *away* from the modiolus.

Figure 2.4: As Suggested by Davis (1958), When the Basilar Membrane is Deflected Upwards, the Stereocilia on Each Hair Cell are Deflected Away from the Modiolus (i.e. away from the limbus).

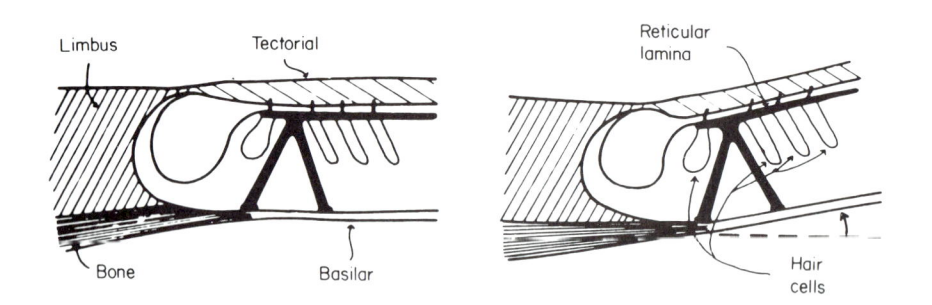

Source: Davis (1958).

Hair Cell Anatomy

Cochlear hair cells are divided into two types, known as inner and outer hair cells. Inner hair cells are situated on the inner, or modiolar, side of the arch of Corti (Figure 2.1B), and are flask shaped (Figure 2.5). Outer hair cells are situated on the side away from the modiolus in three to five rows, and are cylindrical in shape (Figure 2.5). Towards the base of each hair cell there are synaptic structures, where the hair cells make synaptic contact with the afferent auditory nerve fibres. On outer hair cells there are, in addition, large synaptic terminals of the efferent, or centrifugal, innervation of the cochlea, known as the olivocochlear bundle. The

The Physiology of the Cochlea 33

Figure 2.5: Inner and Outer Hair Cells of the Organ of Corti. OCB: fibres of olivocochlear bundle.

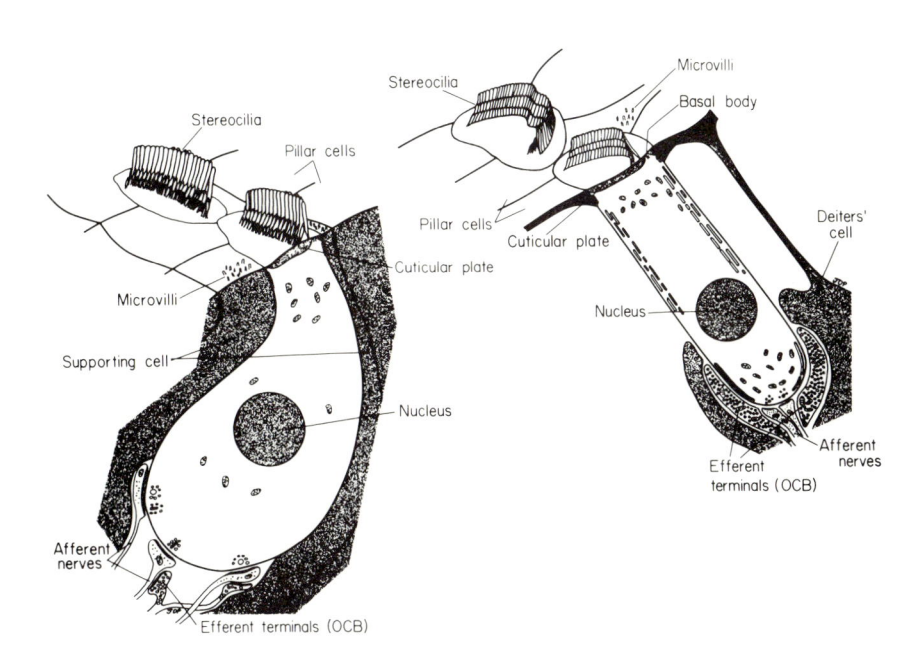

Source: Pickles *et al*. (1984). Illustrations, Birmingham University. © J.O. Pickles, 1984.

central nervous system is able to influence the state of the hair cells by means of this pathway.

The stereocilia on the apical surfaces of hair cells are arranged in a number of rows on each hair cell, with the stereocilia of the different rows graded in height, so that the tallest are on the side away from the modiolus. In the guinea pig there are three rows on each outer hair cell and three or four on each inner hair cell. In primates, however, there may be several rows. The rows on inner hair cells are approximately straight, and on outer hair cells the rows are 'V' or 'W' shaped, with the point or apex of the 'V' or 'W' pointing away from the modiolus. The stereocilia are anchored in a dense plate, known as the cuticular plate, in the apical surface of the hair cell.

The stereocilia themselves are stiff, rigid, structures, composed of actin filaments which run parallel to the long axis of the stereocilium. The actin filaments are bonded together in what has been called a 'paracrystalline array' (Tilney *et al.*, 1980). Each actin filament has certain sites along its length at which it can bond to its neighbours, and this, together with the helical structure of the individual filaments, imposes a certain order both on the positions at which the bonds are made, and on the spatial organisation of the filaments within the stereocilium.

34 *The Physiology of the Cochlea*

Molecular models of the bonding are consistent with our knowledge of the structure of the actin molecule. However, the nature of the cross-bridges is not known. It may be fimbrin, or myosin, both of which have been shown to be present within the stereocilia, and both of which bind to actin (Flock *et al.*, 1982; Macartney *et al.*, 1980). There are about 300 actin filaments in each stereocilium. About 30 of these continue into the rootlet of the stereocilium, which is anchored into the cuticular plate.

We would therefore expect stereocilia to be very rigid structures, and this has been confirmed by micromanipulation experiments, in which the stereocilia have been deflected with a rod. The stereocilia do not bend, but rather pivot at their base, until the force becomes so great that they crack.

The individual stereocilia are not separate structures on the apex of the hair cell, but are joined together by a large number of cross-links which affects their three-dimensional arrangement. Such links are destroyed by osmium fixation, which is probably why they have not been generally reported. Recent results from the author's laboratory, in collaboration with S.D. Comis and M.P. Osborne, have demonstrated cross-links between the stereocilia which are of two types (Pickles *et al.*, 1984). First, the stereocilia of the same row, and the stereocilia of the different rows, are joined together by links which run *laterally* between the stereocilia (i.e. at right angles to the long axis of the stereocilia), particularly near the apical ends of the stereocilia. Figure 2.6A for instance shows links running laterally, between the stereocilia of the tallest row on a guinea pig inner hair cell. They are confined to the upper 40 per cent of the stereocilia. In man, however, it seems that as well as laterally running links between stereocilia near the apex of the stereocilia, there are also lateral links running in a second band nearer the base (Figure 2.6b). Links which run laterally along the rows would tend to make all the stereocilia of one row move together when some are deflected, and the links which run *between* the rows tend to hold the tips of the shorter stereocilia in against the longer stereocilia. This is particularly marked on inner hair cells, where the shorter stereocilia lean in and appear like buttresses supporting the adjacent longer stereocilia (Figure 2.6C).

A second, and particularly important, set of links between the stereocilia, are those which can be seen running upwards, one from the tip of each shorter stereocilium, to join the taller stereocilia in the next row. Figure 2.7A shows such links, running upwards from the tips of the shorter stereocilia, on an outer hair cell. Such links run from the tips of the stereocilia of the middle row, to join the stereocilia of the tallest row, and from the tips of the stereocilia of the shortest row, to join the stereocilia of the middle row. They can also be seen, though less easily, running from the tips of most of the shorter stereocilia on the inner hair cell of Figure 2.6C. They can also be seen in the transmission electron micrograph of Figure 2.7B, as the very fine links running up from the tips of the middle and shortest stereocilia. They appear thicker in the scanning electron micrographs, because the specimens have to be coated with a fine film of metal for scanning electron microscopy. In transmission micrographs, the thickness of the links is about 5 nm, which is of macromolecular dimensions.

Figure 2.6: (A) Lateral Links Running Between Stereocilia on an Inner Hair Cell of the Guinea Pig Organ of Corti. Note that the surface membrane of the stereocilia is particularly rough at the level at which the cross-links are seen. The large blebs near the tips of the stereocilia are probably artefactual. (B) In man, there are lateral links in a second band towards the base of the stereocilia, as well as near the tips. Inner hair cell, middle turn. (C) On inner hair cells the shorter stereocilia lie in towards the longest stereocilia at a particularly sharp angle. The tip of each shorter stereocilium is pointed, and gives rise to a fine, short, upwards-pointing link, which runs up to join the stereocilium of the next row (arrows). Cross-links running laterally between stereocilia of the same row are also visible (arrowheads). Guinea pig. Scale bars: 100 nm.

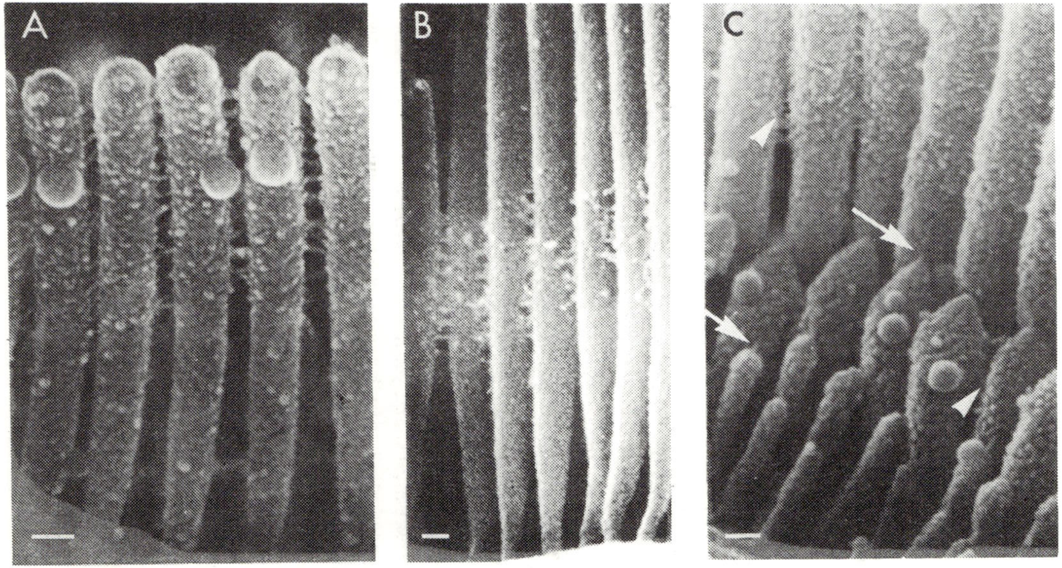

36 *The Physiology of the Cochlea*

Figure 2.7: (A) Upwards-pointing Links Running from the Tips of the Shorter Stereocilia on an Outer Hair Cell of the Guinea Pig Cochlea (arrows). Each stereocilium gives rise to only one of these links, and they are seen only on the shorter stereocilia of each hair cell.
(B) Transmission electron micrograph shows firstly dense links running between the different rows of stereocilia, particularly near the tips of the stereocilia of the middle and shortest rows (arrowheads). Secondly, the fine, hypothesised transducer links are seen, running from the tips of the shorter stereocilia, to join the adjacent longer stereocilia (arrows and inset). Scale bars: 100 nm.

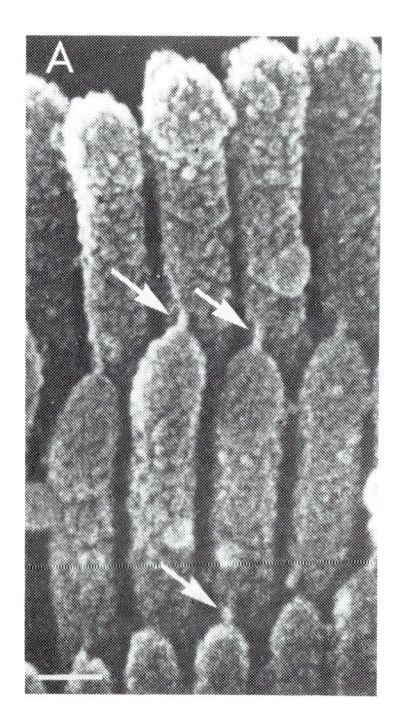

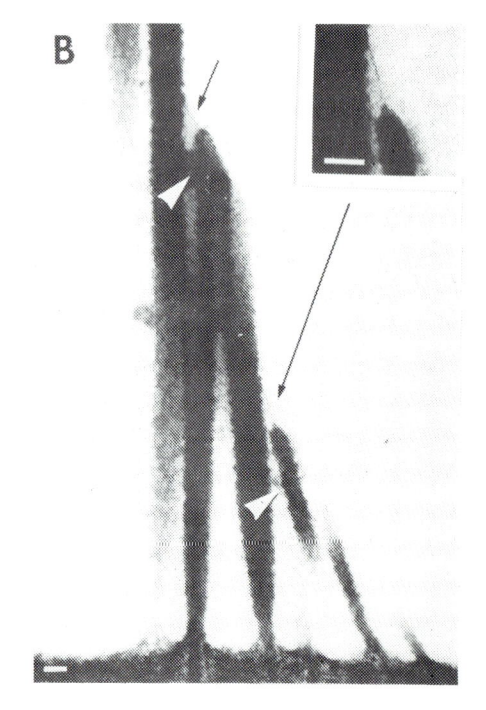

From their position on the stereocilia, we expect distortion of these fine, upwards-pointing links, to be involved in sensory transduction. A hypothesis which shows how deflection of the whole bundle of stereocilia might produce sensory transduction is shown in Figure 2.8. The dense, black links running between the rows hold the tips of the shorter stereocilia in towards the surface of the adjacent longer stereocilia of the next row. This means that when the whole bundle is pushed,

Figure 2.8: A Hypothesis Explaining How Deflection of the Whole Bundle of Stereocilia is Coupled to Distortion of the Hypothesised Transducer Region at the Tips.

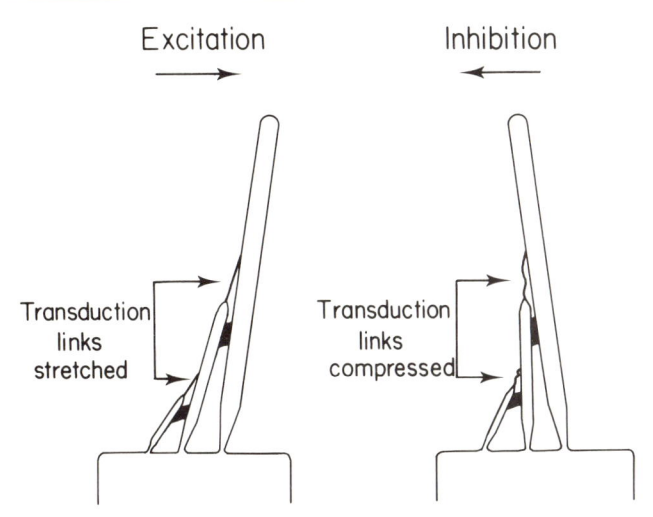

there is a relative sliding movement, in a vertical direction, between the tips of the shorter stereocilia and the adjacent longer stereocilia. This relative movement, it is suggested, would be detected by the fine, upwards-pointing links, running from the tips of the shorter stereocilia. If the bundle of stereocilia is pushed in the direction of the longest, which is the direction known to produce excitation, then the links would be stretched. If the bundle were pushed in the opposite direction, in the direction of the shortest, the links would be compressed. It is suggested that stretch of the links would open ion channels in the membrane, so that current could flow into the cell and change its membrane potential.

Hair Cell Physiology

The possible mechanism of the transduction process has been further elucidated by means of micromanipulation experiments, in which the stereocilia have been manipulated by a fine probe, while intracellular recordings have been made from the cells. These experiments have been performed in hair cells of the vestibular system (e.g. of the bullfrog sacculus), but the results are likely to apply to hair cells of the mammalian cochlea as well. Hair cells of the vestibular system, like those of the cochlea, have a bundle of stereocilia projecting from their apical surface. The stereocilia, like those of the mammalian cochlea, are graded in height. Hudspeth and Corey (1977) showed, by micromanipulation of the stereocilia, that deflection of the whole bundle in the direction of the tallest stereocilia was associated with depolarisation of the hair cell. Deflection of the bundle in the opposite direction, in the direction of the shortest, had the opposite effect, and was associated with hyperpolarisation. They showed that the relation between deflection and voltage response was sigmoidal in shape, so that the voltage response

38 The Physiology of the Cochlea

Figure 2.9: Relation Between Deflection of the Stereocilia, and Intracellular Voltage Response, in a Hair Cell of the Bullfrog Sacculus.

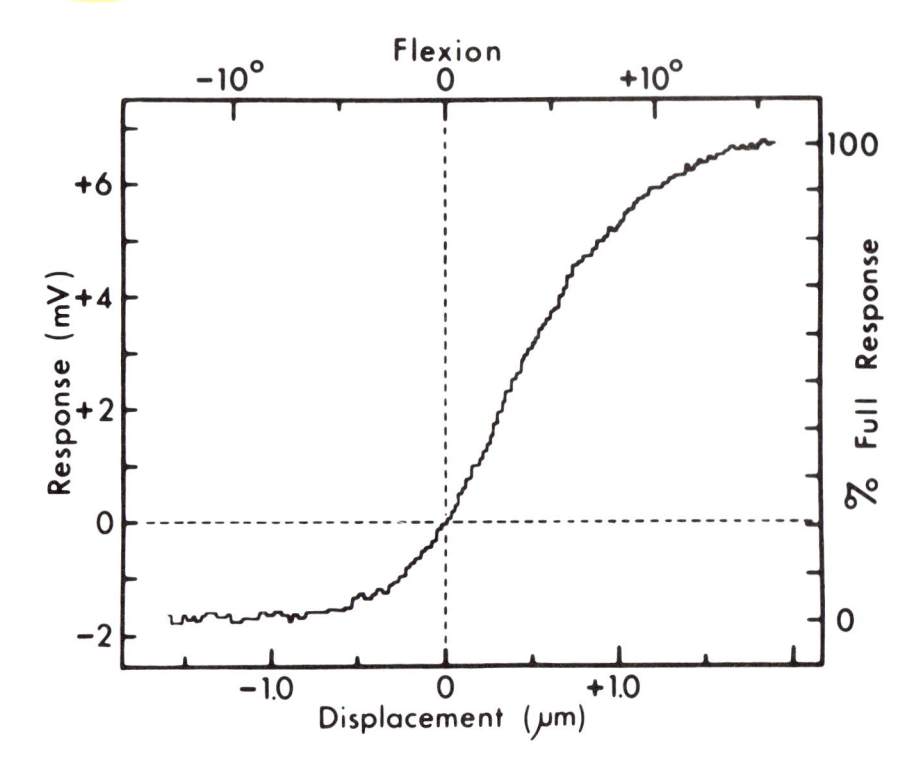

Source: Hudspeth and Corey (1977).

saturated in either direction (Figure 2.9). They also showed that the relation was asymmetric, so that the voltage responses tended to be larger in the depolarising direction, and saturated or limited at greater deflections and voltage responses, than responses in the opposite direction.

By injecting current into the hair cells through an intracellular microelectrode, and measuring the voltage responses produced, Hudspeth and Corey (1977) were able to show that the membrane resistance of the hair cell was low when the hair cell was depolarised, and high when the hair cell was hyperpolarised. It is therefore very likely that when the bundle of stereocilia is pushed in the excitatory direction, membrane channels open, decreasing the membrane resistance, and allowing ions into the cell. Since hair cells are faced with a solution with a positive potential (i.e. the endolymphatic potential, which in the mammalian cochlea has a value of around +80 mV), this means that the inside of the cell will become more positive, or depolarised, when the membrane channels are open. By separate perfusion of the apical membrane of the hair cell, Corey and Hudspeth (1979)

The Physiology of the Cochlea 39

showed that the resistance changes were indeed in the apical membrane of the hair cell, which is the one that contains the stereocilia.

From the currents measured as flowing during the transduction process, and knowledge of the likely conductance value for a *single* channel, Hudspeth (1983) suggested that each stereocilium contains only one transducer channel. In order to find the likely sites at which the transducer channels opened, Hudspeth (1982) used an electrode to explore around the stereocilia on a hair cell while pushing the bundle. He found that the greatest extracellular current flows produced by manipulating the bundle, were in the region where the shorter stereocilia ended. These results are entirely consistent with the hypothesis proposed in the last section: the suggestion that the transduction sites are at the tips of the shorter stereocilia is in agreement with our suggestion that distortion of the link there is responsible for transduction. The suggestion that there is only one transducer channel per stereocilium makes it likely that there is only one transducing structure per stereocilium. Similarly, we have only shown a single upwards-pointing link at that site.

Conclusions Concerning Hair Cell Transduction

The most recent anatomical and physiological evidence is clearly in favour of a simple and direct model of hair cell responses, similar to the 'resistance modulation' or 'battery' model of Davis (1958). In the modern version of this model, deflection of the basilar membrane produces deflection of the bundle of stereocilia on each hair cell, as shown in Figure 2.4. Deflection of the bundle in the direction of the tallest stereocilia produces a stretch of the links running upwards from the tips of the shorter stereocilia, and stretch of these links lowers, by as yet unknown mechanisms, the membrane resistance of the stereocilia in that region. The positive endocochlear potential (+ 80 mV), together with the negative intracellular hair cell potential (−70 mV for outer hair cells), combine to drive K^+ ions, which are present in the endolymph in high concentration, between the endolymph and the inside of the hair cell, so depolarising the hair cell. Deflection of the bundle of stereocilia in the opposite direction will have the opposite effects, increasing the resting hair cell membrane resistance, and so hyperpolarising the cell. The change in membrane potential modulates the release of transmitter at the base of the hair cell, and so modulates the activity of auditory nerve fibres synapsing there. This theory accounts for all the major facts of cochlear function, except for two important ones. Those are the division of the cochlear hair cells into inner and outer hair cells, and the dependence of the sharpness of the mechanical tuning on the state of the hair cells. These points will be considered, when we consider the responses of hair cells to sound, and theories behind the sharp tuning.

Hair Cell Responses to Sound

Inner Hair Cells

The very great majority of auditory nerve fibres (95 per cent in the cat, according to Spoendlin) make their synaptic contacts with inner hair cells. Therefore, until

40   The Physiology of the Cochlea

information appears to the contrary, it is reasonable to suppose that the job of inner hair cells is to detect the movement of the basilar membrane, and transmit the information to the central nervous system.

The responses of inner hair cells to sound were first measured by Russell and Sellick (1978). They showed that inner hair cells had resting potentials of about −45 mV. Sound produced both a.c. and d.c. responses intracellularly. These voltage responses were very sharply tuned, as sharply tuned as auditory nerve fibre responses and, as we now know, the mechanical response of the basilar membrane (Figure 2.3A). This suggests that the frequency selectivity of the hair cells is entirely dependent on the frequency selectivity of the mechanical response of the cochlear partition, and that hair cell responses depend on the mechanical responses in a simple and direct way. At one frequency, called the characteristic frequency, each hair cell gives its threshold response at very low sound intensities. This occurs when the peak of the mechanical travelling wave lies over the hair cell under investigation. As with the mechanical response, the sound intensity necessary to produce a threshold response rises sharply on either side of the characteristic frequency, although in an asymmetric manner, with a long, high-intensity, 'tail' to low frequencies.

The basis of the a.c. and d.c. responses of the cochlea, and the relation between them, can be understood from the input-output function for hair cells shown in Figure 2.9. An alternating input will give an alternating, although distorted, a.c. voltage response. Because the input-output function is asymmetric, there will be a d.c. component in the voltage response.

Underlying the asymmetric voltage response, there will be an asymmetric resistance change in the hair cell, which can similarly be divided into an alternating and a steady component. With sound stimuli, the alternating variation in the voltage response was too fast to be detected. However, Russell and Sellick, by injecting currents down their recording electrode and measuring the size of the voltages produced, were able to measure the steady component of the change in resistance. They showed that, during sound stimulation, the mean membrane resistance of the cell fell, in proportion to the magnitude of the d.c. voltage response. This result is entirely in agreement with the hypothesis that the intracellular voltage responses result from modulating the resistance of the apical membrane of the hair cell, as a result of the travelling wave.

The intracellular voltage responses of inner hair cells will modulate the release of transmitter at the base of the hair cells. This will modulate the firing of auditory nerve fibres, in phase with the movement of the basilar membrane. There will be a.c. and d.c. components to this modulation corresponding to the a.c. and d.c. components of the voltage response, so auditory nerve fibres will show an increase in mean firing rate during sound stimulation, as well as a tendency for the action potentials, when they occur, to occur in certain phases of the sound stimulus.

At this point, a complexity in the responses to a.c. stimuli should be mentioned. The modulated resistance at the apex of the hair cell allows a modulated current to flow through the hair cell. The voltage response in the hair cell, which determines the amount of transmitter released, will depend on the resistance the hair

The Physiology of the Cochlea 41

cell offers to current flow to ground. In other words, if the resistance of the basal membrane of the hair cell is low, the hair cell will offer little resistance to current flowing to ground, and the intracellular voltage responses will be small. The basal surface membrane of the hair cell acts as a capacitor, and so will have a small impedance (i.e. resistance) to high-frequency a.c. signals. This means that high-frequency stimuli will produce only small intracellular a.c. voltage responses. Therefore, there will be little phasic release of transmitter to high frequency sounds, and for those stimuli, most of the action potentials will have to be initiated by the d.c. component of the voltage response.

Outer Hair Cells

If nearly all the afferent auditory nerve fibres are connected to inner hair cells, and the inner hair cells detect the motion of the basilar membrane, it is reasonable to ask the question: what do outer hair cells do? Since outer hair cells have been more difficult to record from than inner hair cells, most of our ideas about their function must come from indirect evidence. The best answer we have on the basis of current knowledge, and a rather surprising one, is that outer hair cells govern the mechanical movement of the basilar membrane, and that they are necessary for its sharp frequency tuning.

This hypothesis is initially suggested by the finding that outer hair cells seem to be the most vulnerable elements of the cochlea, and by the finding that the very sharp mechanical tuning of the cochlea is similarly extremely sensitive to disruption.

Figure 2.10B shows the tuning curves of a set of auditory nerve fibres, in a guinea pig that had been treated with the ototoxic antibiotic kanamycin. This antibiotic is known to damage outer hair cells selectively when used in the correct doses. In the frequency region indicated, the outer hair cells, but not the inner hair cells, had been affected. Where the outer hair cells had been damaged, the tuning curves had lost their low-threshold, sharply-tuned, tips. In fact, the tuning curves became rather similar to those shown for the mechanical tuning of the basilar membrane during deterioration of the cochlea, culminating in death, of Figure 2.3B. If we suppose that the tuning of auditory nerve fibres is determined by the tuning of inner hair cells, and that this itself is determined by the tuning of the basilar membrane mechanics, we are left with the idea that the effect of the kanamycin may have been to affect the sharp mechanical tuning of the cochlea. While that hypothesis has not yet been tested directly, there are some pointers which we can consider.

First, there is evidence showing that certain factors which affect outer hair cells also affect the mechanics of the cochlea. One way in which the mechanical state of the cochlea can be monitored in a very sensitive way is to measure the sound energy the cochlea reflects back into the ear canal. If this is done, it can be shown that the energy reflected back is altered by stimulation of the efferent nerve supply, known as the olivocochlear bundle, which runs from the brainstem to the outer hair cells (Siegel and Kim, 1982). Activation of this nervous pathway must have changed the state of the outer hair cells in some way, and this suggests that the outer hair cells, in some way as yet unknown, affect the mechanical vibration. Secondly, the outer hair cells outnumber inner hair cells by over three to one. However, current electrophysiological evidence suggests that their intracellular d.c. voltage responses are small at high frequencies, presumably because their input-output functions (c.f. Figure 2.9). are very nearly symmetrical (Russell and Sellick, 1983). Moreover, their intracellular a.c. responses will also be small at these frequencies, since the capacitance of the cell wall will have a low resistance at high frequencies, and the current flowing through the apical membrane will be readily shunted to ground. Since both types of voltage response will be small in outer hair cells, the degree of synaptic activation will also be small. In fact, the outer hair cells will be acting merely as current shunts. This would explain the way they are responsible for the large extracellular current producing the cochlear microphonic. However the generation of the large current will require a significant input of energy to the cochlea, and this, together with the large number of outer hair cells involved in its generation, suggests that it must have some important function.

One hypothesis that has been suggested is that the outer hair cells, by feeding energy back into the mechanical stage, will be able to increase the sharpness of mechanical tuning of the basilar membrane (e.g. Kim *et al.*, 1980). It is known that in a mechanical resonator, very sharp degrees of resonance or tuning require very small degrees of damping. One way to achieve this in an electronic circuit is to have very low resistances in the circuit. However, that is often impractical, and the usual solution is to add 'negative resistance' or 'negative damping' into the circuit by including an amplifier. It is suggested that in the cochlea the return of amplified energy to the mechanics might act in a similar way. One of the dangers that any electronic circuit designer has to be aware of, is that in such a case the circuit may become unstable, and oscillate. Such oscillations have indeed been shown in the cochlea. Kemp (1979), who sealed a microphone into the ear canal, showed that many subjects produced a low-level, continuous, acoustic oscillation. Masking tests, and tests of the ability of the oscillator to respond to intermodulation products produced between the components of a complex acoustic signal, suggest that the mechanism responsible is situated *after* the stage of transduction (Kemp, 1979). The fact that in experimental animals the response was vulnerable to cochlear damage in the same way as are hair cells, suggests that hair cells may be involved in the response.

We do not yet know the mechanism by which outer hair cells may return mechanical energy to the cochlear partition. One intriguing hypothesis is that the stereocilia of outer hair cells are motile. The stereocilia and cuticular plate contain actin and myosin (Macartney *et al.*, 1980; Flock *et al.*, 1982), which are of course the active constituents of muscle. It is possible that the change in membrane potential and perhaps Ca^{2+} concentration resulting from deflection of the stereocilia, produce an active movement of the stereocilia, with the right phase shift to build up an oscillation. However, one overriding objection to that hypothesis is the speed of the response; seals and dolphins can hear up to 200 kHz, and this suggests that the actin-myosin interaction will have to build up to within 2.5 μs, and be broken down over a similar period. This is far faster than actin-myosin interactions generally occur. A more conservative hypothesis is that the feedback of energy results from a direct physical process. Speculations here include distortion of cell membranes resulting from water following ion flows as a result of osmosis, or as yet unknown energy pumping in the actin paracrystal. A hypothesis favoured by the author is that the voltage drop across the organ of Corti produced by the cochlear microphonic, moves electrically polarised structures in the organ and tectorial membrane, as a result of direct electrostatic attraction.

Although we do not expect motile proteins to affect the mechanics of the cochlear partition on a cycle-by-cycle basis, there is nevertheless a possibility that they affect the tonic background against which the travelling wave occurs. It is quite likely that the stiffness of the stereocilia is one of the factors governing the pattern of the mechanical travelling wave. It has recently been shown that the stiffness of stereocilia can be increased many fold by increasing the Ca^{2+} content of the bathing medium, which in turn increases the Ca^{2+} concentration intracellularly (Orman and Flock, 1983). This effect is likely to have been produced by an interaction of the actin in the hair cell with a protein such as myosin. If the efferent fibres of the olivocochlear bundle alter Ca^{2+} entry into the hair cells, then the efferent pathway would be able to control the tonic mechanical state of the cochlea.

Auditory Nerve Fibre Responses to Sound

About 95 per cent of auditory nerve fibes innervate inner hair cells. No reports have reliably shown a subpopulation of responses that could arise from the few fibres innervating outer hair cells. We must therefore suppose, until evidence is presented to the contrary, that the published records relate to the majority of the fibres, arising from inner hair cells.

Auditory nerve fibres are only excited by sound. Single stimuli never produce inhibition of activity, except as a rebound following a period of excitation. One of the most important properties of the response is its frequency tuning. This is clearly shown by the tuning curve or frequency threshold curve. As in Figure 2.3, the stimulus intensity is adjusted until a criterion, or threshold, amount of activity is detected, and the threshold is plotted as a function of stimulus frequency. Figure 2.10A shows a set of tuning curves for auditory nerve fibres arising from different frequency regions of the cochlea, or in other words having different best or characteristic frequencies. Those with low characteristic frequencies have relatively symmetrical tuning curves, at least on logarithmic scales of frequency. However, in high frequency fibres, an asymmetry in the tuning curves becomes apparent, and the tuning curves can be divided into a sharply tuned, low-threshold, tip region, and a broadly tuned, high-threshold, tail. As far as we can tell, these tuning curves are similar in shape to the tuning curves of inner hair cells, and the basilar membrane mechanical response, except perhaps in the details of the tail region.

The thresholds of the great majority of auditory nerve fibres lie in the bottom

44 *The Physiology of the Cochlea*

Figure 2.10: (A) Tuning Curves Are Shown for Auditory Nerve Fibres Arising from Different Frequency Regions of a Normal Cochlea. (B) When outer hair cells are damaged with kanamycin, the tuning curves of auditory nerve fibres lose their low thresholds and sharp tuning.

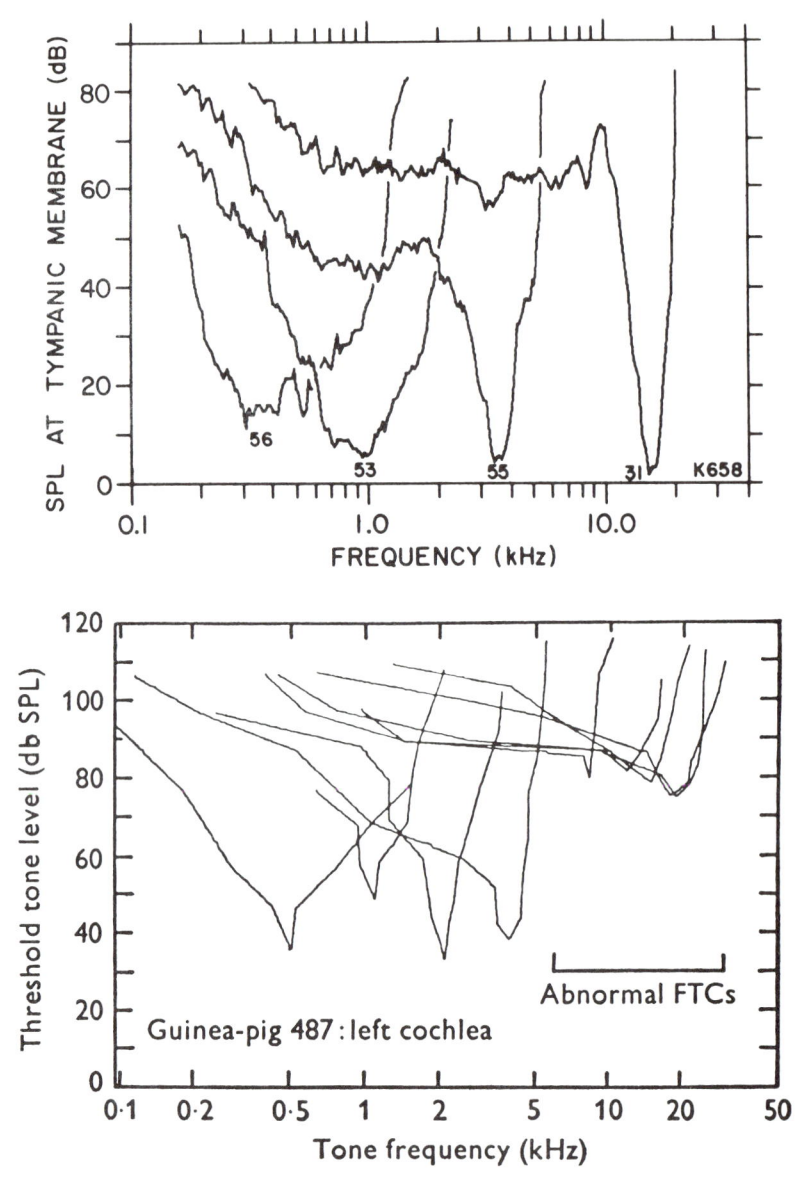

Sources: (A) Kiang, N.Y.S. (1980) *Journal of the Acoustical Society of American, 68*, 830-5. (B) Evans, E.F. and Harrison, R.V. (1975) *Journal of Physiology, 256*, 43-4P.

The Physiology of the Cochlea 45

Figure 2.11: Plots of Stimulus Intensity Versus Auditory Nerve Fibre Firing Rate, are Shown for Different Frequencies of Stimulation. The different frequencies of stimulation are shown as a parameter on the curves. CF = characteristic frequency.

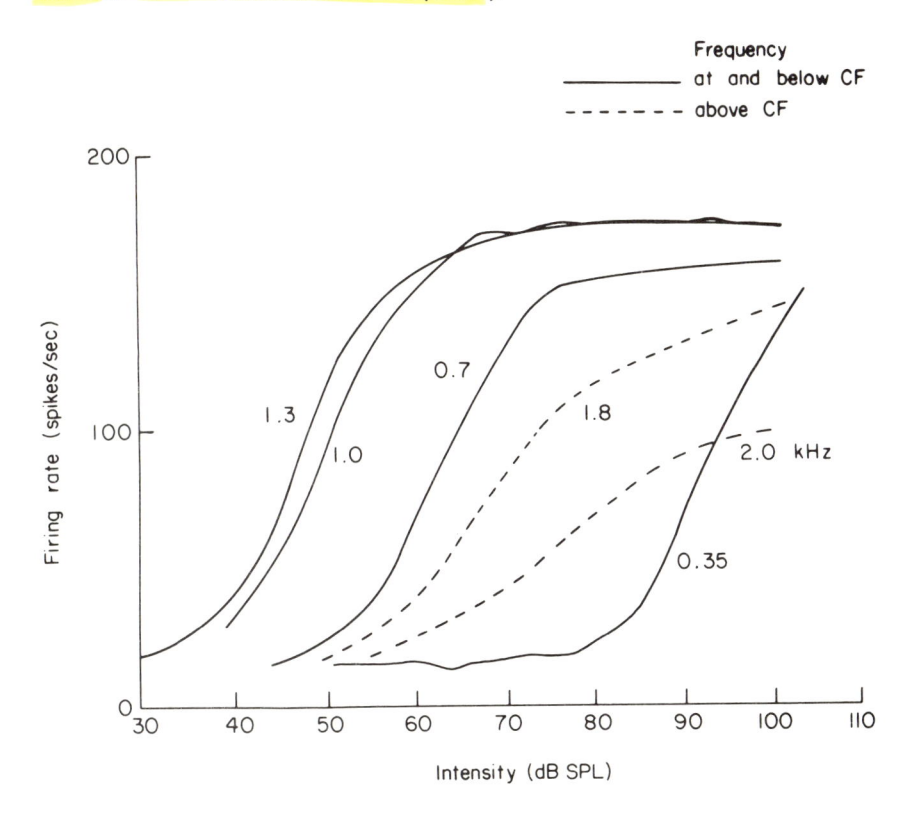

Source: Sachs, M.B. and Abbas., P.J. (1974) *Journal of the Acoustical Society of America*, 56, 1835-47.

10–15 dB of the intensity range, near the animal's absolute threshold. The thresholds of the others are scattered over the rest of the range, a few having thresholds of 80 dB SPL or more. If the stimulus intensity is increased from below a fibre's threshold, the firing rate at first increases slowly, and then steeply, to finally level out at a maximum, or saturated, rate (Figure 2.11). The stimulus intensity range from threshold to saturation is usually only 20–50 dB. The curves at different frequencies all follow a sigmoidal form, although of course with different starting intensities as a result of the frequency selectivity of the fibre. However, the rate-intensity functions for frequencies above the characteristic frequency have shallower slopes.

When action potentials are initiated by an auditory sinusoid, they are initiated preferentially during one half cycle of the stimulus. This is known as 'phase locking',

The Physiology of the Cochlea

and is related to the existence of a.c. receptor potentials in inner hair cells, and the associated phasic release of transmitter at the synapse. Like the a.c. receptor potentials, the amount of phase-locking declines with increasing stimulus frequency, so that for frequencies above 5 kHz, no phase-locking is observed.

Since the mechanical travelling wave peaks at different places along the cochlea for different frequencies of stimulation, stimuli of different frequency will activate spatially separate sets of auditory nerve fibres. This is known as the place coding of frequency. On the other hand, the phase locking of action potentials can also theoretically convey information about the frequency of the stimulus. This is known as the temporal coding of frequency.

We can now understand the responses of auditory nerve fibres to some complex stimuli, such as speech sounds. As a result of their frequency tuning properties, auditory nerve fibres respond to speech sounds rather as bandpass filters would, responding maximally when the stimulus has a lot of energy in their frequency range. When action potentials do occur, they will be phase-locked to the individual cycles of the frequency-filtered stimulating waveform, for components under 5 kHz, which covers most of the speech range. Therefore, such stimuli will be coded by both place and temporal coding.

Response of Auditory Nerve Fibres to Electrical Stimulation

In order to understand the operation of the prosthesis, it is obviously important to measure the responses of auditory nerve fibres to electrical stimulation of the cochlea. There have been surprisingly few studies of this important topic, following the pioneering work of Kiang and Moxon (1972).

Kiang and Moxon (1972) electrically stimulated the cochleae of cats. The cats had previously been treated with the ototoxic antibiotic neomycin, to destroy the hair cells. This was done in order to ensure that the effects would be produced only by direct stimulation of the auditory nerve fibres, as presumably would happen in human beings with severe losses, rather than by electrophonic effects.

Tuning Curves

First, they measured the intrinsic tuning properties of auditory nerve fibres to sinusoidal electrical stimulation. They showed that the tuning curves to electrical stimuli were very nearly flat, with very little variation in the tuning properties. Most fibres had minimum thresholds for sinusoidal stimuli of around 100 Hz (constant peak-to-peak current), rising very slowly for higher and lower frequencies of stimulation (Figure 2.12). Glass (1983) has since confirmed this result, and shown that the low and high frequency slopes of the 'tuning curves' were about 4 dB/octave. This is very much less than the slopes of tuning curves to auditory stimuli, which have low frequency slopes of 80–250 dB/octave, and high frequency slopes of 100–600 dB/octave. Therefore, auditory nerve fibres show very little intrinsic frequency selectivity to stimulus frequency. If there is to be any place coding of frequency, ways must be found of confining the stimulus current to limited regions

The Physiology of the Cochlea 47

Figure 2.12: 'Tuning Curves' to Sinusoidal Electrical Stimuli Show Much Less Frequency Selectivity than do Tuning Curves to Acoustic Stimuli (compare with Figure 2.10A).

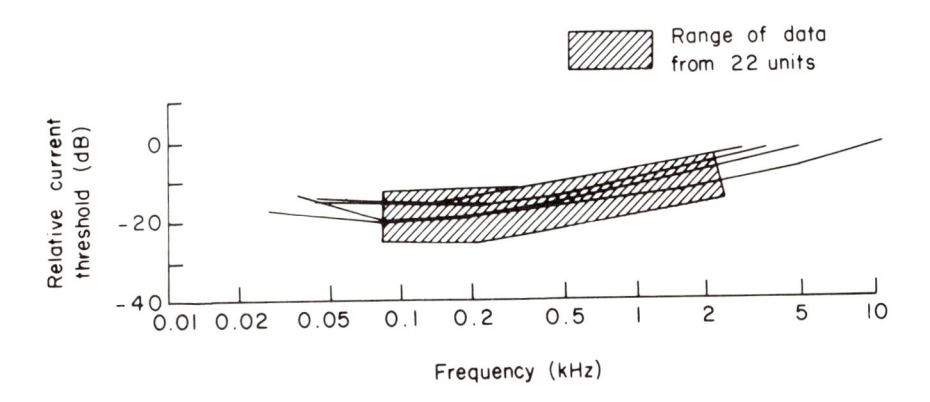

Source: Kiang and Moxon (1972).

of the cochlea, depending on the stimulus frequency. Current spread can be controlled best with bipolar stimulation. Although human data suggest that bipolar stimulation of different regions of the cochlea produces sensations with different frequency qualities, animal electrophysiological experiments have not so far found any large differences in the responses of auditory neurons, depending on the site of bipolar stimulation (Glass, 1983).

Dynamic Range

Another difference between acoustical and electrical stimulation of the cochlea is seen in the dynamic range, or the range of intensity from threshold to the maximum response. Whereas the dynamic range to auditory stimuli is usually 20–50 dB, that to electrical stimuli is only 2–15 dB (Figure 2.13). This problem is compounded, since the different auditory nerve fibres all seem to have very similar thresholds to electrical stimuli. This means that the intensity of an electrical stimulus has to be very precisely controlled, lest all the auditory nerve fibres be fully on, or fully off.

Temporal Coding

In one way, however, auditory nerve fibres seem able to convey more detailed, rather than less detailed, information in response to electrical stimuli. Phase-locking to sinusoidal electrical stimuli is more precise, so that action potentials are initiated over a narrower extent of the stimulus cycle. Temporal coding of the stimulus is therefore improved, although the frequency limit for activation by sinusoidal current (generally up to 2 kHz or so) means that the frequency range is smaller than with acoustic stimuli (up to 5 kHz). If the central nervous system were able

48   *The Physiology of the Cochlea*

Figure 2.13: Rate-intensity Functions for an Auditory Nerve Fibre Show Much Steeper Slopes to Electrical Stimuli, than to Acoustic Stimuli.

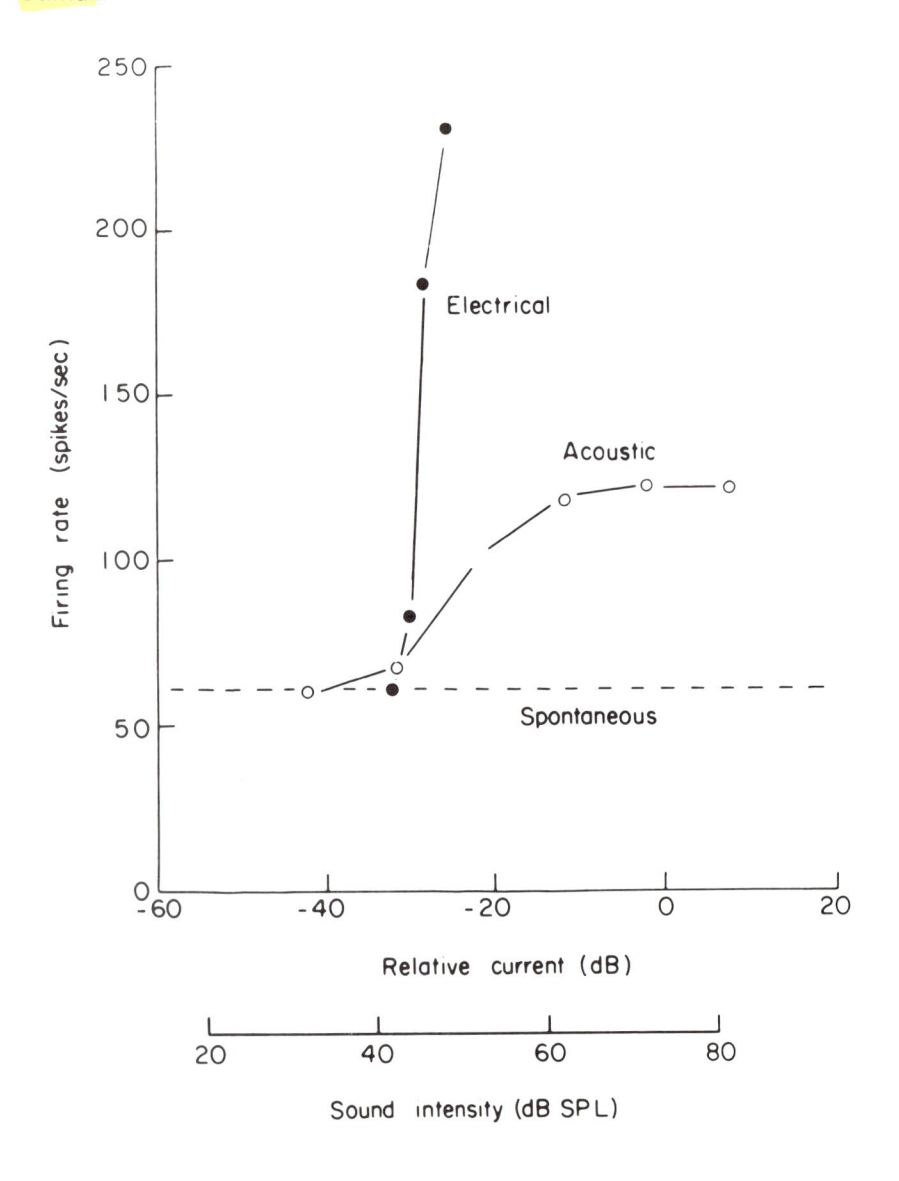

Source: Kiang and Moxon (1972).

to make use of such temporal information, which is controversial, it is possible that some of the deficiencies of electrical stimulation might be compensated for.

References

von Bekesy, G. (1960) *Experiments in Hearing*, Wiley, New York
Corey, D.F. and Hudspeth, A.J. (1979) *Nature, 281*, 675–7
Davis, H. (1958) *Laryngoscope, 68*, 359–82
Flock, A., Bretscher, A. and Weber, K. (1982) *Hearing Res., 6*, 75–89
Glass, I. (1983) *Hearing Res., 12*, 223–37
Hudspeth, A.J. (1982) *J. Neurosci., 2*, 1–10
—— (1983) *Ann. Rev. Neurosci., 6*, 187–215
—— and Corey, D.P. (1977) *Proc. Nat. Acad. Sci. USA, 74*, 2407–11
Kemp, D.T. (1979) *Arch. Otorhinolaryngol., 224*, 37–45
Kiang, N.Y.S. and Moxon, E.C. (1972) *Arch. Otol. Rhinol. Laryngol., 81*, 714–30
Kim, D.O., Molnar, C.E. and Matthews, J.W. (1980) *J. Acoust. Soc. Am., 67*, 1704–21
Macartney, J.C., Comis, S.D. and Pickles, J.O. (1980) *Nature, 288*, 491–2
Orman, S. and Flock, A. (1983) *Hearing Res., 11*, 261–6
Pickles, J.O. (1982) *An Introduction to the Physiology of Hearing*, Academic Press, London and New York
—— Comis, S.D. and Osborne, M.P. (1984) *Hearing Res., 15*, 103–12
Russell, I.J. and Sellick, P.M. (1978) *J. Physiol., 284*, 261–90
—— (1983) *J. Physiol., 338*, 179–206
Sellick, P.M., Patuzzi, R. and Johnstone, B.M. (1982) *J. Acoust. Soc. Am., 72*, 131–41
Siegel, J.H. and Kim, D.O. (1982) *Hearing Res., 6*, 171–82
Tilney, L.G., DeRosier, D.J. and Mulroy, M.J. (1980) *J. Cell Biol., 86*, 244–59

3   COCHLEAR ANATOMY AND HISTOPATHOLOGY

Lars-Goran Johnsson

Design and implantation of cochlear prostheses should be guided by knowledge of the normal and pathological anatomy of the labyrinth. The purpose of this chapter is to provide the pathologist's view of the problems in implantation and artificial stimulation of the cochlea in deaf patients. The reader is referred to recent review articles on the subject (Miller and Sutton, 1980; Aran, 1983).

Two different modes of artificial stimulation of the cochlear nerve are used; the single electrode which is inserted into the scala tympani, with a ground electrode located in the middle ear; and the multipolar devices which aim at discrete stimulation of nerve fibres in the osseous spiral lamina, with multiple pairs of electrodes usually embedded in a silicon matrix, which may be moulded in the shape of scala tympani.

Our present knowledge of temporal bone pathology in man and experimental animals allows the most important matters to be considered by implant designers and surgeons to be set out below.

Histopathological Considerations

Injury

The overriding objective should be to keep surgical insult to remaining cochlear and neural structures to a minimum. A prosthesis remaining outside the cochlea should be used whenever possible, in order to avoid further injury to its tissues.

Neuronal Degeneration

(1) Most implant candidates can be expected to have a severely reduced population of cochlear nerve fibres. The degeneration is a continuous process and is most severe in the distal (dendritic) processes in the osseous spiral lamina, especially in the basal turn.

(2) Almost all patients can be expected to have some nerve fibres remaining in the osseous lamina, and numerous ganglion cells in the modiolus.

(3) Generally the surviving fibres in osseous lamina will be located primarily in the apical and possibly in the middle turn. These fibres pass through the modiolus and lie close to the medial wall of scala tympani in the basal turn.

(4) Almost all patients can be expected to have a relatively large number of vestibular nerve fibres remaining, but the fibres of the macula of the saccule are likely to be degenerated.

Implant Design and Location

(1) Prosthesis design and insertion should be based on laboratory studies with

microdissections of the human labyrinth.
(2) Almost all intracochlear prostheses are likely to accelerate neural degeneration, especially if mechanical damage occurs during insertion.
(3) The least traumatic prosthesis is one of extracochlear type. (Placed on the round window, it may be functionally as effective as one inserted in the cochlea (Aran et al., 1983; Cazals et al., 1984a. Hochmair-Desoyer et al., 1980).)
(4) The long-term effect of electrodes placed in contact with the otic capsule is not known.
(5) Holes drilled in the otic capsule cause injury to its endosteum and extensive intralabyrinthine bone formation, followed by damage to sensory and neural structures. Drilling just close to the endosteum may also cause growth of intracochlear bone.
(6) The least traumatic intracochlear device is a short implant in scala tympani inserted through the round window.
(7) The round window and scala tympani can be occluded by osteoneogenesis resulting from extensive otosclerosis and severe labyrinthitis, which often are associated with exceptionally severe cochlear nerve degeneration. Preoperative X-rays (tomograms) can reveal such abnormal bony growth.
(8) The long-term outlook for the effectiveness of multipolar 'tonotopical' prostheses is probably poor because of the continuing degeneration of the distal processes of cochlear neurons.
(9) The last place where a regular nerve fibre arrangement may remain is in the modiolar wall of scala tympani, and not on the underside of the osseous lamina.
(10) Prostheses filling the scala tympani are likely to cause more injury than slender types. Special care should be taken to spare the endosteum and the collecting venules on the wall and floor of scala tympani from injury.
(11) Prostheses extending more than 10–13 mm into scala tympani should be avoided. Unless special precaution is taken in design and insertion, they tend not to conform to the shape of the cochlear spiral, and to cause rupture of the cochlear duct in the first half of the basal turn.
(12) The implant should preferably be designed so that it can be removed if necessary without causing extensive damage to the labyrinth.

Unfavourable Sites

(1) The modiolus, because the bone removal involved in surgery results in new bone formation and neuronal injury.
(2) The apical turn, even though the nerve fibres are likely to have survived there, because injury involved in placing an implant there through the otic capsule or by inserting it deeply is likely to be severe.

Unacceptable Sites

(1) Scala vestibuli, because of injury to Reissner's membrane, resulting in enhanced nerve degeneration.

52 *Cochlear Anatomy and Histopathology*

(2) The cochlear nerve in the auditory canal is accessible through a retrolabyrinthine route (Silverstein, *et al.* 1982). This approach has not been tried for the purpose of stimulating the nerve. The spread of current to adjacent structures from electrodes in such a location is likely and there are also risks of intracranial complications.

The Cochlear Nerve, Distribution and Degeneration

It is important for the implant surgeon to understand the basic arrangement of cochlear innervation and the degeneration pattern of the first-order neurone. For a review of nerve degeneration in the human temporal bone the reader is referred to a number of articles covering findings in specimens from patients with various forms of deafness (Ghorayer *et al.*, 1980; Johnsson, 1974; Johnsson and Hawkins, 1972, 1976; Kerr and Schuknecht, 1968; Lawrence and Johnsson, 1972; Lindsay, 1973; Lindsay and Hinojosa, 1978; Otte *et al.*, 1978; Schuknecht, 1974). An extensive review of the anatomical and pathological aspects of implantation has been published in German (Spoendlin, 1979a).

Cat Type I Cells

The ultrastructure of cochlear neurons, their distribution and pattern of degeneration after nerve sectioning have been most thoroughly studied by Spoendlin (1971, 1978, 1979b) in the cat. In this animal about 95 per cent of the neurons have large myelinated cell bodies with thickly myelinated processes connecting the inner hair cells with the cochlear nucleus. These particular cells are referred to as Type I.

Cat Type II Cells

The remaining neurons are referred to as Type II. They supply the outer hair cells and are small, usually unmyelinated, with unmyelinated processes. Spoendlin (1971) at first thought that they were resistant to degeneration because they did not disappear after section of the nerve. He later suggested (Spoendlin, 1979b, 1981) that the Type II cells have few or no central processes in the auditory nerve, and that they therefore do not degenerate when the eighth nerve is severed. Spoendlin's hypothesis has created controversy because it would leave the outer hair cells apparently without connection with the brainstem, and perhaps without function (Tumarkin, 1982). Fortunately, recent investigations indicate that the Type II hair cells do send processes to the brainstem (Kiang *et al.*., 1982).

Degeneration

The Type I cells may be particularly sensitive to metabolic disturbances, but both Types I and II do degenerate after sectioning of their processes in the internal and auditory canal and/or osseous spiral lamina. The part separated from the cell body degenerates rapidly and, in addition, there is a slow transganglionic or retrograde Wallerian degeneration. A small number of the Type I neurons resist retrograde degeneration after section of the auditory nerve. They lose the myelin sheath around the cell body, while their processes remain myelinated. These altered Type I neurons, formerly classified as Type III, are now called Type Ia (Spoendlin, 1979b). They apparently have the ability to ramify and grow to produce neuroma-like agglomerations of spiral fibres next to the inner hair cells along the entire length of the cochlea. The organ of Corti does not degenerate after eighth nerve sectioning, provided the blood supply is not disturbed (Rawdon-Smith and Hawkins, 1939; Schuknecht, 1953; Schuknecht and Woellner, 1955; Spoendlin, 1971, 1978, 1979b).

The Nerve in Man

It is not clear to what extent the structure and arrangement of the cochlear neurones in man correspond to those of the cat and other experimental animals. From the data available at present, it appears that the majority of the spiral ganglion cell bodies in man may be of the unmyelinated or partly myelinated type, although most of their processes presumably are fully myelinated. There are about 30,000–35,000 neurons in the human cochlea (Guild, 1932; Rasmussen, 1940). The total number presumably varies somewhat from individual to individual, and may also depend on the length of the cochlea. In the modiolus the cochlear nerve fibres fan out to the different turns, so that the fibres in the periphery of the nerve trunk supply the basal turn, and fibres for the middle and apical turns lie more centrally in the nerve trunk. Most of the nerve fibres reach Corti's organ along a more or less radial course in the osseous spiral lamina, where their arrangement is fairly orderly (Johnsson and Hawkins, 1972) and, in all likelihood, specific for pitch (Figure 3.1). Also, in man more than 90 per cent of the nerve fibres presumably supply the inner hair cells (Nomura, 1976). All fibres lose their myelin sheath at the habenula perforata before they reach the basilar membrane and Corti's organ. The 'dendritic' fibres, with their main portion located in the osseous spiral lamina, should preferably be referred to as *distal* or *peripheral processes*, and the 'axonal' fibres, with their main portion in the internal auditory canal, as *proximal* or *central processes*.

Profound Deafness

Most forms of profound deafness are caused by primary injury and degeneration of hair cells (Johnsson, 1974). This form of hearing deficit is, or should be, referred to as sensorineural hearing loss, because it almost invariably leads to a progressive secondary nerve degeneration which is most pronounced in the lower half of the basal turn. Initially the nerve network in the spiral lamina remains quite dense (Johnsson *et al.*, 1981, 1984), but most patients with deafness that has lasted for several years can be expected to have very few nerve fibres in the spiral lamina of the basal turn. In the apical turn, on the other hand, numerous nerve fibres may survive in the spiral lamina for decades and perhaps for a lifetime. Their proximal processes, as emphasised earlier, are located in the middle of the nerve trunk, close to scala tympani in the basal turn.

54 *Cochlear Anatomy and Histopathology*

Figure 3.1: Dissection Showing Close Relation Between Osseous Lamina (OL) and Darkly Stained Round Window Membrane. In a normal right ear the arrow indicates the best location and direction for implant insertion. Posterior pole of oval window to left, posterior ampulla in lower left corner. SD, saccular duct; S, saccule; DR, ductus reuniens. OsO_4.

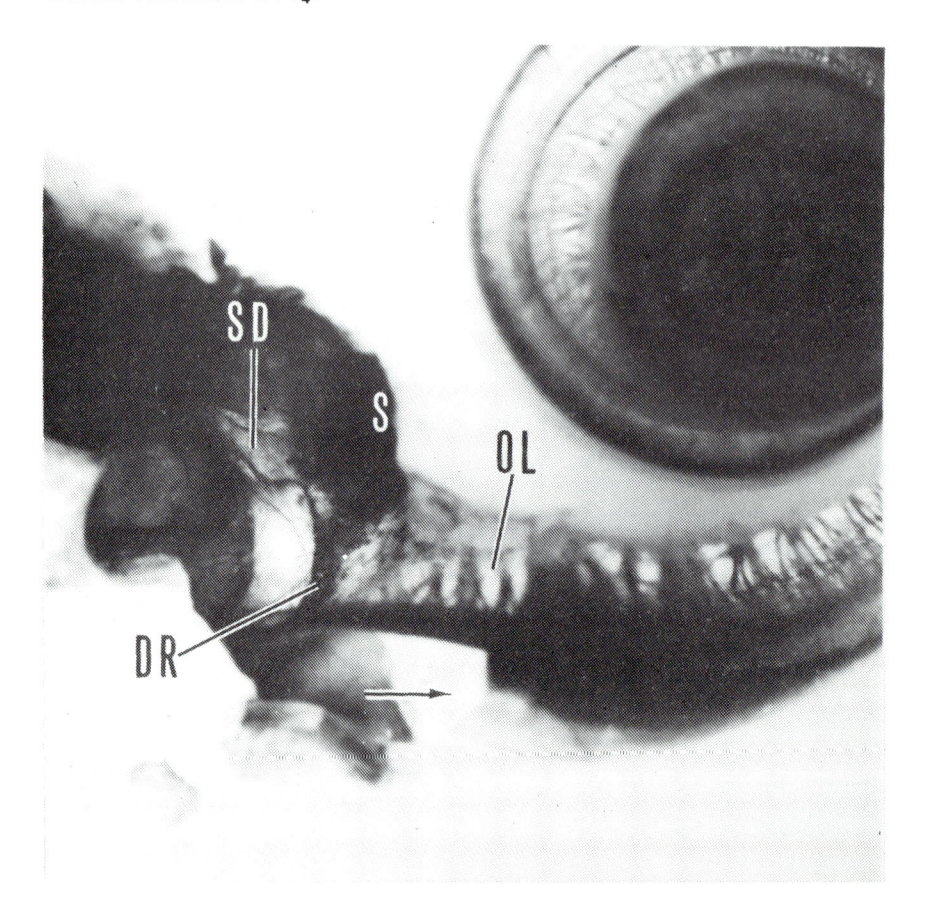

Delayed Effect of Hair Cell Loss

In monkeys treated with ototoxic drugs we have often observed a markedly uneven, patchy sensorineural degeneration in the basal turn (Johnsson and Hawkins, unpublished data). Scattered islands of supporting cells of Corti's organ remain and are each supplied by bundles of nerve fibres which are interspersed with areas of more or less complete nerve degeneration in the spiral lamina. Similar degeneration patterns are rare in our human material, but they do occur occasionally from various causes, including ototoxicity (Johnsson *et al.*, 1981).

Patients who have become deaf after receiving ototoxic drugs initially have a severe sensory, i.e. hair cell degeneration, with an almost normal density of nerve fibres in osseous spiral lamina (Johnsson et al., 1981, 1984). Within a few years, however, the secondary nerve degeneration becomes so severe that a tonotopical stimulation of the fibres in osseous lamina is likely to be impossible (Johnsson et al., 1981; Tange and Huizing, 1980).

Ganglion Cell Survival

Neural or predominantly neural forms of hearing loss where the nerve degeneration is primary are uncommon in our material (Johnsson, 1974; Johnsson and Hawkins, 1972). They are seen, for example, after certain forms of viral infection of the perilymphatic space (Lindsay, 1973a), and they lead to severe primary degeneration of the spiral ganglion cells and their processes.

The early secondary nerve degeneration involves mainly the distal processes of the first-order neuron both in man (Egami et al., 1978; Hinojosa and Marion, 1983; Johnsson et al., 1981, 1984; Lawrence and Johnsson, 1972; Lindsay, 1973a and b; Nadol, 1977, 1980; Otte et al., 1978; Schuknecht, 1974; Ylikoski et al., 1981) and in experimental animals (Kellerhals et al., 1967; Liberman and Kiang, 1978). It usually begins at the peripheral end, especially in the case of ototoxicity, and progresses toward the modiolus (Johnsson et al., 1984). Thus, despite severe degeneration in the peripheral part of the osseous lamina, one can still find nerve bundles of more or less normal diameters entering the lamina along the modiolar wall of scala tympani (Johnsson et al., 1981, 1984). The cochlear nerve itself in the internal meatus can still be of almost normal size, even in deafened ears (Ylikoski et al., 1978). Actual ganglion cell counts (Hinojosa and Marion, 1983; Ibrahim and Linthicum, 1980) suggest that more than 50 per cent of cochlear ganglion cells can survive for a long time in profoundly deaf ears. On the other hand, studies of comparable material from Schuknecht's temporal bone collection showed a greater reduction of the number of ganglion cells (Kerr and Schuknecht, 1968; Otte et al., 1978). Liberman and Kiang (1978) have shown in experimental animals that nerve fibres without distal processes can still be electrically excitable. The vitality and excitability of comparable ganglion cells in human ears are difficult to assess.

It is likely that degeneration occurs also in man at the central terminals of the cochlear fibres, resembling that observed in monkeys (Miller et al., 1980; Stebbins et al., 1969) and other experimental animals after destruction of Corti's organ (Morest, 1981; Powell and Erulkar, 1962; Webster and Webster, 1978). Unfortunately, there is only limited information about such transsynaptic degeneration in human material. Whether maintaining the activity of the nerve fibres by means of artificial stimulation could prevent transsynaptic degeneration is not known.

Importance of Supporting Cells

The secondary type of nerve degeneration in osseous lamina is effectively delayed by the presence of the supporting cells and pillar cells (Johnsson, 1974; Johnsson and Hawkins, 1972, 1976; Otte et al., 1978; Schuknecht, 1953; Spoendlin and

Gacek, 1963). According to Spoendlin (1978), injury to the unmyelinated portion of the nerve fibres inside Corti's organ represents the crucial factor that initiates degeneration. *Therefore, all implantation surgery should aim at preserving the remaining organ of Corti in the deaf ear in so far as possible. Any disruption of the walls of the cochlear duct, notably the basilar membrane or Reissner's membrane, will, in addition to mere mechanical damage, cause contamination of the endolymph with perilymph which, in turn, will cause further damage to Corti's organ* (Duvall and Rhodes, 1967; Lawrence, 1966; Schuknecht and Seifi, 1963) *and accelerates the ongoing secondary nerve degeneration.* After experimentally produced ruptures of Reissner's membrane which, it should be noted, have usually been relatively small, damage to Corti's organ is confined to the region of the rupture, and there is only limited longitudinal spread of the degeneration. One may hope that this also holds true for the human cochlea, if a rupture should occur during implantation surgery.

Vestibular Nerve

In contrast to the cochlea, the vestibular portion of the labyrinth is relatively resistant to insults. Some vestibular organs may survive a labyrinthectomy intended to destroy them. It is not known why the vestibular nerve is resistant to degeneration, when clearly the cochlear nerve is so susceptible (Gacek, 1967). Vestibular neuroepithelia and notably the vestibular nerve fibres tend to demonstrate much slower and less extensive forms of degeneration than their cochlear counterparts. In man the most severe degeneration occurs in the macula of the saccule which often degenerates hand in hand with the cochlea. This is of particular interest since there are indications that the macula responds to acoustical stimulation (Cazals *et al.*, 1980, 1984), and the structure is located relatively close to electrodes in the round window and scala tympani.

The Number of Nerve Fibres Needed

It is not yet known how many nerve fibres are needed to achieve useful auditory sensation by means of artificial stimulation in man. Perhaps only a few nerve fibres are needed to transmit an adequate number of impulses to the brainstem. It is also possible that the stimulus is simply conducted along tissues and fluids.

Investigations by Cazals *et al.* (1980, 1984) suggest that the vestibular end organs or their nerves can respond to acoustical stimulation of deafened ears and transmit information to the auditory cortex. It is of course too early to say whether the vestibular nerve can serve as a useful substitute path in artificially evoking auditory sensation in man.

If non-neural tissue can conduct currents in an effective way, one can hope that there will be little or no long-term deterioration of the hearing levels that may be achieved with the implant.

Animal Models of Human Cochlear Implants

The extent of degeneration associated with cochlear prostheses in animals varies, depending on implant design, technique of insertion, and the length of time the prosthesis has been in place. Mechanical damage to the basilar membrane and osseous spiral lamina, which probably can be avoided by good design and technique, is the greatest stimulus to sensorineural degeneration.

Histological Changes after Animal Implantation

Schindler *et al*. (1977), using moulded, tight-fitting implants filling the entire scala tympani in the basal turn, saw little evidence of increased neural degeneration in neomycin-deafened cats, provided that the osseous lamina, basilar membrane or endosteum was not injured. They state, however, that if hair cells are present they degenerate. Presumably the same would happen to remaining supporting structures, and thus the implant could nevertheless cause additional degeneration with time. If injury does occur, the authors emphasise that the nerve degeneration is limited to the region of damage. Leake-Jones and Rebscher (1983) reported relatively mild cochlear pathology after gentle insertion of multipolar prostheses. One cat, however, showed severe sensorineural degeneration and bone formation nine months afterward.

Thin Electrodes

Severe changes, including osteoneogenesis, were present in Clark's and his coworker's cats, which were implanted with thin electrodes in the basal or apical turn (Clark *et al*., 1975; Clark, 1977).

In their most recent report the Australian team (Shepherd *et al*., 1983) described the histopathology in cats after 80 days of implantation with a slender array of electrodes reaching 6 mm into scala tympani. There was scattered hair cell loss throughout the cochlea, local ganglion cell loss next to the prosthesis, extensive connective tissue formation in scala tympani and new bone formation. The major portion of the ganglion cell population remained intact. Long-term observation of such implanted ears is likely to show more widespread nerve degeneration and bone formation in scala tympani.

Ganglion Cell Loss

Sutton *et al*. (1980) have observed ganglion cell degeneration in monkeys 3-4 months after implantation with tightly fitted prostheses of the moulded type. It is worth noting that slender, 'free-fit' devices also caused ganglion cell degeneration, although there was no visible rupture of cochlear structures. In a later study of longer-term, 'free-fit' implantations, the authors also found varying degrees of ganglion cell loss and osteoneogenesis. After more than two years of survival, few ganglion cells were present, and many of the remaining cells were in the process of degeneration (Sutton and Miller, 1983).

Cochlear Anatomy and Histopathology

Modiolar Electrodes

It is too early to evaluate the extent of injury produced by intramodiolar electrodes (Simmons, 1979). Their insertion involves extensive drilling of the otic capsule and could cause injury to nerves and blood vessels with osteoneogenesis. The bone growth observed in the cochlea of one deaf white cat with intramodiolar electrodes was believed to have been caused by an infection prior to surgery. It may, however, have been the result of disruption of the blood supply or irritation of the endosteum caused by the implantation.

The Effect of Current

Electrical stimulation by itself can cause destruction of Corti's organ adjacent to the electrode (Duckert and Miller, 1982; Fourcin et al., 1979; Leake-Jones et al., 1981). Stimulation by a round window electrode does not prevent or retard secondary nerve degeneration (Cazals et al., 1984).

Animals and Man

One should be cautious in drawing far-reaching conclusions from findings in animals, which may have a labyrinth more resistant to trauma than man's. It appears, as suggested earlier (Sutton et al., 1980), that the labyrinth in the cat may be less subject to trauma than the primate cochlea, including that of man. Even after considerable surgical trauma to vestibular organs and the cochlea (Lawrence et al., 1961), large portions of the sensorineural epithelium appear intact in the cat, when comparable procedures in man, in all likelihood, would cause deafness. In fact, complete deafness in man can occur after a seemingly uncomplicated stapedectomy or after blue-lining the horizontal semicircular canal.

The Effects of Ageing

Although obvious, it is frequently forgotten that the degree of sensorineural degeneration observed depends to a great extent on the interval between the implantation and the time the temporal bones of the animal are obtained. Similarly, the density of the cochlear nerve population of animals with hereditary deafness will depend on the age of the animal at the time of death. If the hair cell loss is complete, which it often is, the secondary nerve degeneration is a continuous process which, for example in white cats and Dalmatian dogs, does not end after a year, which is a common time period used in degeneration experiments. With time the degeneration leads to a severe or complete loss of nerve fibres in osseous lamina. It is likely that some ganglion cells will survive (Johnsson et al., 1973; Mair, 1973).

Electrical Pathways in the Labyrinth

In attempting to stimulate the residual ganglion cells, possible preferential pathways between the electrode and the remaining neuronal elements should be considered (Black and Clark, 1980; Spelman et al., 1980). It is conceivable that the radially disposed nerve canals in osseous spiral lamina can act as spatially arranged conduction pathways to the modiolus.

Myelin Remnants

After nerve degeneration these canals remain patent and contain remnants of myelin sheaths (Johnsson *et al.*, 1982). They are, however, not effectively sealed off from the scalae and are in all likelihood filled with perilymph. As stated earlier, if tonotopical stimulation is attempted, it should be aimed at the modiolar wall in scala tympani or at the base of osseous lamina rather than at the habenula perforata region.

Canals Between CSF and Perilymph

No distinct barrier has been shown to exist between the cerebrospinal fluid and the perilymph. The VIIIth nerve is surrounded by cerebrospinal fluid. Perineural and perivascular spaces probably provide a communication between the subarachnoid space and the modiolus and the canals in osseous lamina (Duckert and Duvall, 1977, 1978; Holden and Schuknecht, 1968). Furthermore, the bony wall of the modiolus facing scala tympani appears to be porous. There is, in other words, a fluid-filled pathway between scala tympani and the brainstem. This path may be wider in deaf patients with nerve degeneration than in individuals with a dense population of neurons filling the modiolus and the canals in osseous lamina.

Implant Sites

The Apical Turn

The apical region of the cochlea seems to offer the implant surgeon an important advantage over the basal turn, viz., the presence of surviving nerve fibres. Therefore, the effectiveness of extracochlear apical electrodes perhaps should be explored in experimental animals. The modiolus, the very last site where neural elements survive (Johnsson *et al.*, 1981, 1982), is not recommended, for reasons already mentioned.

The Basal Turn

The region of the outer margin of the osseous spiral lamina in the basal turn is not particularly suitable for tonotopical stimulation, because that is where the nerve degeneration begins. A multipolar implant in scala tympani should aim at stimulating the thick nerve bundles arranged in order along the body modiolar wall. Although proximity of the electrode to the nerve fibres is important, the surgeon should keep in mind that it also may endanger their survival and can cause new bone formation in their vicinity. From a histopathological point of view, the lower basal turn still appears to be the best intracochlear site for implants, provided that they are suitably short, to avoid damage to endosteum and venules.

Holes in the Bony Cochlea

When the endosteum of the labyrinth is disturbed, the otic capsule frequently responds with new bone formation (Lawrence et al., 1961; Lawrence and Johnsson, 1972; Simmons, 1979). Therefore, implantation surgery should aim at avoiding damage to the otic capsule and its endosteum. For this reason, the drilling of multiple holes in the bony cochlea is particularly objectionable from the pathological point of view.

Surgical Anatomy of the Round Window

For the surgical anatomy of the round window the reader is referred to an article by Gacek (1978). The window niche is often completely or partially covered by a thin membrane, which is derived from middle ear mucosa. This membrane should be removed at surgery. The true window membrane, which is much thicker, is located well anterior to it and is almost always out of sight inside the niche.

The close relationship between the round window membrane and osseous spiral lamina and basilar membrane is shown in Figure 3.2. It is easy to damage the spiral lamina during implantation, even when using short electrodes, and this could lead to rupture of the cochlear duct and new bone formation. Ideally, the implant should be inserted through the inferior half of the round window membrane and pushed anteriorly in a more or less horizontal direction. It is worth noting that in the ears which will be briefly described here this was correctly done, and there was no injury to the osseous lamina (Johnsson et al., 1982).

Surgical Obstacles

Severe labyrinthitis and extensive otosclerosis can cause bone formation in the labyrinth which may occlude scala tympani and the round window (House, 1982; Ibrahim and Linthicum, 1980; Johnsson et al., 1978; Suga and Lindsay, 1977). Polytomography of the labyrinth is helpful in evaluating the patency of scala tympani (House, 1982). Sectional radiography should in any case be performed prior to implantation surgery in order to rule out congenital malformations and aplasias of the labyrinth.

Histopathological Changes

Histopathological findings in only one pair of human temporal bones with cochlear implants have been reported. The reader is referred to a detailed article on the subject (Johnsson et al., 1982). Both implants caused severe mechanical injury to the inner ear. The damage was to a great extent attributable to the length of the implants and to their design, which was relatively crude. Although the changes observed were extreme, they were instructive and in many respects quite

Figure 3.2: Left Cochlea, Showing Normal Dense Nerve Network of Darkly Stained Distal Processes in Osseous Lamina; They Lose Their Myelin Sheaths at Habenula Perforata. R, portion of Reissner's membrane left *in situ*. OC, organ of Corti, seen as two dark bands representing inner and outer hair cells. SL, portion of spiral ligament left *in situ*. ST, scala tympani, with radiating venules, displayed after a segment of osseous lamina has been removed. RW, round window niche. DR, ductus reuniens. OW, oval window. OsO_4.

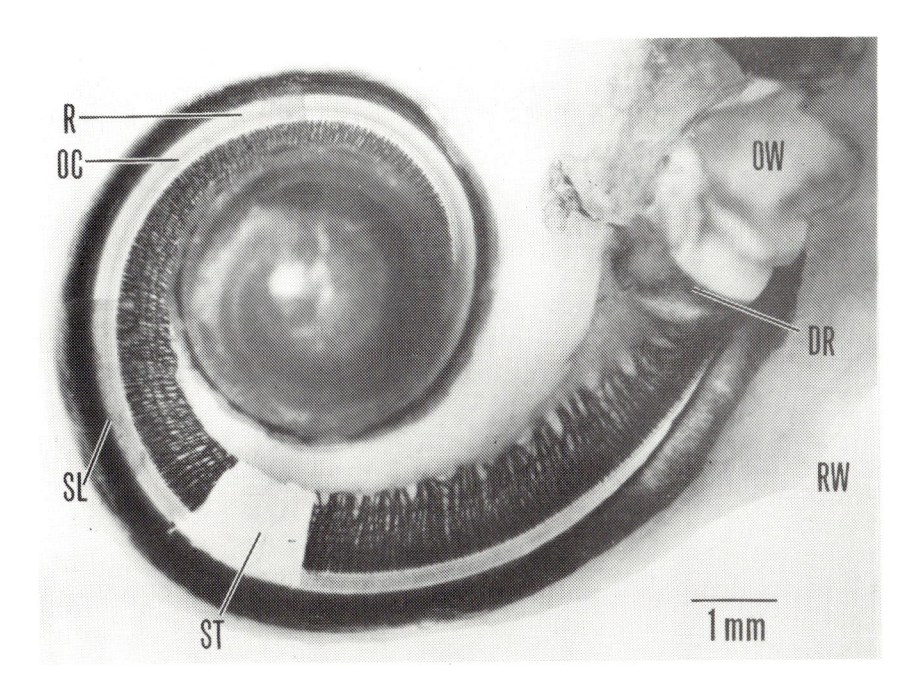

characteristic. Therefore, both temporal bones are illustrated and briefly described here. Recent devices are much less likely to cause injury than that seen in Figures 3.3–3.11.

Temporal Bone Post-mortem

These temporal bones were obtained from a 63-year-old male who suffered from bilateral, complete long-standing deafness. He had had a single platinum wire electrode in the right ear for two years and five silver wire electrodes in the left ear for eight years, both inserted in scala tympani through the round window.

The Round Window

In the round window niche the implants were encapsulated in connective tissue, which appeared to have effectively sealed the window. Both implants were found to have deviated in a more or less symmetrical fashion from their intended course,

62 *Cochlear Anatomy and Histopathology*

Figure 3.3: Right Labyrinth, Showing Single Electrode Entering Scala Media Along Bony Wall, ca. 12 mm from Opening of Niche. Note distortion of basilar membrane in upper half of basal turn. No nerve fibres visible in osseous lamina. At arrow, two patches of Corti's organ. OW, oval window; RW, round window niche; BM, basilar membrane. *Insets.* Scala tympani (seen after osseous lamina removed), circumscribed connective tissues formation around electrode in first curvature. Apical turn with two patches of supporting cells (OC), supplied by myelinated nerve fibres.

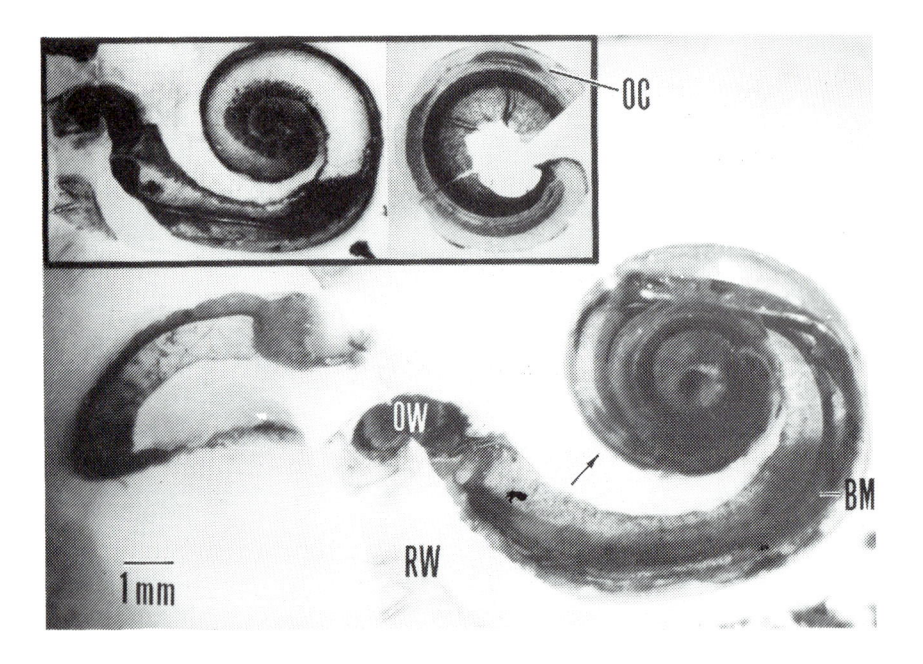

each taking an 'uphill' direction along the curving bony wall of scala tympani in the region about 13 mm from the basal end of the cochlea, where it entered scala media and finally bent posteriorly.

Electrode Penetrated Scala Media

In the right ear, where the implant extended farther into the basal turn, the cochlear duct in the upper half of the basal turn had been displaced by the implant. In the left ear, there was extensive new bone formation around the electrodes. The bending of the implant was clearly dictated by the shape and the geometry of the basal turn and is evidently characteristic for implants of this type and length.

In the right ear, two islands of Corti's organ remained in the upper end of the basal turn and in the apical turn, respectively. Each was supplied by several bundles of nerve fibres in the osseous spiral lamina. In the left ear, which had cochlear

Cochlear Anatomy and Histopathology   63

Figure 3.4: Horizontal Section of Scala Tympani, Lower Half of Basal Turn, Showing Loose Avascular Connective Tissue Formation Around Electrode, E, Which has Been Removed. There is a dense sleeve of fibroblasts around the electrode (cf. Figure 3.3). H and E after initial OsO_4 staining.

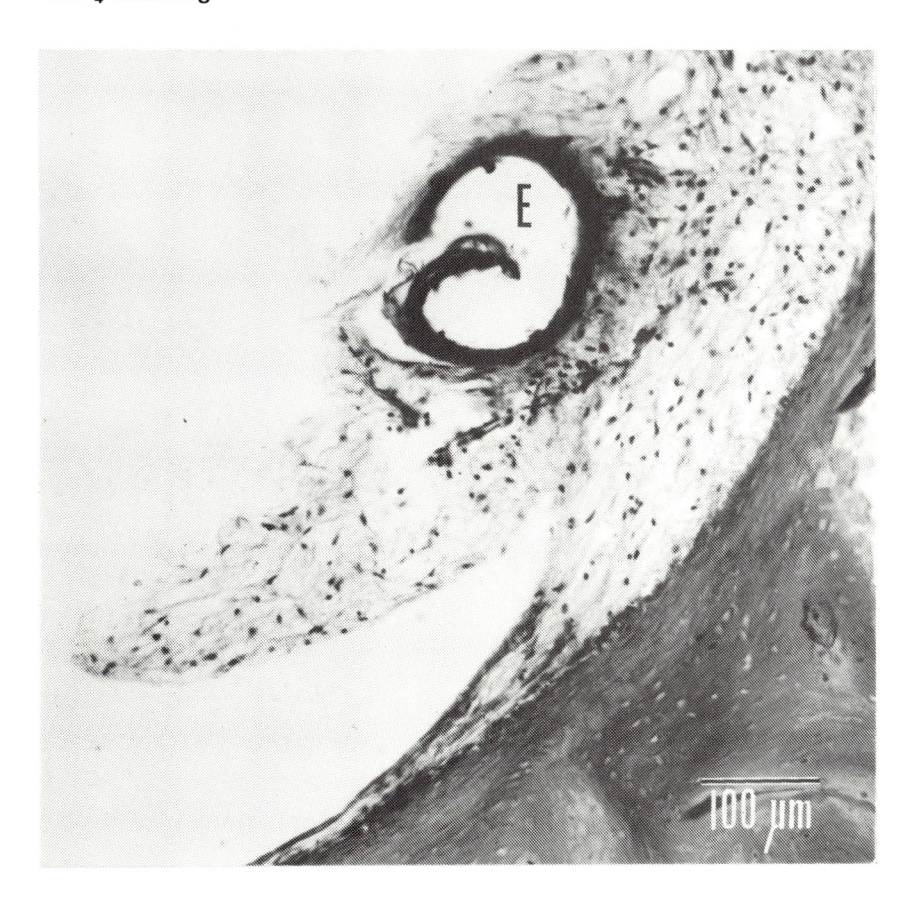

Source: Johnsson et al. (1982).

hydrops, no nerve fibres were present in the osseous spiral lamina.

Ganglion Cell Loss

There was an extensive loss of ganglion cells in both ears, the degeneration of the distal processes being much more pronounced than that of the proximal processes. In view of the severity of the neural degeneration and the fact that a rupture of the cochlear duct must have occurred in both ears during surgery, it is safe to assume that the ongoing nerve degeneration had been aggravated by the implants.

Figure 3.5: Higher Magnification of Two Patches of Corti's Organ (OC) Seen in Figure 3.3 at Arrow, Showing the Close Relation Between Remaining OC and Survival of Nerve Fibres in Osseous Lamina. OsO_4.

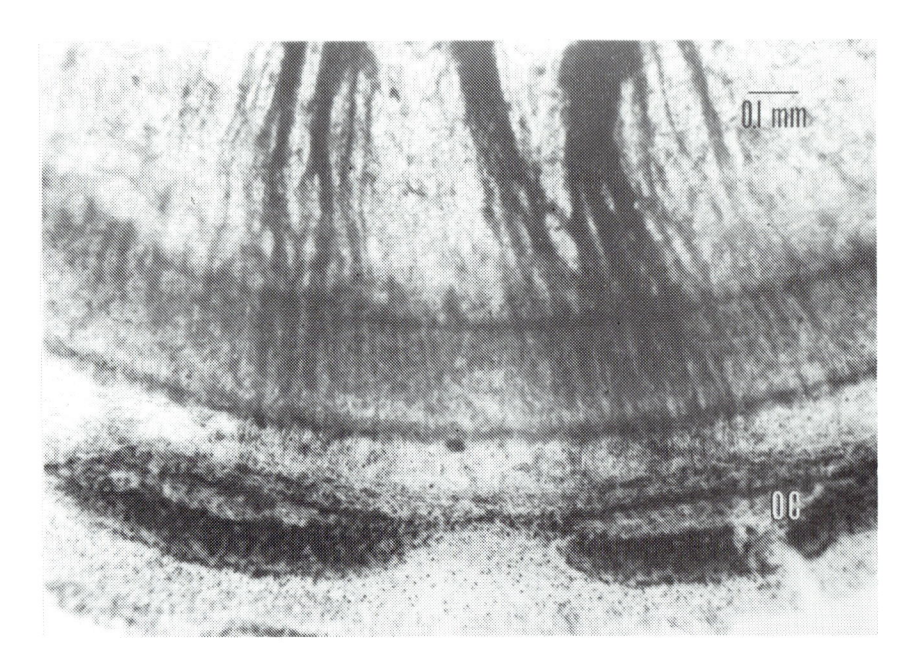

Source: Johnsson et al. (1982).

New Bone Formation

The degree of osteoneogenesis in scala tympani in the left ear was remarkable. Two phases of the process could be discerned. At first, there was growth of a poorly vascularised connective tissue, which then underwent metaplasia and became ossified.

Bilateral Vestibular Pathology

An unexpected finding was the almost complete destruction of the posterior membraneous ampulla and canal in both ears. This was in all probability the result of the close proximity of the implant to these structures. The finding is of great interest and may indicate that even external cochlear electrodes located on the otic capsule could induce bone growth, particularly if drilling has been done close to the endosteum in preparing the site for the electrode.

Cochlear Anatomy and Histopathology   65

Figure 3.6: (A) Horizontal Midmodiolar Section after Dissection of Right Ear (Figure 3.3). Several ganglion cells with their proximal processes seen above the fundus of the internal meatus. (B) Higher power magnification of area indicated by lines in upper half of basal turn. OsO_4, H and E.

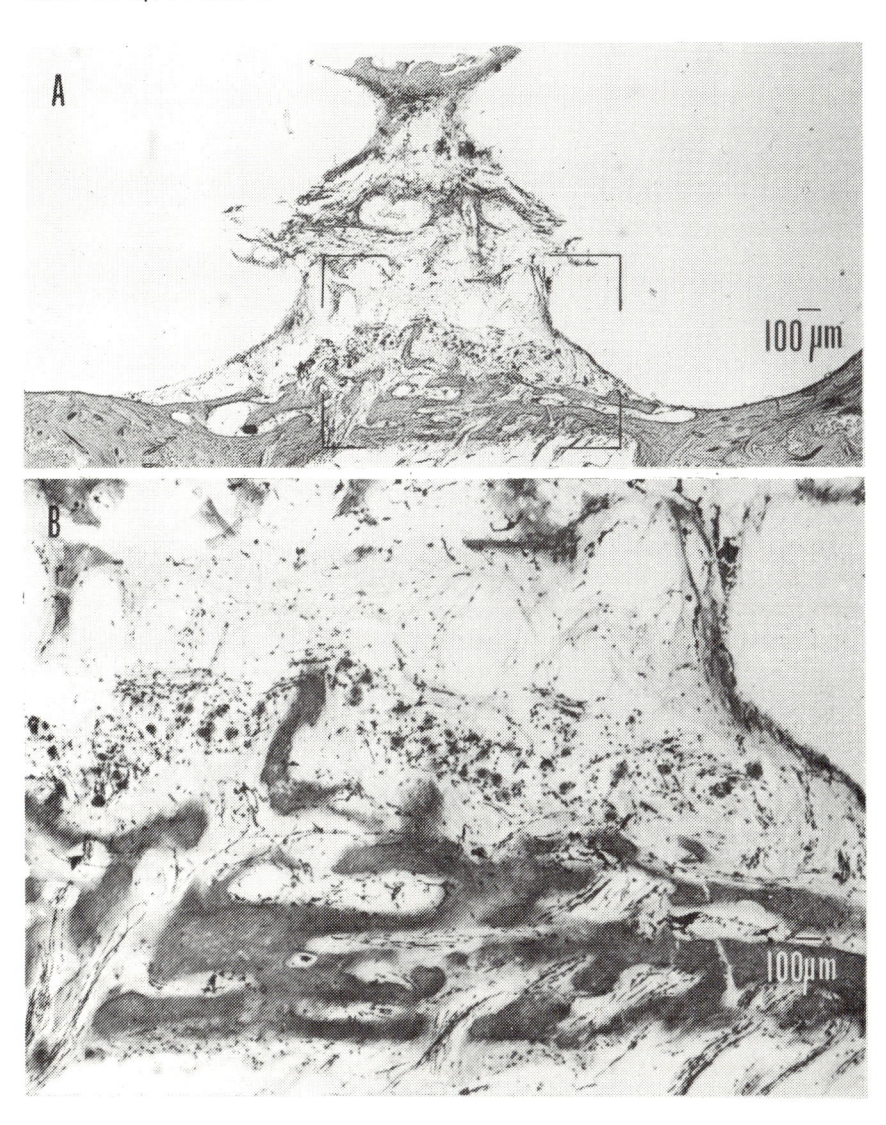

Source: Johnsson et al. (1982).

66 *Cochlear Anatomy and Histopathology*

Figure 3.7: Left Cochlea Showing Similar Location of Distal End of Electrode as in Figure 3.3. Note absence of Corti's organ and nerve fibres in osseous lamina, OL. OW, oval window. E, bundle of 5 electrodes in round window niche surrounded by cuff of connective tissue. OsO_4.

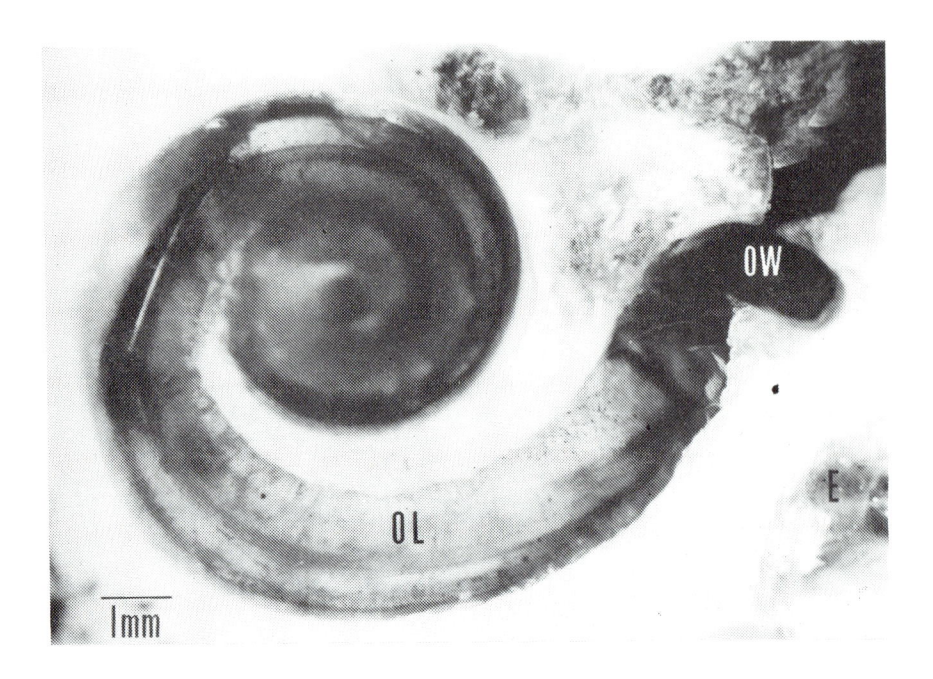

Electrolysis of Implants

Little is known about possible electrolysis of implants. The left ear of the case reported (Johnsson *et al.*, 1982) showed obvious argyrosis with darkening of the tissues around the implant.

Tissue samples in the form of small pieces of spiral ligament from both ears were examined with the electromicroprobe. Samples from both ears showed silver to be present. A control sample from the non-implanted ear of another patient did not contain silver. A sample of the patient's brain showed no silver content. No attempt was made to determine the amount of metal found or to pursue the matter further. The observations are presented here as a warning that electrolysis of electrodes may occur, and toxic metals may thus spread into surrounding tissues. Care should be taken in coating electrodes properly and in keeping the exposed metal surfaces as small as possible.

Cochlear Anatomy and Histopathology 67

Figure 3.8: Multiple Electrodes in Figure 3.4 Uncovered by Removal of Ectopic Bone in Scala Tympani. Implant was lying in a narrow tunnel inside the bone (arrow) surrounded by loose connective tissue. OsO_4.

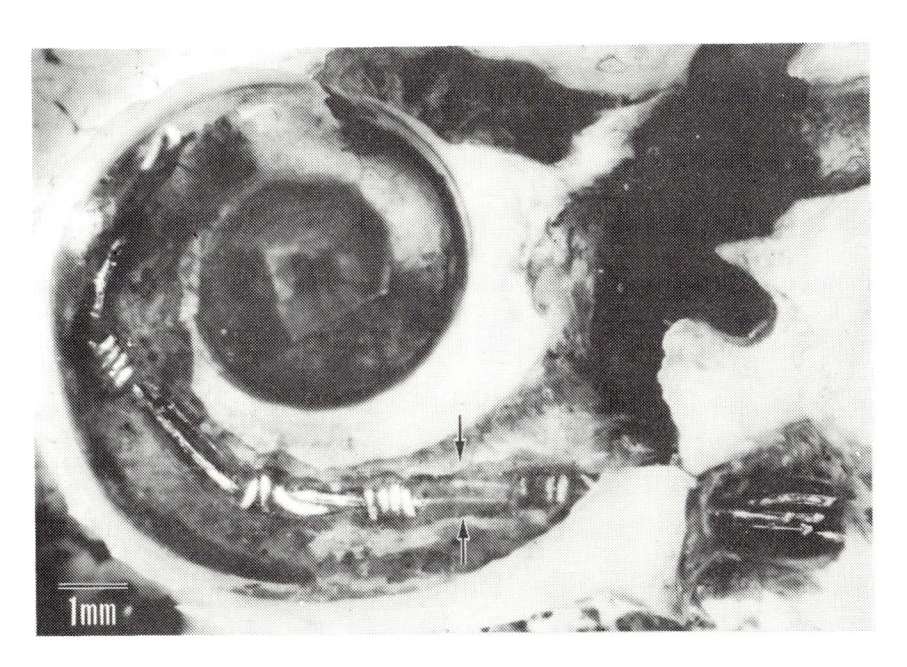

Source: Johnsson *et al.* (1982).

Future Temporal Bone Studies

It is absolutely essential that the temporal bones from all patients with cochlear implants be properly examined post mortem. Such examinations will provide useful information for improving both implant design and surgical techniques. Not only should each patient be persuaded to sign a temporal bone pledge, but the next-of-kin should be fully informed about the importance of this examination for otological research and progress.

Do Not Remove the Electrode

Because the cochlea contains a hard implant, the bones cannot be sectioned. The implant should not be extracted from the cochlea. Especially if it is long its removal can further damage cochlear tissues, so that the position of the implant in relation to surrounding structures can no longer be determined. Microdissection and surface preparations combined with conventional histology as employed in this study (Johnsson *et al.*, 1982) is a good way of examining the temporal bones from these particular patients (Hawkins and Johnsson, 1975). Furthermore, the strategy of

Figure 3.9: Horizontal Midmodiolar Section of Left Ear, Figure 3.7. A few scattered ganglion cells remain at the base of modiolus (oblique arrows). Note formation of connective tissue in scala tympani (vertical arrows) which in the basal turn is in the process of becoming ossified. OsO_4, H and E.

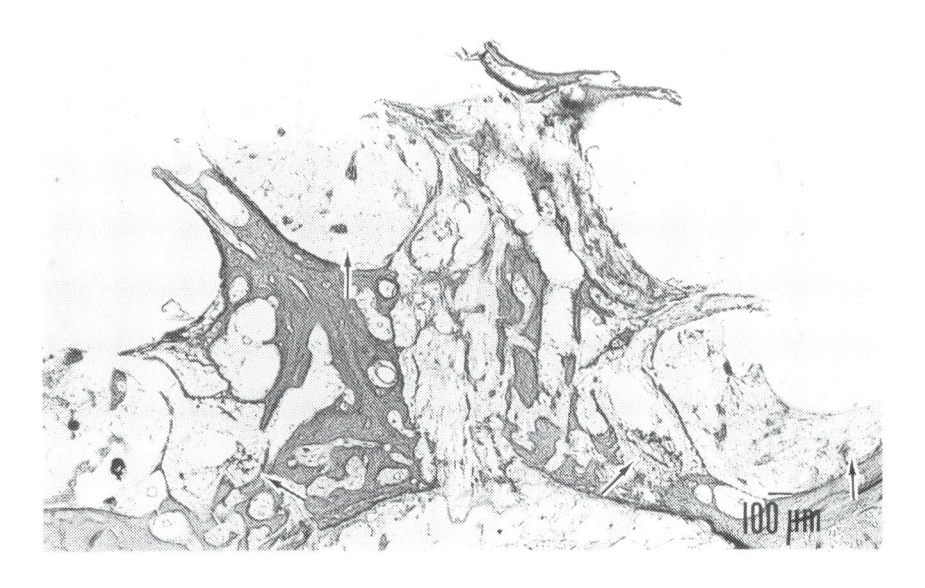

Source: Johnsson et al. (1982).

studying the first-order neurons in surface preparations of the osseous spiral lamina as well as in celloidin sections of the modiolus gives a more complete and reliable picture of the condition and distribution of the remaining neurons than would examination of celloidin sections alone. The microdissection technique also permits the use of transmission and scanning electron microscopy, plus X-ray microanalysis of tissue with the electron probe.

Photography in Situ

An alternative technique (P. Burgio, 1983, personal communication) is to remove that portion of otic capsule lying above the implant in the basal turn after fixation. The bone is drilled to a thin shell under saline irrigation and then removed. After the implant has been photographed *in situ* under the dissection microscope and gross anatomical changes have been noted, the prosthesis is carefully removed. In specimens where short implants or round window electrodes are present electrodes can be extracted directly, taking precautions to avoid injury to the middle and inner ear structures. The temporal bone is then processed by conventional histology. It may also be helpful to determine the position of the implant by taking an X-ray of the specimen.

Cochlear Anatomy and Histopathology 69

Figure 3.10: Higher Magnification in Polarised Light of Scala Tympani in Lower Half of Basal Turn (left side of Figure 3.7). Curved outline of the original wall to the left. Note formation of new, immature trabecular bone.

Source: Johnsson et al. (1982).

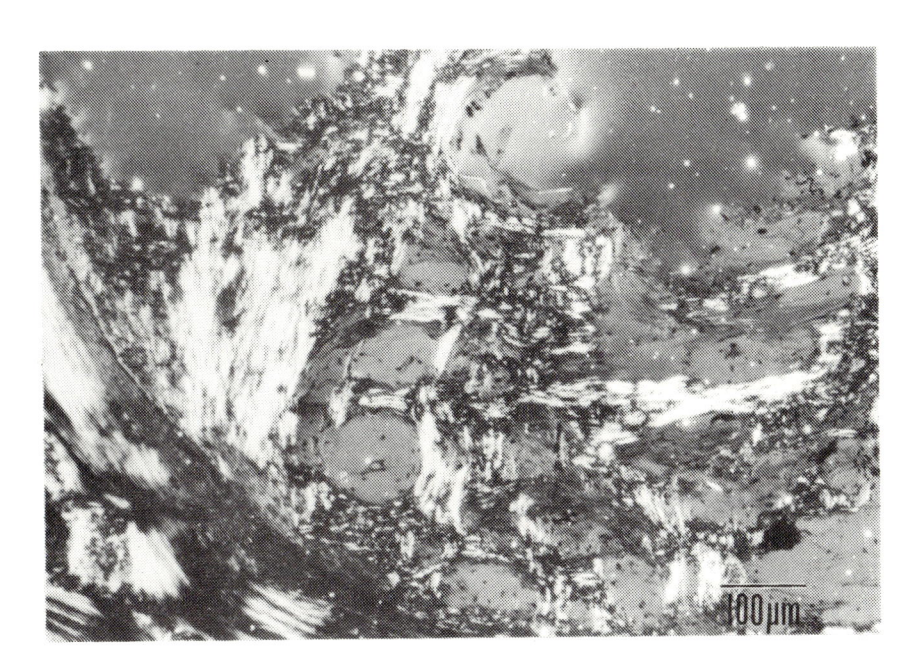

Figure 3.11: (A) Macula Utriculi, and (B) Macula Sacculi, From Right Ear, Figure 3.3. Note marked degeneration of saccular network, while the utricular network is of more or less normal density. OsO_4.

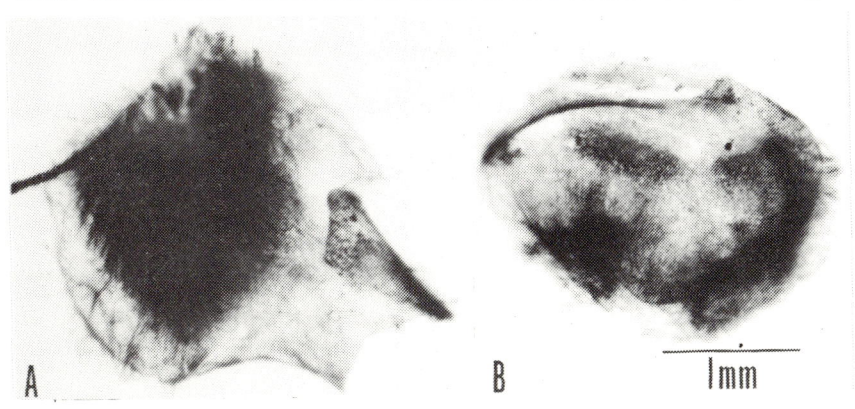

Source: Johnsson et al. (1982).

Nerve Fibre Counts

At least in selected cases, the cochlear and vestibular nerve should be dissected out from the internal auditory canal and examined in cross sections. Nerve fibres should be counted and their number should be related to the number of ganglion cells. The brainstem should be carefully fixed and at least the cochlear nuclei should be studied for transsynaptic degeneration.

The effect of the implant on the middle ear and the mastoid process should also be investigated. The electrodes should be removed from these parts and the mastoid process separated from the labyrinthine bone block for conventional histology.

It is too early to assess correctly all the problems involved in cochlear implantations from the histopathological point of view. A prosthesis in a patient's ear should remain functional at least for several years, if not for a lifetime. Such conditions are difficult to mimic in animals. There, even at best, the period between surgical implantation and histopathological examination of the ear will be comparatively short. Time is an important factor in evaluating the effect of a prosthesis on the human labyrinth, where it must remain for a much longer period if its potential for injury is to be fully assessed.

The ever-present problem is still that the prosthesis tends to cause degeneration of the very nerve fibres it is designed to stimulate, and that the long-term outlook for successful tonotopical stimulation remains poor.

Acknowledgements

This investigation was supported by a grant from the Research Fund of the American Otological Society, Inc., by USPHS Program Project Grant NS-05785 and Research Grants NS-05065 and NS-12706 from the National Institute of Neurological and Communicative Disorders and Stroke, and by Paulo Säätiö and Finska Läkaresällskapet, Helsinki.

The author is indebted to Professor J.E. Hawkins, jr and Dr J-M. Aran for their advice and critical reading of the manuscript.

References

Aran, J-M. (1983) Auditory neural protheses. *Int. J. Neurosci.*, May; *19* (1–4): 59–64.
──── Wu, Z.Y., Charlet de Sauvage, R., Cazals, Y. and Portmann, M. (1983) Electrical stimulation of the ear: Experimental studies. *Ann. Otol. Rhinol. Laryngol.*, Nov–Dec; *92* (6Pt1): 614–20.
Barn, D.E. and Rubel, E.W. (1983) Differential effects of age on transneural cell loss following cochlea removal in chickens. In *Abstr. Sixth Midwinter Res. Meet.*, Association for Research in Otolaryngology, p. 5
Black, R.C. and Clark, G.M. (1980) Differential electrical excitation of the auditory nerve. *J. Acoust. Soc. Am.*, *67*, 868–74
Cazals, Y., Aran, J-M. and Charlet de Sauvage, R. (1984) Artificial activation and degeneration of the cochlear nerve in guinea pigs. *Arch. Otolaryngol.* In press
──── Erre, J-P. and Guilhaume, A. (1980) Acoustic responses after total destruction of the cochlear receptor: brainstem and auditory cortex. *Science, 210*, 83–5

———, ———, ———, Guilhaume, A. and Aurousseau, C. (1984) Vestibular acoustic reception in the guinea pig: A saccular function. *Acta Otolaryngol.* In press
Clark, G.M. (1977) An evaluation of per-scalar cochlear electrode implantation techniques. An histopathological study in cats. *J. Laryngol. Otol., 91*, 185-99
———, Kranz, H.G., Minas, H. and Nathan, J.M. (1975) Histopathological findings in cochlear implants in cats. *J. Laryngol. Otol., 89*, 495-504
Duckert, L.G. and Duvall, A.J., III (1977) Cochlear communication routes in the guinea pig: Internal acoustic meatus and modiolus. *Trans. Am. Acad. Ophthalmol. Otolaryngol., 84*, 198-212
——— (1978) Cochlear communication routes in guinea pig — spiral ganglia and osseous spiral lamina: An electron microscope study using microsphere tracers. *Otolaryngology*, 434-46
——— and Miller, J.M. (1982) Acute morphological changes in guinea pig cochlea following electrical stimulation. A preliminary scanning electron microscopic study. *Ann. Otol. Rhinol. Laryngol., 91*, 33-40
Duvall, A.J., III and Rhodes, V.T. (1967) Ultrastructure of the organ of Corti following intermixing of fluids. *Ann. Otol. Rhinol. Laryngol., 76*, 688-708
Egami, T., Sando, I. and Sobel, J.H. (1978) Noise-induced hearing loss. A human temporal bone case report. *Ann. Otol. Rhinol. Laryngol., 87*, 868-74
Fourcin, A.J., Rosen, S.M., Moore, B.C.J., Douek, E.E., Clarke, G.P., Dodson, H. and Bannister, L.H. (1979) External electrical stimulation of the cochlea: Clinical, psychophysical, speech-perceptual, and histological findings. *Br. J. Audio., 13*, 85-107
Gacek, R.R. (1967) Afferent auditory neural system. In A.B. Graham (ed.), *Sensorineural Hearing Processes and Disorders*. Henry Ford Hospital, International Symposium, Little, Brown and Co., Boston, MA, pp. 49-59
——— (1978) Further observations on posterior ampullary transection for positional vertigo. *Ann. Otol. Rhinol. Laryngol., 87*, 300-5
Ghorayer, B., Sarwat, A. and Linthicum, H.F. (1980) Viable spiral ganglion cells in congenital and acquired profound hearing loss. *J. Laryngol. Otol., 94*, 367-76
Guild, S.R. (1932) Correlations of histological observations and the acuity of hearing. *Acata Otolaryngol., 17*, 207-49
Hawkins, J.E., jr and Johnsson, L-G. (1975) Microdissection and surface preparations of the inner ear. In C.A. Smith and J.A. Vernon (eds.), *Handbook of Auditory and Vestibular Research Methods*. Charles C. Thomas, Springfield, pp. 5-52
Hinojosa, R. and Marion, M. (1983) Histopathology of profound sensorineural deafness. *Ann. N. Y. Acad. Sci., 405*, 459-84
Hochmair-Desoyer, I.J., Hochmair, E.S., Rischer, R.E. and Burian, K. (1980) Cochlear prostheses in use: Recent speech comprehension results. *Arch. Otolaryngol., 229*, 81-98
Holden, H.B. and Schuknecht, H.F. (1968) Distribution pattern of blood in the inner ear following spontaneous subarachnoid hemorrhage. *J. Laryngol. Otol., 82*, 321-9
House, W.F. (1982) Surgical considerations in cochlear implantation. *Ann. Otol. Rhinol. Laryngol., 91*, Suppl. 91(2), Pt. 3, 15-20
Ibrahim, A.A. and Linthicum, F.H. (1980) Labyrinthitis ossificans and cochlear implants. *Arch. Otolaryngol., 106*, 111-13
Johnsson, L-G. (1974) Sequence of degeneration of Corti's organ and its first-order neurons. *Ann. Otol. Rhinol. Laryngol., 83*, 294-303
——— and Hawkins, J.E., jr (1972) Sensory and neural degeneration with aging, as seen in microdissection of the human inner ear. *Ann. Otol. Rhinol. Laryngol., 81*, 179-84
——— and ——— (1976) Degeneration patterns in human ears exposed to noise. *Ann. Otol. Rhinol. Laryngol., 85*, 725-39
———, ———, Kingsley, T.C., Black, F.O. and Matz, G.M. (1981) Aminoglycoside-induced cochlear pathology in man as seen in microdissection. *Acta Otolaryngol. (Stockh)* Suppl. 383
———, ——— and Linthicum, F.H., jr (1978) Cochlear and vestibular lesions in capsular otosclerosis as seen in microdissections. *Ann. Otol. Rhinol. Laryngol., 87*, Suppl. 48
———, ———, Muraski, A.A. and Preston, R.E. (1973) Vascular anatomy and pathology of the cochlea in Dalmation dogs. In A.J.D. de Lorenzo (ed.), *Vascular Disorders and Hearing Defects*, University Park Press, Baltimore, pp. 249-95
———, ———, Rouse, R.C. and Linthicum, F.H., jr (1982) Cochlear and otoconial abnormalities in capsular otosclerosis with hydrops. *Ann. Otol. Rhinol. Laryngol.* Suppl. 97, 91
———, ———, Weiss, J-M. and Federspil, P. (1984) Total deafness from aminoglycoside overdosage: Histopathological case study. *Am. J. Otolaryngol.* Submitted

——, House, W.F. and Linthicum, F.H. (1982) Otopathological findings in a patient with bilateral cochlear implants. *Ann. Otol. Rhinol. Laryngol.* Suppl. 91(2), Pt. 3, 74–89

——, Rouse, R.C., Hawkins, J.E., jr, Kingsley, T.C. and Wright, C.G. (1981) Hereditary deafness with hydrops and anomalous calcium phosphate deposits. *Am. J. Otolaryngol.*, 2, 284–98

Kellerhals, B., Engström, H. and Ades, H.W. (1967) Die Morphologie des Ganglion spirale Cochleae. *Acta Otolaryngol. (Stockh.)*, Suppl. 226

Kerr, A. and Schuknecht, H.F. (1968) The spiral ganglion in profound deafness. *Acta Otolaryngol. (Stockh.)*, 65, 586–98

Kiang, N.Y.S., Rho, J.M., Northrop, C.C., Lieberman, M.C. and Ryugo, D.K. (1982) Hair-cell innervation by spiral ganglion cells in adult cats. *Science*, 217, 175–7

Lawrence, M. (1966) Histological evidence for localized radial flow of endolymph. *Arch. Otolaryngol.*, 83, 406–12

—— and Johnsson, L-G. (1972) The role of the organ of Corti in auditory nerve stimulation. *Ann. Otol. Rhinol. Laryngol.*, 82, 464–72

——, Walsh, D. and McCabe, B.F. (1961) Fluid barriers within the otic capsule. *Trans. Am. Acad. Ophthalmol. Otolaryngol.*, 65, 246–59

Leake-Jones, P.A. and Rebscher, S.J. (1983) Cochlear pathology with chronically implanted scala tympani electrodes in cochlear prostheses. *Ann. NY Acad. Sci.*, 405, 203–23

——, Walsh, S.M. and Merzenich, M.M. (1981) Cochlear pathology following chronic intracochlear electrical stimulation. In *Proc. West Coast Cochlear Prosthesis Conf. Ann. Otol. Rhinol. Laryngol.* Suppl. 82, 90(2), Pt. 3, 6–8

Liberman, M.L. and Kiang, N.Y.S. (1978) Acoustic trauma in cats: Cochlear pathology and auditory-nerve activity. *Acta Otolaryngol. (Stockh.)*, Suppl. 358

Lindsay, J.R. (1973a) Histopathology of deafness due to postnatal viral disease. *Arch. Otolaryngol.*, 98, 258–64

—— (1973b) Profound childhood deafness. Inner ear pathology. *Ann. Otol. Rhinol. Laryngol.*, 82, Suppl. 5

—— and Hinojosa, R. (1978) The acoustic ganglion in profound sensorineural deafness. In R. Naunton and C. Fernández (eds.), *Evoked Electrical Activity in the Auditory Nervous System*, Academic Press, New York, pp. 301–21

Mair, I.W.S. (1973) Hereditary features in the white cat. *Acta Otolaryngol. (Stockh.)*, Suppl. 314

Miller, J.M. and Sutton, D. (1980) Cochlear prosthesis: Morphological considerations. *J. Laryngol. Otol.*, 94, 359–66

Miller, J., Sutton, D. and Webster, D.B. (1980) Brainstem histopathology following chronic scala tympani implantation in monkeys. *Ann. Otol. Rhinol. Laryngol.*, Suppl. 66, 89, 15–17

Morest, D.K. (1981) Degeneration in the brain following exposure to noise. In R.P. Hamernik, D. Henderson and R. Salvi (eds.), *New Perspectives on Noise-Induced Hearing Loss*, Raven Press, New York, pp. 87–93

Nadol, J.B. jr (1977) Electron microscopic observations in a case of longstanding profound sensorineural deafness. *Ann. Otol. Rhinol. Laryngol.*, 86, 507–17

—— (1980) Electron microscopic findings in presbyacusic degeneration of the basal turn of the human cochlea. *Otolaryngol. Head Neck Surg.*, 87, 1818–36

Nomura, Y. (1976) Nerve fibers in the human organ of Corti. *Acta Otolaryngol.*, 82, 17–24

Ota, C.Y. and Kimura, R.S. (1980) Ultrastructural study of the human spiral ganglion of the human spiral ganglion. *Acta Otolaryngol.*, 89, 53–62

Otte, J., Schuknecht, H.F. and Kerr, A.G. (1978) Ganglion cell populations in normal and pathological human cochleae. Implications for cochlear implantation. *Laryngoscope*, 88, 1231–46

Powell, T.P.S. and Erulkar, S.D. (1962) Transneuronal cell degeneration in the auditory relay nuclei of the cat. *J. Anat. Lond.*, 96, 249–68

Rasmussen, A.T. (1940) Studies of the VIIIth cranial nerve of man. *Laryngoscope*, 50, 67–83

Rawdon-Smith, A.F. and Hawkins, J.E., jr (1939) The electrical activity of a denervated ear. *Proc. R. Soc. Med.*, 32, 496–507

Schindler, R.A., Merzenich, M.M., White, M.W. and Björkroth, B. (1977) Multielectrode cochlear implants. Nerve survival and stimulation patterns. *Arch. Otolaryngol.*, 103, 691–9

Schuknecht, H.F. (1953) Lesions of the organ of Corti. *Trans. Am. Acad. Ophthalmol. Otolaryngol.*, 57, 366–82

—— (1974) *Pathology of the Ear*. Harvard University Press, Cambridge

—— and Seifi, E.A. (1963) Experimental observations on the fluid physiology of the inner ear. *Ann. Otol. Rhinol. Laryngol.*, 72, 687–721

—— and Woellner, R.C. (1955) An experimental and clinical study of deafness from lesions of the cochlear nerve. *J. Laryngol. Otol., 69*, 75-97

Shepherd, R.K., Clark, G-M., Black, R.C. and Patrick, J.F. (1983) The histopathological effects of chronic electrical stimulation of the cat cochlea. *J. Laryngol. Otol., 97*, 333-41

Silverstein, H. and Norrett, J. (1982) Retrolabyrinthine total vestibular neurectomy. In D.E. Brackmann (ed.), *Neurological Surgery of the Ear and Skull Base*, Raven Press, New York, pp. 303-15

Simmons, F.B. (1979) Electrical stimulation of the auditory nerve in cats. Long term electrophysiological and histological results. *Ann. Otol. Laryngol., 88*, 533-9

Spelman, F.A., Clopton, B.M., Pfingst, B.E. and Miller, J.M. (1980) Designs of the cochlear prosthesis: Effects of the flow of current in the implanted ear. *Ann. Otol. Rhinol. Laryngol., 89*, Suppl. 66(2), Pt. 2, 8-10

Spoendlin, H. (1971) Degeneration behavior of the cochlear nerve. *Arch. klin exp Ohr Nas Kehlkopfheilk, 200*, 275-91

—— (1978) The afferent innervation of the cochlea. In R.F. Naunton and C. Fernández (eds.), *Evoked Electrical Activity in the Auditory Nervous System*, Academic Press, New York, pp. 21-41

—— (1979a) Anatomisch-pathologische Aspekte der Elektrostimulation des ertaubten Innenohres. *Arch. Otorhinolaryngol., 223*, 1-75

—— (1979b) Neural connections of the outer hair cell system. *Acta Otolaryngol., 87*, 381-7

—— (1981) Differentiation of cochlear afferent neurons. *Acta Otolaryngol., 91*, 451-6

Spoendlin, H.H. and Gacek, R.R. (1963) Electromicroscopic study of the efferent and afferent innervation of the organ of Corti in the cat. *Ann. Otol. Rhinol. Laryngol., 72*, 660-86

Stebbins, W.C., Miller, J.M., Johnsson, L-G. and Hawkins, J.E. jr (1969) Ototoxic hearing loss and cochlear pathology in the monkey. *Ann. Otol. Rhinol. Laryngol., 78*, 1007-25

Suga, F. and Lindsay, R. (1977) Labyrinthitis ossificans. *Ann. Otol. Rhinol. Laryngol., 86*, 17-30

Sutton, D. and Miller, J.M. (1983) Cochlear implant effects on the spiral ganglion. *Ann. Otol. Rhinol. Laryngol., 92*, 53-8

——, Miller, J.M. and Pfingst, B.E. (1980) Comparison of cochlear histopathology following two implant designs for use in scala tympani. *Ann. Otol. Rhinol. Laryngol.*, Suppl. 66(2), Pt. 2, 11-14

Tange, R.A. and Huising, E.H. (1980) Hearing loss and inner ear changes in a patient suffering from severe gentamacin ototoxicity. *Arch. Otorhinolaryngol., 228*, (2): 113-21

Tumarkin, A. (1982) Bimodal hearing, the controversial second filter, and the mystery of missing OHC afferents. *J. Laryngol. Otol., 96*, 297-308

Webster, D.B. and Webster, M. (1978) Cochlear nerve projections following organ of Corti destruction. *Otolaryngol., 86*, 342-53

Ylikoski, J., Belal, A.J. and House, W.F. (1981) Morphology of human cochlear nerve after labyrinthectomy. *Acta Otolaryngol. (Stockh.), 91*, 161-71

——, Collan, Y. and Palva, T. (1978) Pathologic features of the cochlear nerve in profound deafness. *Arch. Otolaryngol., 104*, 202-7

4 COCHLEAR IMPLANT DESIGN AND CONSTRUCTION

Stephen J. Rebscher

Introduction

The design, fabrication and application of cochlear prostheses has advanced through the combined efforts of several research teams throughout the world. Each of these teams has considered the problems of mechanical and electronics engineering, biomaterials, manufacturing methods, basic sciences and surgical techniques prior to design of an implant system. A high level of understanding and exchange of information between specialists in each of these disciplines is essential to the success of an implant device. As the application of cochlear prostheses begins to move from the research laboratory to the clinic, it is important that each person working with these patients has an understanding of the design considerations involved in each system. With this background the clinical professional will be better prepared to assist the patient and to contribute to future development. This chapter concerns basic concepts of biomaterials selection and engineering considerations in addition to the description of prostheses developed at the University of California, San Francisco (UCSF) and other centres.

Design Considerations

In 1979 the group at the University of California, San Francisco (UCSF) under the direction of Dr Michael M. Merzenich in collaboration with Dr Gerald E. Loeb at the National Institute of Health (NIH), prepared to design the present generation of devices by outlining the following engineering objectives for the prosthesis. During the following two years each of these objectives presented unique problems in materials selection, design, modelling and fabrication techniques before implantation of the first patient in 1981. A brief description of this system is shown in Figure 4.1.

Reliability

The cochlear implant, and future neuroprostheses, present particularly difficult problems in long-term reliability. With relatively high impedance stimulating contacts, operating at low current levels these devices are acutely sensitive to insulation failures. This problem is compounded in the multichannel array by the proximity of many leads within a miniature flexible electrode. In addition electronic components of wholly implanted systems must be well protected for long-term use. Hermetic sealing techniques developed by the pacemaker industry have proven directly applicable in the manufacture of cochlear prostheses.

Implant Design and Construction 75

Figure 4.1: This Schematic Illustrates the Major Components of the UCSF Cochlear Implant System. The connector base is attached to the skull with bone cement. The electrode and driving components are assembled within the base and secured by a screw. Connection for the electrode, antenna array, cable and receiver each consist of platinum-iridium contacts held in a silicone pad. Tightening the screw after assembly of the system applies pressure to the pads which excludes moisture and prevents future condensation. In an experimental series patients are implanted with the percutaneous cable for a period of 12–14 weeks. Following this period the connector is opened and the cable is removed.

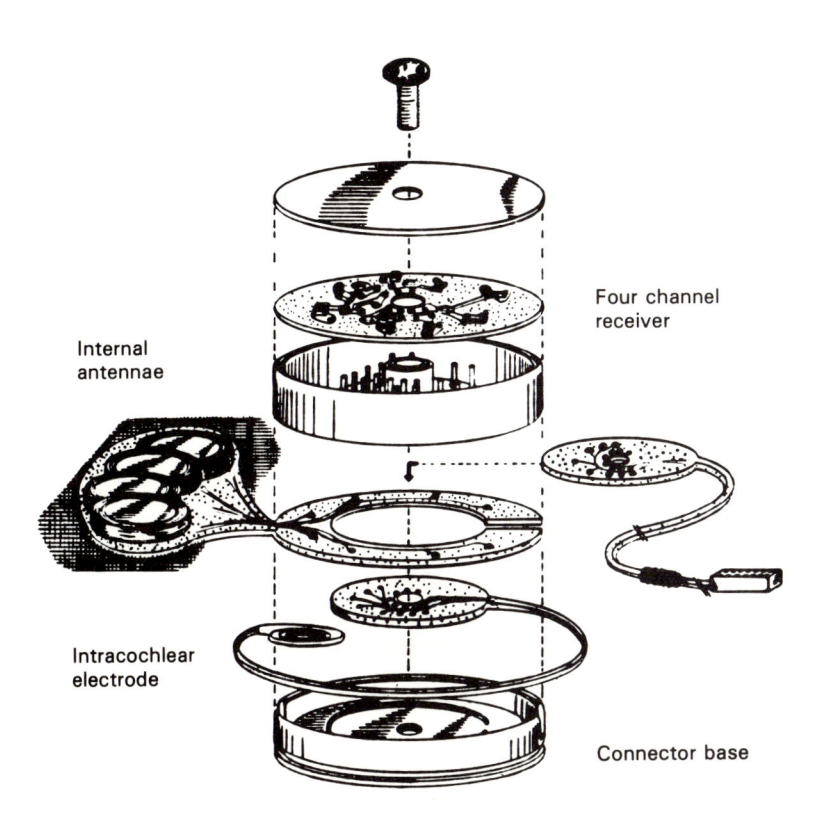

Four channel receiver

Internal antennae

Intracochlear electrode

Connector base

Biocompatibility

Biocompatibility of materials is a complex issue because of the large number of materials needed, the different sites at which they will be implanted, and the necessity that a viable population of neurons be maintained surrounding the implant site. Lengthy animal studies are necessary to test materials within the cochlea both for their intrinsic compatibility and for their performance with electrical stimulation. The difficulty of *in situ* testing is tremendously increased by the fragility and inaccessibility of the cochlea. The wide range of biomaterials currently employed in cochlear implant systems and other medical devices is reviewed below.

Safety Issues

In addition to the direct response of tissue to the implant two safety problems are of major concern. First, traumatic damage to intracochlear structures may occur during surgical insertion of the electrode array. This damage usually occurs as the electrode rises in the scala tympani after passing the first half of the basal turn, and results in penetration of the basilar membrane or fracture of the osseous spiral lamina. These effects have been reported in both cadaver temporal bone studies by O'Reilly (1981) and in autopsy studies of a cochlear implant patient (Johnsson *et al.*, 1982). To avoid this class of injury, it was necessary to design an electrode with predictable mechanical properties allowing unobstructed movement in the horizontal plane of the cochlear spiral but which prohibits flexing of the electrode tip in the vertical plane. Reducing the direct danger of chronic electrical stimulation by surrounding tissues is the second area of study. Noble metal electrodes of large surface area must be designed which will not be actively corroded by long-term stimulation, and which will not reach charge density levels at which irreversible electrolytic reactions with body fluids will release toxic products.

Functional Multichannel Stimulation

To utilise the tonotopic organisation of the cochlea in producing perceptions of changing pitch, an intracochlear electrode needs several discrete stimulating sites. To localise this stimulation each site should contain a bipolar pair of electrodes whose region of current spread does not exceed the distance between adjacent channels.

Surgical and Percutaneous Connectors

It is clear that future development in both transcutaneous transmission design and speech-processing strategies will improve cochlear implant performance. These benefits will only be efficiently available to current patients if an implantable connector is integrated into the system and interchangeability maintained in future designs. A surgical connector to fulfil this requirement must be capable of making low impedance multiple connections without leakage to adjacent channels in a simple and repeatable way. An additional benefit of such a connector is the option to use a temporary percutaneous, direct wire connection for laboratory psychophysical testing, *in vivo* electrode evaluation and simulation of various speech processing strategies.

Biomaterials

Black (1981) defines biomaterials as 'materials of natural or man made origin used to direct, supplement or replace the function of living tissue'. A tremendous variety of compounds are presently used in implanted devices with new materials and applications being developed and used each year. Present and future cochlear implant systems require components from several material groups because of the diverse mechanical and electrical properties dictated by cochlear morphology, physiology and the functional requirements of the prosthesis.

In the past materials were considered appropriate for implantation if they generated a minimal response in tissues following implantation. These materials were considered *biocompatible*. However, the current trend in biomedical engineering is toward a broader view with careful consideration of not only the host response but also the response of the material to the host, the site specificity of the host response, differences in response due to size, shape and surface finish of the implant and finally the overall function of the system in the intended biological environment. It should be noted that most material evaluation has been based on histology of test implant sites, while the physiology of these tissues is a much more sensitive indicator of their interaction with a foreign body. This is particularly important in the development of neural prostheses because the surrounding neural elements must not only survive in the presence of the implant but also must remain physiologically responsive.

A look at contemporary implant devices provides a useful insight to the wide range of characteristics which are needed in biomaterials (for reviews of clinically applied materials see D.F. Williams, 1981a). Implanted devices currently act as bone and tendon replacements to transmit loads; they function as bearings in the many joint replacements applied in the orthopaedic field, and as fluid control devices in heart surgery, cranial shunts and bladder control devices. Cosmetic implants may be simply space filling as in the breast, nose and ear implants or be protective as well as in the cranial plate or burr hole covers. Devices which produce electrical stimuli are growing in number and include the pacemaker, bladder control devices, bone growth stimulators, chronic pain reduction devices and the auditory and visual prostheses. In many of these examples metals, ceramics, polymers and specialised conductors have complementary roles and all are used in currently applied cochlear prostheses.

This section presents the fundamental concepts considered in the selection of materials for the cochlear prosthesis and an overview of the materials currently used in implantable devices.

Biological Environment

The biological environment surrounding an implanted device presents two different

78   Implant Design and Construction

features. First, the body is an active, aggressive biological system which may attack a foreign body by fluid or chemical erosion, cellular processes and high mechanical stress. However, the body is also homeostatic in terms of temperature and composition. In addition to the normal environment encountered by an implant variations are encountered due to ageing, disease, pregnancy, inflammation or allegeric responses. Ideally these variations should be considered when choosing materials for implantation.

Biological Reaction to Implanted Material

After identifying the physical characteristics required in a device the primary consideration in selection of materials is the history of each material in previous surgical applications. The body's normal reaction to the chronic presence of a foreign body includes a wide range of inflammatory responses. Less frequently observed, but potentially more serious, are the possibilities of allergic sensitivity, infection and carcinogenesis. Properly to evaluate the biological response to a given device the site-specific response to the entire implant system must be seen in addition to the history and testing of each material component.

The Inflammatory Reaction. Inflammation is a non-specific response to tissue damage. Physical trauma, infection, foreign body presence, necrosis and immune responses all stimulate varying degrees of inflammation. Often several of these factors will be present in the tissues immediately surrounding an implant which complicates the objective evaluation of host/implant response.

The first clinical signs of inflammation include redness, swelling, heat and pain. The redness results from local dilation of capillary beds and increased permeability of the endothelial lining of these capillaries. At the same time platelets and erythrocytes become sticky and begin sludging, which causes swelling around the site of injury. Swelling may also be increased if the lymphatic channels are blocked by damaged cell components. Heating may result from increased cellular activity or the presence of pyrogenic agents from bacterial toxins or foreign debris.

As the capillaries dilate and become more permeable to fluids cellular components in the circulation begin to congregate in the injured area and pass from the vessels into surrounding tissue. The first of these cells, the neutrophils, begin entering injured tissue within minutes to phagocytise debris from damaged cells and invading organisms. Neutrophils incorporate these particles into compact, dense vacuoles which are degraded by enzymes. Neutrophils enter tissue for only about 24 hours following an injury and live only a few days after this infiltration. This is an important factor in the response. The presence of a large number of neutrophils surrounding an implant after several weeks indicates an ongoing irritation or challenge from the foreign body. If the prosthesis does not continue to elicit neutrophil infiltration the number of these cells will quickly decline and larger monocytes will invade the tissue to become macrophages. These cells are more characteristic of a static reaction to foreign body and will phagocytise cell, bacterial and foreign body particles. Monocytes are very active and fuse to form multinucleated giant cells up to 80 μm in diameter. These giant cells also have a relatively short life, but will accumulate in large numbers if either a great deal of debris is created or the particles cannot be digested by degradative enzymes within the cells. In the normal inflammatory process these cells, as well as fragments from dead neutrophils and macrophages are expelled by the lymphatic system. In the final stages of the inflammatory response, tissue rebuilding occurs as newly vascularised granulation tissue replaces damaged tissue. During this rebuilding active fibroblasts produce large amounts of collagen and mucopolysaccharides to form a fibrous, fluid-filled capsule around an implanted device or a scar in place of injured tissue. Thus the steps observed in the body's response to an injury or to the implantation of a prosthesis are very similar. The main difference is that the response to a foreign body becomes chronic at some point in the process while the normal response reaches an end point at the formation of scar tissue. The point at which progress stops and the response becomes chronic determines whether the material present in the implant will be tolerated over a long term.

Allergic Sensitivity. An allergic response has also been demonstrated in some patients with implanted devices. The response may be either site specific or generalised as particles and dissolved material from an implant are distributed throughout the body by the lymphatic system. An antibody/antigen mediated response enhances the inflammatory process and may be diagnosed by the presence of eosinophilic cells which preferentially phagocytise antibody/antigen complexes.

Determining the role played by allergic sensitivity in the overall reaction to an implanted device has proven difficult. It would be even more difficult in a complex device, such as the cochlear implant, which is fabricated from many materials. Polymers, as a group, have been suspected of causing very few sensitivities; however various metals appear to create more serious reactions. Contact dermatitis has been observed in tests with nickel, chromium, gold, cobalt and platinum. Sensitivities to cobalt and nickel appear to be the most severe. Cobalt is the main alloying metal in the Co-Cr and Co-Cr-Mo metals, such as Vitallium. Stainless steel 316L, which contains nickel, is commonly used for implanted devices. Failures, and subsequent removal of joint prostheses have been statistically correlated with allergic sensitivities in some of these implants (Evans *et al.*, 1974).

Carcinogenesis. There appear to be two basic forms of carcinogenesis associated with implants. The first, foreign body carcinogenesis, is independent of the chemical composition of the implanted device. These tumours appear to be generated by long-term irritation of the tissue surrounding the implant and may be caused by increased metabolic activity in cells adjacent to the device, surface properties of the foreign body, or generalised trauma and loss of circulation. The frequency of tumour generation seems to be directly proportional to the size of the implant and inversely proportional to the porosity. It is interesting to note that most foreign body tumours are associated with well-tolerated implants. The second form is related directly to materials found in implant devices. The wear or dissolution products of some metals may act indirectly as carcinogens, as procarcinogens linking to a carcinogenic organo-metallic complex or as co-carcinogens with other compounds. Nickel appears to be the most active metal associated with tumour formation. It should be emphasised that although there is strong evidence that some implanted metals may be carcinogenic the number of tumours reported associated with implanted devices is extremely small and none of these tumours has been observed to metastasise to remote sites.

Infection. The potential for infection in tissue surrounding an implanted device is a function of not only the surgical technique and sterility of the device prior to implantation but also may be affected by the materials and even the physical shape and form of the prosthesis. Both nickel and cobalt are mildly cytotoxic and appear to inhibit the action of phagocytic cells essential to the immune system.

The physical form of an implant may affect its susceptibility to infection. Shapes which include fluid filled, acellular spaces create an excellent environment for the proliferation of bacteria within the fibrous capsule surrounding the device. Merritt *et al*. (1979) studied the effect of porosity in implants and found that implant sites infected during or just after surgery showed a greater infection rate for porous materials, while sites inoculated four weeks after surgery showed greater infection in non-porous or dense materials. The difference in these results appears to lie in whether the host or bacteria are first to invade a porous material.

It must be emphasised that infection adjacent to an implanted device is very difficult to resolve and will often necessitate the removal of the device. The design and materials of an implant must be chosen to minimise this. In addition, the surgical approach, sterile field and contamination control during implant surgery must be carefully planned and these plans judiciously observed. Although no cases of infection have been reported involving the central nervous system, this possibility is present and requires additional care in the design of any neural prosthetic implant and the cochlear implant in particular.

Current Biomaterials

Polymers. The current application of polymers in prosthetic devices includes a diverse range of compounds and applications. Many of these materials are commonly used in household or industrial products and with the exception of clean production techniques and ultrafiltration to remove possible contamination, are applied without modification in the production of implantable devices. Dacron, Teflon, acrylic, silicones and epoxies are historic examples of widely applied polymers which were found to exhibit acceptable biological performance and have been extensively used in medical devices. Ultra-high-molecular-weight polyethylene (UHMWPE), polyurethane and Parylene are less common compounds developed by other industries which have also proven very useful in implantable systems.

Polymers have three properties which make them extremely well suited to both production and application of implantable devices. First, the fully polymerised compounds elicit minimal reactions in tissues (Bruck, 1973, reviewed the biocompatibility and use of polymers in implantable devices). It is important to note, however, that many of the monomer precursors of these compounds are highly toxic or sensitising. Second, because of their stable, covalent bonding, these

Table 4.1: Physical Properties of Common Polymers. The properties of many polymers may be altered by additives, fabrication techniques and curing methods. The values listed represent those for commonly applied biomedical formulations

	Parylene C[a]	Teflon[b]	Silicone	Epoxy	Urethane
Tensile strength (PSI)	13,000	3,400	800–1,000	4,000–13,000	500–10,000
Elongation to break (%)	200	300	100	3–6	100–1,000
Water absorption % in 24 hours	0.01	0–0.01	0.12	0.08–0.15	0.02–1.5
Melting temperature (°C)	280	330	300	220	170
Resistivity ohms/cm	9×10^{16}	$10^{16} – 10^{18}$	2×10^{15}	$10^{12} – 10^{17}$	to 10^{15}

Notes: a. Registered trademark Union Carbide Corp. b. Registered trademark E.I. DuPont.
Source: Adapted from Loeb et al. (1977).

polymers are extremely resistant to corrosion and chemical attack. Last, and very important, these compounds can be easily and precisely formed to a wide range of shapes and volumes with specifically assigned properties. Many polymers act as excellent electrical insulators and are utilised in this way in many neuromuscular and electrical stimulating devices. Table 4.1 summarises the characteristics of several currently used medical polymers. Because of their positive biological performance and ease of fabrication there is a growing interest in the development of conductive polymers which could replace metal electrodes. A limitation presented by all polymers is their lack of hermeticity in applications requiring an encapsulating seal. Epoxy was used as the original encapsulating material for cardiac pacemakers but has been replaced by truly hermetic metal/glass/ceramic encapsulation.

Teflon. Teflon (PTFE) is a fluorinated polymer which forms extremely long chains with common molecular weights of 6–10 million. To minimise contamination, Teflon prepared for use in medical devices is polymerised in water. Teflon is extremely hydrophobic, has a melting point above 250°C and displays an extremely low coefficient of friction. It is used industrially in highly corrosive environments because it is resistant to chemical attack. Along with its chemical inertness the hydrophobic nature of Teflon may explain its minimal tissue reaction, particularly in blood. Because of its low thrombogenicity Teflon is used in many vascular grafts and valve prostheses as well as vascular suture applications. Several attempts have been made to utilise the low friction of Teflon surfaces in joint replacements. However, in this application the low tensile strength of the material permits rapid wear. The wear particles produce chronic irritation which is probably due more to their shape and size than normal chemical composition. Teflon is also used in reconstructive surgery, as an artificial dura in neurosurgery and as valves in hydrocephalic shunts. Homsy (1981) reviewed the applications and biocompatibility of Teflon.

Implanted Teflon provokes a fine layer of granulation tissue and a fibrous capsule surrounding the implant within one to four weeks. When implanted in bone, a layer of collagen separates the bone from the implant. A few giant cells have been observed within the connective tissue layer even after several years. In cell culture Teflon appears to produce no negative effects. Because Teflon collects static electricity it should be handled with extreme care to avoid the attraction of contaminating particulates.

Teflon is most frequently used in cochlear implants as an insulation layer for electrode leads. Groups at Stanford University, Nucleus Ltd. in Australia, the Hochmairs in Austria and Dr Chouard in Paris all use Teflon-insulated electrode leads. This application has been generally successful although the material is prone to pin holes and separation from leads because it does not bond to the wire.

Polyethylene. Polyethylene is a common polymer currently used in many products from plastic bags to the slippery bases of snow skis. The plastic is manufactured by the direct polymerisation of pure ethylene gas. The lengths of these chains effect the strength and properties of the final product. The most popular uses of polyethylene in medical devices include many forms of tubing and wear-resistant, low-friction contact surfaces in total joint replacement prostheses. For the latter, ultra-high-molecular-weight polyethylene (UHMWPE) is used. These long-chain polymers have greater density, low friction, and produce less wear products than either metal to metal or metal to Teflon surfaces.

Bruck (1973) and Hastings (1981) reviewed the clinical experience with polyethylene in more than ten thousand cases over fourteen years. They report acceptable tissue reaction to polyethylene particles of modest size and no reported cases of neoplastic formation or other severe problems connected with its use.

Dacron. Like polyethylene, Dacron is a common polymer used in many popular products. Dacron, or polyester, is manufactured by pulling continuous filaments from a melt (King *et al.*, 1981) and weaving these into a wide variety of fabrics. The compound consists of repeating units of polyethylene terephthalate often referred to as PET (Guidoin *et al.*, 1977).

The wide variety of medical applications for Dacron fabrics has generated a large number of very specialised weaves. The functional effects of different weave patterns of Dacron in several implant sites have been compared (Eskin *et al.*, 1978; Guidoin *et al.*, 1977; Sawyer *et al.*, 1979). Clearly the type of fabric desired is dependent upon the site in which it is applied and the structural role which it is to play. Three types of Dacron fabric are used in the UCSF cochlear implant system. First, a fine weave fabric is used to support the 0.5 mm platinum-iridium connector balls on the electrode lead pad. In this application the Dacron prevents the balls from sinking into the Silastic pad which has little inherent resistance to penetration. Second, a very coarse weave mesh (hole size greater than 1 mm) is moulded into, and extends from, the internal receiver antenna structure to allow adhesion of the coil unit to the skull with bone cement. Third, a fine Dacron felt is attached around the distal end of the percutaneous cable to act as a barrier to infection tracking along this conduit from the cable exit site centrally. In this role, the matted felt allows ingrowth of soft connective tissue from the dermal layers which acts as a barrier to invading bacteria from the exit site. A similar covering of Dacron felt has been applied successfully in cardiac assist lines (Myojin and Von Recum, 1978) and parenteral feeding catheters. Dacron generates a mild inflammatory reaction when implanted chronically with a small number of persistent giant cells. We have found that this reaction is greatly increased by the presence of small particles which may be produced in cutting or manipulating Dacron fabrics, particularly the felts, and should be avoided by careful sonication and rinsing. Dacron sleeves or skirts can be either moulded directly into the prosthesis or attached with the use of Silastic Medical Adhesive Type A.

Silicones. Silicone-based elastomers are the material of choice for many implant applications. The ability to form, extrude and polymerise silicone rubbers into a large variety of shapes and consistencies enables the fabrication of varied prostheses. The relatively low viscosity silicone elastomer can be easily injected into a complex mould without damaging fine electrode lead wires. The material has also been used extensively in prostheses for plastic surgery, neurosurgical ventricular shunts, catheters for parenteral feeding and as replacement joints for fingers. Van Noort and Black (1981) reviewed the use of silicones in medical devices.

The most common silicones applied medically are produced by the Dow Corning Corporation under the trade name Silastic. There are many different types of Silastics available, ranging from room temperature vulcanising medical adhesive, putty-like gels which are extruded or shaped and then heat cured to fluid elastomers which polymerise with a tin or platinum-based catalyst. All of these are polymerised from units of dimethylsiloxane and achieve molecular weights in millions. During curing many cross linkages occur and are modified by the presence of vinyl and phenyl side groups added to alter the basic properties of the Silastic.

As mentioned earlier, the properties of Silastic seem suited to long-term medical applications. Cured Silastic is stable both in the presence of heat and in harsh or oxidative environments. It retains its flexibility and elasticity for many years, even at low temperatures. Silastic is an excellent ion barrier and electrical insulator. Water will pass readily through Silastic in its vapour phase but cannot condense if pressures are maintained above atmospheric pressure. This property is used in the UCSF surgical connector to protect the connection of electrode leads to hermetically sealed receiver electronics.

In general the biological performance of Silastic is excellent. Parenteral catheters and Silastic-over-Dacron grafts show low thrombogenicity and atraumatic, chronic placement of properly cured Silastic (MDX 4210) cochlear inserts in cats have shown almost no reaction to the material (Leake-Jones and Rebscher, 1983). In several human patients we have implanted RF receivers coated with Silastic (MDX 4210) and later found a thin fibrous tissue capsule had formed over the implant when the structures were exposed after several months. This agrees with findings of Van Noort and Black (1981). We have also observed yellowing and slight swelling of some samples of Silastic after long-term contact with blood. It is believed this represents the uptake of lipids by the polymer and varies from patient to patient. Two factors appear significantly to affect the compatibility of Silastic implants. First, the presence or absence of filler substances may affect overall reaction to the material (Chawla, 1978). Fillers, which give an off-white, opaque appearance are added to many silicone rubbers (Silastic 382 is an example) to increase their strength. The presence of fillers causes greater thrombogenic response and may decrease overall compatibility. Second, the presence of additives and catalysts, particularly in free units, may seriously affect the compatibility of the final product. This can be a problem in the clinical use of Silastic Medical Adhesive type A which releases acetic acid as it cures and is frequently used intraoperatively. The problem can also be manifest in any Silastic prosthesis in which complete curing cycles have not been carefully monitored or in which excess catalyst has been employed.

Polyurethane. As a viscous, clear liquid, uncured polyurethane resembles a filler-free silicone elastomer. After proper curing the polyurethanes are extremely resistant to abrasion and damage caused by repeated flexion. Some formulations display elongation factors up to 1,000 per cent and tensile strength as high as 10,000 PSI (Boretos, 1981). With strength and the ability to withstand continual flexing as prime considerations polyurethane is used in artificial hearts.

Although the prepolymers of polyurethane are toxic the cured polymer demonstrates excellent biological performance. In contact with blood polyurethane generates less clotting than Silastic 382 and will not absorb lipids as silicones often will. Electrically conducive carbon powder may be added to either polyurethane or Silastic to form a flexible bioelectric conduit or connector.

Polymethylmethacrylate. Polymethylmethacrylate (PMMA) is a fast-setting adhesive polymer which is frequently used to secure dental and orthopaedic devices. For this reason it is often referred to as dental acrylic or bone cement. The compound may be machined or drilled and attains great strength within 10 to 15 minutes after mixing. It is thus very useful as a mouldable setting or fixture.

Historically, the use of PMMA has been somewhat controversial. It appears now that most problems associated with the use of acrylic cement can be directly attributed to residual monomers of methylmethacrylate, catalyst or modifiers (Charnley, 1970; Dillingham *et al.*, 1975; deWijn and Van Mullen, 1981). Packaging which ensures the correct proportion of each compound as well as thorough mixing, has greatly reduced these problems. The cement is well tolerated, at least on a gross level, by thousands of orthopaedic, dental and plastic surgery patients. However, the use of large quantities of PMMA should be avoided for two reasons. First, the polymerisation of the plastic is highly exothermic. A large mass of orthopaedic bone cement can exceed a temperature of 70°C, which will cause significant local necrosis. Second, the presence of any non-essential foreign body in the area of the implant should be avoided to minimise the overall foreign body reaction and infection risk.

Parylene and other Insulation Coatings. The problems of protecting electronic circuits in the harsh, fluid environment of the body have been addressed by hermetic-sealing techniques. A continuing concern is how reliably to insulate electrical leads which exit these packages and interface with target tissues. This problem is largely dependent on the class of device. For instance, in cardiac pacemakers the electrode surface areas are so large (and the resulting electrode impedance low) that the minor current leakage at connectors or pin-hole insulation flaws will not significantly affect the device's performance. The same situation appears to hold for bone growth stimulators, some muscle stimulators and even spinal and cortical pain reduction devices. However, the smaller electrodes required to stimulate discrete sectors of nerve in the cochlea, or elsewhere, require leakage-free connections and leads. In the past Teflon has been used as an insulating coating on medical devices. Unfortunately it is often difficult to produce a pin-hole free Teflon coating, there is no adhesion between wire surfaces and the Teflon coating and the material cannot be easily added to devices during fabrication due to the high temperatures which must be used. In search of an insulator for chronically implanted microelectrodes, Loeb *et al.* (1977) reported the

86 Implant Design and Construction

use of Parylene-C with excellent success. Parylene is a vapour-deposited polymer developed by Union Carbide during the early 1960s and used since then primarily in the electronics industry, although it is currently being employed in a growing number of medical devices. The properties of the polymer include: (1) uniform, conformal thickness, (2) pin-hole free deposition, (3) high tensile strength (10,000–13,000 PSI), (4) high resistivity (6–9 x 10(16) ohm/cm), (5) very low water absorption and (6) excellent performance in the biological environment. These characteristics are to a large degree a function of the deposition techniques employed in applying the polymer.

Parylene is vapour deposited at room temperature (Figure 4.2) from para-xylylene monomers. These monomer subunits are generated from the dimer di-para-xylylene at elevated temperature outside the deposition chamber. Because the monomers require many collisions (an average of 10,000) before each polymerisation occurs, the coating is built up slowly, reducing the incidence of pin holes. There is no surface tension or shrinkage as Parylene polymerises because the deposition occurs at room temperature without a liquid phase. In practice, this produces very uniform coatings over irregularly shaped objects and allows the coating of electronic components which could not withstand the elevated temperatures of other coating systems. The high tensile strength of Parylene-C offers an extra margin of reliability in the handling and manipulation of electrode leads during the fabrication of intracochlear electrodes and makes Parylene an excellent coating where stabilisation of electronic components and fine wire bonds, etc., is needed. A comparison of Parylene-C and other medical polymers in Table 4.1 indicates two additional benefits of this coating. First, Parylene has a very high resistivity. This makes possible its use in very thin layers (1–2 μm), which is particularly important in high density devices. Second, these characteristics of Parylene make it preferable to epoxy as an encapsulating material or as a barrier coating within a hermetically sealed package.

Although Parylene-C is rapidly becoming an important polymer in a wide variety of medical and medical-electronic devices there are some difficulties associated with its use. First, because Parylene does not bond to metal an organic layer is deposited prior to its application. At UCSF we have used the polyimide Pyre-ML as a preliminary layer prior to Parylene coating. A new coating developed by Hahn et al. (1983) involves direct deposition of a polymethane coating from methane gas in a glow discharge system. This coating may act as an excellent substitute for binding Parylene or as a reliable layer in itself.

Ceramics. The use of implantable ceramics began during the 1970s with orthopaedic joint replacements. Although the majority of ceramic applications remain in this field, its excellent properties are being utilised in a growing number of devices. The biological performance of dense alumina (Al2O3) ceramic is superior to metals and many polymers whereas the strength of ceramic rivals that of implantable metals. Coupled with their high strength, many ceramics are extremely wear resistant and produce only one-tenth the wear of products of a metal/polymer combination in a full joint replacement (Griss and Heimke, 1981). For consideration

Figure 4.2: Schematic Illustration of the Parylene Coating Process Developed by Union Carbide Corporation, NY. The process begins with the vaporisation of powdered di-para-xylylene. In the second stage higher temperature is used to split this dimer to the monomer para-xylylene. In a vacuum, at room temperature, these monomer subunits contact the object to be coated and polymerise to form a strong homogeneous layer.

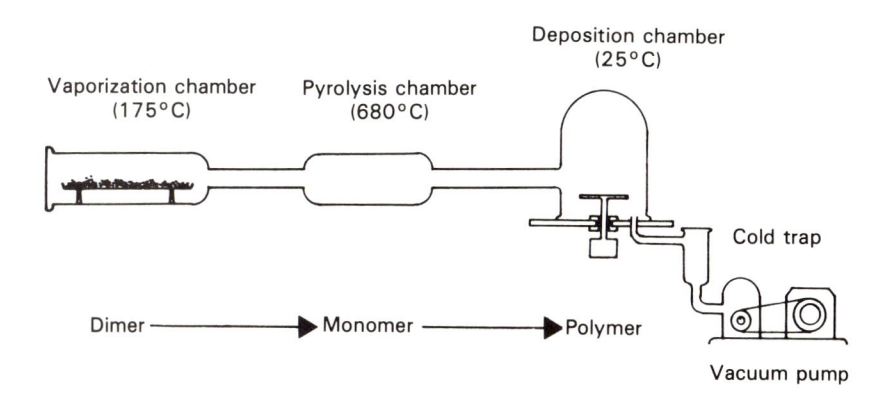

in use with electronic devices, ceramics offer very high resistivity and complete hermeticity. In addition, a ceramic-enclosed package is transparent to radio frequency energy which allows bidirectional telemetry of information without the use of exterior antennae. Finally, ceramics are available in almost any size or configuration and in a variety of compositions with significantly different properties.

Most ceramics consist of aluminium oxide (99.7 per cent) with trace amounts of magnesium oxide. This powder can be either pressed into forms or mixed as a slurry, moulded and dried to a preformed shape for firing. The firing, at 1,500–1,700°C, creates a highly ordered crystalline structure of ionic bonds which gives it high strength (Black, 1981; de Groot, 1981). After firing the ceramic will retain its full strength when implanted or immersed in saline (Krainess and Krapp, 1978).

To increase the affinity of bone surrounding orthopaedic and middle ear ossicle replacements, calcium, silicon and phosphate salts may be added to the ceramic (Blencke et al., 1978). These salts appear to stimulate growth by providing the mineral constituents required for new bone formation and by creating porosity within the implant surface as the salts dissolve. The growth of new bone around such bioactive ceramic can be observed in 8–10 days following implantation. Unfortunately ceramics which contain large amounts of soluble salts lose 30–50 per cent of their original strength after implantation (Osterholm and Day, 1981).

As mentioned above the biological performance of ceramics is considered to be exceptional. Cells in culture are not affected by the presence of solid pieces of alumina and readily adhere to it. Following implantation of ceramic devices a very thin fibrous membrane surrounds the prosthesis in most cases (Harms and Mausle, 1979) with bone appearing almost to attach to the implant in some cases (Heimke *et al.*, 1978). The only reported reactions to ceramic occur when fine particles are produced by wear processes or presented in cell culture. *In vivo* these particles are localised in the fibrous tissues surrounding the implant and produce a very mild reaction.

The single problem which has prevented the widespread use of ceramics in neural prosthetic devices is that of effectively forming a hermetic seal to encapsulate electronic components. Attempts to 'weld' two halves of a ceramic enclosure with a narrow laser or electron beam result in fine cracks along the joint. Unfortunately, the temperatures required to fuse the ceramic as a whole (1,500–1,700°C) are too high for any electronic components to survive. An alternate which may prove effective is to fuse rings of titanium on to each half of the ceramic capsule during the initial firing. The titanium rings can then be welded together after electronic assembly with sufficient heat sinking to avoid cracking the ceramic.

Carbon. Carbon, either in its elemental form or as silicon carbide, is used in an increasing number of medical devices. Current applications include carbon-coated cardiac valve and vascular replacements, tendon replacements, percutaneous connectors and dental implants. The success of carbon in each of these devices is due to both its strength in certain crystalline forms and biological properties. Haubold *et al.* (1981) discuss the use of carbon in medical devices.

When applied by glow discharge or sputtering methods, carbon forms a thin (less than 1.0 μm) coating which bonds tenaciously to titanium and other metals. Utilising a film of carbon deposited in this way, metal cardiac valves are less thrombogenic and resistant to fluid erosion. Cochlear implant groups at the Universities of Zurich and Utah have used carbon connectors as percutaneous skin ports. These connectors appear to resist infection because the surrounding skin forms a seal with the carbon pedestal. Covalently bound carbon fibres are readily available commercially and have been incorporated in tendon replacements and other applications where high strength with flexibility is needed.

The possibility of galvanic corrosion must be carefully considered when using carbon. Carbon itself is extremely passive and will corrode less noble metals (Thompson *et al.*, 1979). Titanium, being adjacent to carbon on the galvanic scale, appears to be immune to such attack while stainless steels suffer pitting corrosion. The response of cobalt/chromium alloys is intermediate between these and appears to be acceptable but not preferred.

Metals Suitable for Chronic Implantation. The surgical use of metals as long-term implants has a long and interesting history. Originally silver, brass, copper, nickel-plated steel and aluminium were used with mixed success (Williams, 1981b). Stainless steel (18–8 alloy, 18 per cent chromium and 8 per cent nickel) was first used in the 1920s to obtain greater strength with reduced corrosion. Soon the addition of molybdenum and more complex alloys further reduced the problems of limited strength and corrosion resistance. Titanium was first used as an implant material in 1940. What is particularly interesting about these metals is that their seemingly negative properties often have been utilised to advantage. Two examples of this are silver and copper. Silver exhibits a mild toxicity which is beneficial in reducing the incidence of infection in some applications; a similar gradual dissolution of copper in intrauterine devices may be responsible for its efficacy in the prevention of pregnancy. In metals for use in the cochlear implant we are interested only in those with stable biological performance.

Stainless 316L, cobalt-chrome alloys and titanium alloys (6AL4V) are the principal materials used in devices requiring high strength, wear resistance or hermetic integrity. Vitallium (62.5 per cent Co, 30 per cent Cr, 5 per cent Mo and 0.5 per cent C) is a common cobalt alloy used in dental implants, fracture fixation and joint replacements. There are many other Co alloys with various proportions of Co, Ni, Cr and Mo together with trace amounts of other elements to yield specific properties. Stainless 316L is mostly used in bone fixation and other applications where maximum strength and low fatigue failure are needed for relatively short time periods. Because of its corrosion resistance and light weight, titanium has become popular and is used in bone fixation, dental implants, artificial joints, heart valves and pacemaker encapsulation.

Corrosion of Implanted Metal. The ability to resist corrosion is essential both in terms of maintaining the strength and function of the metal and in preventing potentially toxic release of heavy metal ions. Williams (1981b,c) discusses the corrosion properties of titanium and cobalt alloys and Sutow and Pollack (1981) reviewed the characteristics of stainless steels in detail. In general it is the surface oxide layers which determine corrosion resistance and not the properties of the metal itself. As an example titanium in its elemental form is extremely reactive and forms at least three oxides at different valences. It is this oxide layer, up to 150 Å thick, which provides resistance to corrosion under a variety of physiological conditions.

Physical stresses may act to breakdown, or actually remove, this oxide layer and increase corrosion. In addition, stainless steel is susceptible to corrosion in a reduced oxygen or increased chloride environment, both of which can occur either in fine pits or in scratches on the interface between two parts of a device and lead to pitting or crevice corrosion. Stainless steel is also susceptible to galvanic attack by more noble metals. With these points in mind, stainless steel should be finely polished, should not be designed with fine crevices or multiple parts and should not be used in conjunction with other metals. Titanium is excellent in these respects because it is not subject to corrosion in a reduced oxygen or increased chloride environment and rarely exhibits pitting or crevice corrosion. Because titanium rapidly forms a new oxide layer the loss of corrosion resistance due to stress or fatigue appears to be much less than in stainless steel or cobalt/chromium alloys. The corrosion resistance of Vitallium, and other cobalt/chromium alloys, generally falls between that of stainless steel and titanium and it appears that some Co alloys may be used with titanium without significant galvanic effects.

90   *Implant Design and Construction*

Toxicity of Metal Alloys. In general the alloys discussed above (Stainless 316L, Vitallium, cobalt/chromium alloys and Ti6Al4V) have shown acceptable tissue responses in a wide range of patients and applications. Minimal tissue response is usually observed surrounding stainless steel implants unless severe corrosion or wear has taken place. Vitallium exhibits excellent compatibility in most cases as does titanium and Ti6Al4V. In terms of corrosion-induced tissue response Stainless 316L required a 7 per cent replacement rate, CoCrMo 5 per cent and CoCr 0 per cent in one study (Sutow and Pollack, 1981).

A controversy surrounds the use of alloys containing nickel, chromium and cobalt. All three of these elements damage cells in culture and all have been shown to cause hypersensitisation in some patients. Nickel and cobalt cause haemolysis in elemental form and nickel has possibly been associated with tumour formation. Problems associated with nickel dissolution are also more difficult to trace because the resulting compounds are more soluble and are thus more quickly distributed throughout the body. In view of these problems some researchers feel that titanium alloys should be used for any implant for which they can be engineered while others point to over 40 years of clinical use of cobalt, chrome and nickel alloys with very few problems and no directly related tumours. Unfortunately, titanium is both more difficult to machine, form and hermetically seal than cobalt/chromium alloys or stainless steel, making titanium implants both more difficult to engineer and more costly to the consumer.

Metals for Electrical Stimulation. The concepts and efforts involved in developing an ideal stimulating electrode material have been well documented (Brummer and Turner, 1977a,b,c; Brummer and McHardy, 1977; McHardy *et al.*, 1980; Robblee *et al.*, 1980). Electrodes stimulating through large surface areas, such as pacemaker electrodes or bone growth stimulators, may be made from stainless steel. However the use of smaller contact surfaces, particularly as required in the multichannel cochlear implant, requires a much greater ability to pass large amounts of charge through small surface area electrodes. The limiting factors are the real electrode surface area (determined by the geometric area and the surface texture) and the charge per phase which can be passed without electrolytic dissolution or gas formation. These limits are more important in a neural prosthesis than in either of the two previous examples because neurones in close proximity to the electrode must survive if discrete zones of stimulation are to be created.

Dissolution and gas formation may cause adverse tissue reaction in several ways. Most direct of these are toxic effects of metallic ions and extreme shifts in local pH generated by release of H^+ and OH^+ ions. Several other toxic ion species may be released including chlorates, metal oxides and denatured organics. To minimise these problems, all current intracochlear electrodes utilise either platinum or platinum-iridium alloy electrodes. Platinum itself has a gassing limit approximately ten times that of stainless steel (300 $\mu C/cm^2$ compared with 40 $\mu C/cm^2$) whereas pure iridium (in its activated state) demonstrates a gassing limit another order of magnitude greater than platinum (i.e. 4,000–5,000 $\mu C/cm^2$). Unfortunately pure iridium is very difficult to work with and cannot be formed easily into electrode contacts or leads. To overcome this problem several groups are currently studying methods by which iridium, or its oxide, could be coated onto platinum or platinum-iridium electrodes.

With current technology committed to platinum-iridium contacts, two principles must be considered. First, the contact surface area must be as large as possible by geometric design and surface roughening. Second, the signal driving the active and ground electrodes must be charge balanced (i.e. each phase of a signal must be followed by a symmetrical inverse phase so that all chemical reactions undergone in the first phase will be completely reversed during the second). This is accomplished by capacitively coupling each pair of electrodes. A future method of generating even higher currents without dissolution or gassing may be to use oxide-coated electrodes which act more like capacitors by inducing current through the film while the metal electrode itself is never involved in any oxidation-reduction reactions.

Encapsulation and Hermetic Sealing of Implanted Electronics

Any electronic circuits or components which are implanted in the body must be protected from the harsh environment which surrounds them. Small amounts of moisture containing ions or combined with soluble salts present on the surface of components, will lead to rapid failure. It is the presence of contaminating ions on circuitry which leads to eventual failure in systems encapsulated in Silastic, Parylene or epoxy, which are all good ion barriers. The effects of outward leakage must also be considered in sealing implanted devices. Solder, flux and some components have toxic, soluble compounds or elements which can leach out into the body. In this case the polymer coatings mentioned above are useful as a barrier against the contamination of tissues surrounding the prosthesis.

Because of the small numbers of experimental units needed, most early cochlear implant devices were also based on the epoxy encapsulation methods. Michelson and Schindler (1981) implanted several devices sealed in epoxy and beeswax in alternating layers (Figure 4.3). This, with an added coating of Silastic to avoid attack of the epoxy, could be expected to last many years if carefully applied. The House device incorporates a copper receiver coil with no electronic components within an epoxy capsule (House, 1982; House et al., 1981). The Hochmairs (Burian et al., 1980, 1981; Hochmair et al., 1979; Hochmair-Desoyer et al., 1983) have successfully used epoxy moulded receivers in their multichannel experiments.

However, with the longevity of components improving, and the possibility of truly 'lifetime' implants close at hand, the goal of most medical device manufacturers has been hermetically sealed units. The receiving electronics of cochlear implant systems developed at UCSF, Nucleus Ltd. of Australia, and Biostim Inc. are all hermetically sealed in titanium with ceramic feedthrough seals, and the prototype multichannel receivers being developed at Stanford University will be sealed in essentially the same way (Figure 4.4).

92 *Implant Design and Construction*

Figure 4.3: Epoxy Encapsulation of an Early UCSF Implanted Receiver. The polymer absorbs water which may interact with residual salts on electronic circuits to form a conductive path leading to device failure. Capillary forces along the electrode leads may carry body fluid to the receiver components with the same result. These problems have led to general acceptance of hermetic sealing.

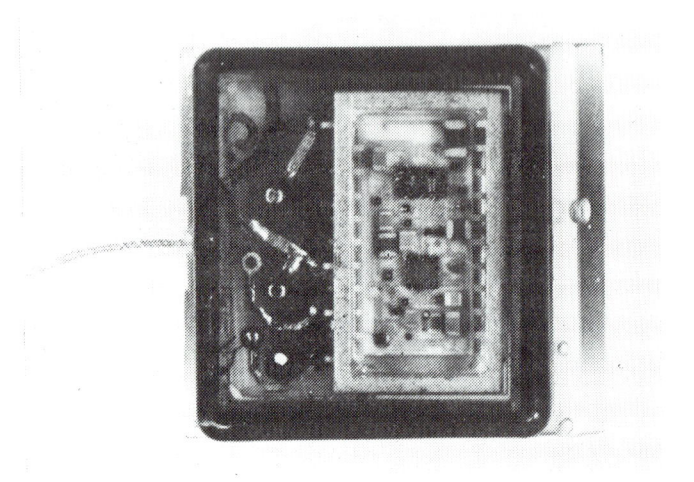

Figure 4.4: Titanium Receiver Capsule with 24 Hermetically Sealed Platinum Feedthroughs (Astroseal Inc., El Monte, CA). The feedthrough pins are directly connected to the electronic components within the capsule as the receiver is assembled.

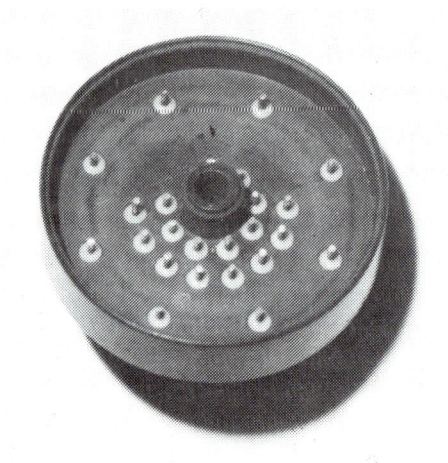

There are two sealing problems which must be overcome in the design of long-life package for these devices. First, feedthroughs permitting antenna input and electrode output must be leaktight and, second, the capsule must be hermetically sealed after installation and testing of the electronic components. The common sealing materials for feedthroughs in the electronics industry are various glass compounds. Unfortunately, these sealing glasses contain a high percentage of toxic lead and are relatively soluble in body fluids. Ceramic seals offer biocompatibility and hermetic sealing but are difficult to use with titanium alloys. A second strategy for achieving a hermetic titanium receiver with a large number of ceramic feedthroughs is presently being evaluated at UCSF and has been used commercially by the Australian manufacturer Nucleus Ltd. In this technique all the feedthrough pins (platinum in this case) are sealed into a flat plate of ceramic and this plate is brazed onto a titanium shell. The drawback with this is the toxicity of the brazing compounds and the danger of galvanic corrosion generated in small crevices at the junction of the braze and the shell.

The final step in a hermetic package is the closure after assembly of the electronic components. In a titanium shell this is accomplished with either electron beam or laser welding in a vacuum or inert atmosphere with heat sinks provided to protect the electronics.

At UCSF the goal for the next generation of receivers is to build hermetically sealed units completely from ceramic. The Hochmairs in Vienna are working on a similar project. The advantage of an all-ceramic package lies in its transparency to radio frequency signals, allowing the antenna structures to be sealed along the electronic components in one unit. In terms of long-term reliability and tissue compatibility as a function of implant volume, this design offers great benefit.

Barrier Coatings

The use of a conformal coating over completed electronic components and circuits is widespread in the electronics and medical device industries. A thin film, or thicker casing of silicone rubber, Parylene or epoxy will help to stabilise the components mounted on a circuit or hybrid substrate as well as provide short-term protection from moisture and salts normally present in the environment or found in an implantable device due to the failure of a hermetic seal.

Epoxy coating adds a thick layer over components which imparts tremendous strength to an assembly, but not without serious drawbacks. First, an epoxy coating several millimetres thick is heavy. This has particular significance in a free-floating device such as a pacemaker or the internal receiver developed by Nucleus Ltd in Australia. Second, epoxy shrinks during its polymerisation process. This shrinkage can break the connections of fine wires to exposed chip components. Last, filling the internal volume of a hermetically sealed package makes accurate leak detection more difficult because there is no space for a gas to be absorbed and released during the detection phase of the procedure. Parylene is an excellent conformal coating for use as a barrier layer. A 2–3 μm coating of Parylene provides greater moisture protection than several millimetres of epoxy and there is no shrinkage or surface tension associated with its deposition. In practical

94 *Implant Design and Construction*

application it requires that masks and jigs must be used to ensure that Parylene coats only the interior, electronic surfaces of the device during the deposition. Parylene has also been used as an exterior coating with a 'window' left uncoated to act as a ground in monopolar pacemaker systems. This concept could be applied in the development of a monopolar cochlear implant system, thereby reducing the number of electrical feedthroughs needed in the receiver can itself. Silicone-based conformal coatings offer a compromise between Parylene and epoxies. These coatings can be applied by hand, without masking jigs, and do not change in volume as they cure. Unfortunately silicones provide only slightly superior moisture protection than epoxy and create the same problems in leak test assurance. Caution must be exercised when cleaning assemblies conformally coated with silicone rubbers because these materials swell rapidly in some organic solvents, particularly freon and aromatic hydrocarbons. This can disrupt fine solder leads and wire bonds, leading to failure which may be intermittent. For this reason all silicone rubber containing devices should be cleaned only in a mixture of detergent and water. It should be noted that the area on the package to be welded must be kept entirely free of Parylene, or other coatings, as these will prevent the formation of a good quality weld joint.

Surgical and Percutaneous Connection to the Cochlear Implant

Once a successful interface has been achieved between the electrode and its target tissue, a reliable connection to the stimulus generating source must be made. Many strategies have been used by the pacemaker industry and other manufacturers to attach leads to an implanted or external signal source. However, in no other field is the need for an effective, reliable implanted connector as great as in neural prostheses. This is apparent when one compares the functional complexity of a neural stimulating device with that of other implanted systems. In a conventional pacemaker, one or two low impedance electrodes are driven by a stimulus generated within the implanted device. The entire pacemaker can be effectively replaced, along with its electrodes, when necessary. In comparison, the cochlear implant and other neural prostheses must have many relatively small, high impedance, contact surfaces to achieve discrete spatial stimulation and physically to fit within the very small dimensions of the structures to be stimulated. These devices will be very sensitive to any leakage or shunting at the connector. The susceptibility to trauma which characterises most neural stimulation sites also necessitates a reliable, implanted connector, providing the option of leaving implanted electrodes in position while the electronic portion of a device is replaced.

Percutaneous Connection to Implanted Electrodes

The advantages of an implanted driving system for the cochlear implant are clear. A subcutaneous device greatly reduces the risk of infection and maintenance associated with any chronic percutaneous opening. However, the use of a percutaneous connector is desirable in research projects where direct access to each electrode is needed. In such patients data may be derived from the electrode as well as transmitted through it. This information can include precise measurement of the electrode status *in situ* and complex measurements of the fields created by one or more bipolar electrode pairs using others as recording electrodes. These types of measurement have played an important role in the design and refinement of the intracochlear electrode and provide insight regarding the perceptual processes whereby patterns of stimulation produce psychophysically measured sensation in the patient.

Although direct connection offers advantages for the clinical investigation of electrically stimulated hearing, it also presents several problems. First is the risk of infection at the exit site of the connector. The initial risk of such an infection is minimal but increases as epithelium lining the inner surfaces of the exit site sloughs and accumulates to generate a medium for bacterial growth. In most reported cases, mild infection which has occurred has been resolved with application of topical or systemic antibiotics; however, in some the spread of infection has necessitated the removal of the entire prosthesis. The situation becomes more complex when a percutaneous connector is removed and replaced with a wholly implanted driving system. In this case the exit site is closed, which effectively traps bacteria and cellular debris within the wound. This irritation would normally be resolved through immune response but the continued presence of the foreign body allows a sanctuary for the remaining bacteria and prevents successful resolution of the infection. Experience with orthopaedic joint replacements indicates that the only way to eliminate infection in the presence of a foreign body is to remove the device and reimplant the patient after the infection is completely resolved. This may be impossible for cochlear electrodes if the scala tympani is occluded by scar tissue. For this reason the percutaneous connector strategy developed at UCSF relies on two concepts. First, the exit site is situated across the scalp at the opposite ear from the one implanted to provide a long pathway for infection originating at the exit site. Second, a thin, flexible cable is used to reduce irritation and is removed 10–12 weeks post surgery before cell debris accumulates to support bacterial growth. A Dacron cuff placed just below the skin acts as a barrier to infection and is rapidly incorporated in connective tissue to anchor the cable. With this strategy patients at UCSF have exhibited no symptoms of infection either during percutaneous connection or after implantation of an RF receiver.

The second problem with percutaneous connections is that of lead breakage or leakage of fluid into the connector. As mentioned earlier, Eddington *et al.* (1978) and Dillier *et al.* (1980) have had success sealing a percutaneous plug. The pedestal holding the connector is made from pyrolitic carbon. Conductive fluids are excluded by layers of epoxy and Silastic. The bottom layer of Silastic acts as an elastic stress relief for the fine electrode leads. In the UCSF design the continuous cable exiting the skin to a remote plug eliminates the need to seal these contacts against moisture.

Design of the UCSF Cochlear Implant System

Introduction

As described in the introduction to this chapter the development team at UCSF has designed and implanted several generations of intracochlear electrodes (Loeb *et al.*, 1983; Merzenich *et al.*, 1984; Michelson and Schindler, 1981). The first of these devices were single-channel electrodes built in moulds made from actual casts of human temporal bones. These electrodes were stimulated via percutaneous miniature plugs or epoxy-encapsulated RF receivers. Subsequent multichannel arrays were also made in this way. The present devices incorporate developments which address each of the goals detailed previously. It is important to note that patients currently are divided into two groups in the UCSF project. The first group, termed experimental patients, receive a temporary percutaneous cable for three months of extensive testing. Following this period these patients receive a transcutaneous RF receiver through a minor surgery. The second group, clinical patients, are implanted with the receiver immediately and are involved in testing and development to a minor degree.

Dimensions and Physical Characteristics

Figure 4.5 is a scanning electron micrograph of the UCSF intracochlear electrode spiral. The 16 platinum-iridium (Pt90Ir10) contacts can be seen on the upper and inner surfaces of the spiral. The carrier which forms the bulk of the electrode, and supports the contacts and their leads, is moulded Silastic (Dow MDX 4-4210). The mould to form the electrode (Figure 4.6) was constructed to fit a mathematical model of the cochlear spiral generated by measuring several temporal bone castings. This strategy has been adapted because it is felt that too close a fit may result in occlusion of perilymph flow within the scale tympani which may lead to neural degeneration in these areas (Leake-Jones and Rebscher, 1983). The electrode array is formed in one place with its connector pad (Figure 4.7). The finished electrode is designed to be inserted 24 mm past the round window. The segment of the electrode from the round window to the 15 mm point is 1 mm in diameter and tapers rapidly to 0.75 mm diameter for the remainder of its length.

The remaining physical properties of the electrode concern its flexural behaviour. As mentioned previously trauma may occur during insertion due to either upward movement of the electrode tip, resulting in damage to the osseous spiral lamina or basilar membrane, or by direct irritation of the endosteum lining the scala. In both cases the characteristics of the metal electrode leads dominate the flex patterns of the array while elasticity is added by the silicone rubber carrier.

To prevent upward bending of the tip of the electrode the contact leads are formed into a vertically oriented rib (Figure 4.8). This vertical rib is very resistant to flexion out of the horizontal plane, but bends easily in the spiral plant. Two factors contribute to this vertical stiffness. First, each contact wire is flattened 0.001×0.003 in. or 0.0075×0.0025 in.) producing a lead which is very difficult to bend in the 'long' axis. Second, each of these flattened leads is positioned vertically in the rib with respect to the other similarly oriented leads. When the arrangement of

Implant Design and Construction 97

Figure 4.5: Scanning Electron Micrograph of the UCSF Intracochlear Electrode. The 16-contact electrode array tapers from 1.0 mm diameter at the base of the cochlea to 0.75 mm at the apex. The electrode array is inserted 24 mm into the scala tympani with the pair of electrodes at the tip stimulating the 500–800 Hz region of the cochlea. The 16 contacts are formed from platinum-iridium (90:10) and moulded into a clear silicone rubber carrier.

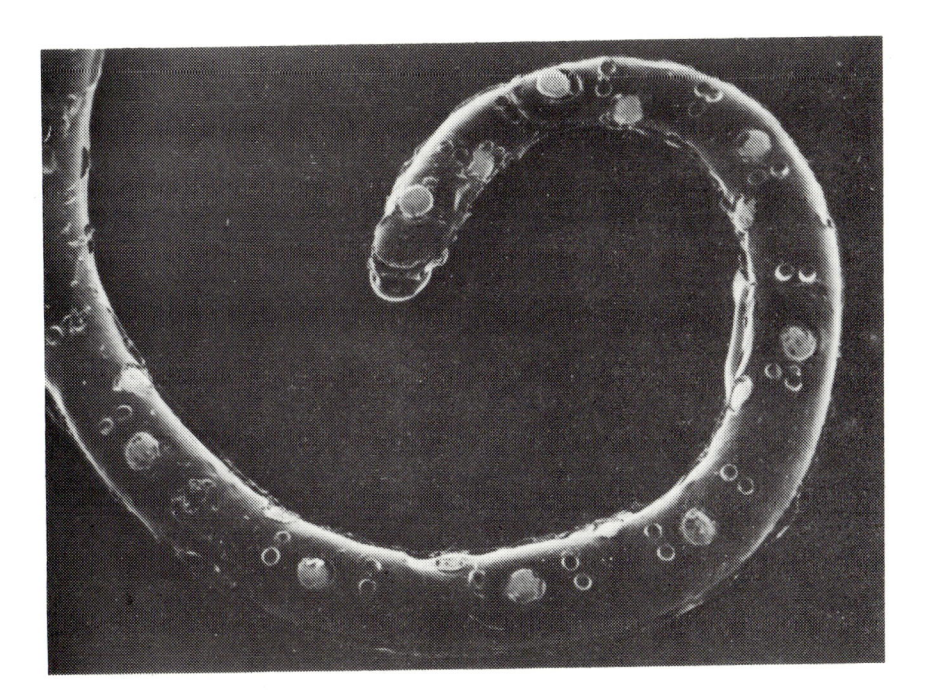

all the leads is completed, the central rib consists of the 16 leads stacked perpendicular to the plane of the spiral. Insertion tests in many human cadaver temporal bones have shown that this rib successfully prevents upward flexing of the electrode tip and the damage which may accompany such flexing. The second mode of damage associated with insertion trauma in these devices is a more subtle scraping or irritation of the scala lining. Only when the Silastic electrode carrier is moulded as a precise spiral form will its elastic memory keep the tip of the array from pressing on either the medial or lateral wall of the scala tympani during insertion. This feature is also essential in overcoming the friction encountered during electrode insertion.

Multichannel Electrode Configuration
To allow the use of the UCSF electrode in research and development of future multichannel devices the contact surfaces have been placed in eight bipolar pairs.

98 *Implant Design and Construction*

Figure 4.6: The Electrode Fabrication Mould Was Built at UCSF Utilising a Computer-controlled Milling Machine Programmed to Match Precisely Measurements Derived from Metal Castings of Human Cadaver Temporal Bones. Each half of the cochlear spiral can be removed from the mould to allow use of specially cut spirals of different size or for the opposite ear.

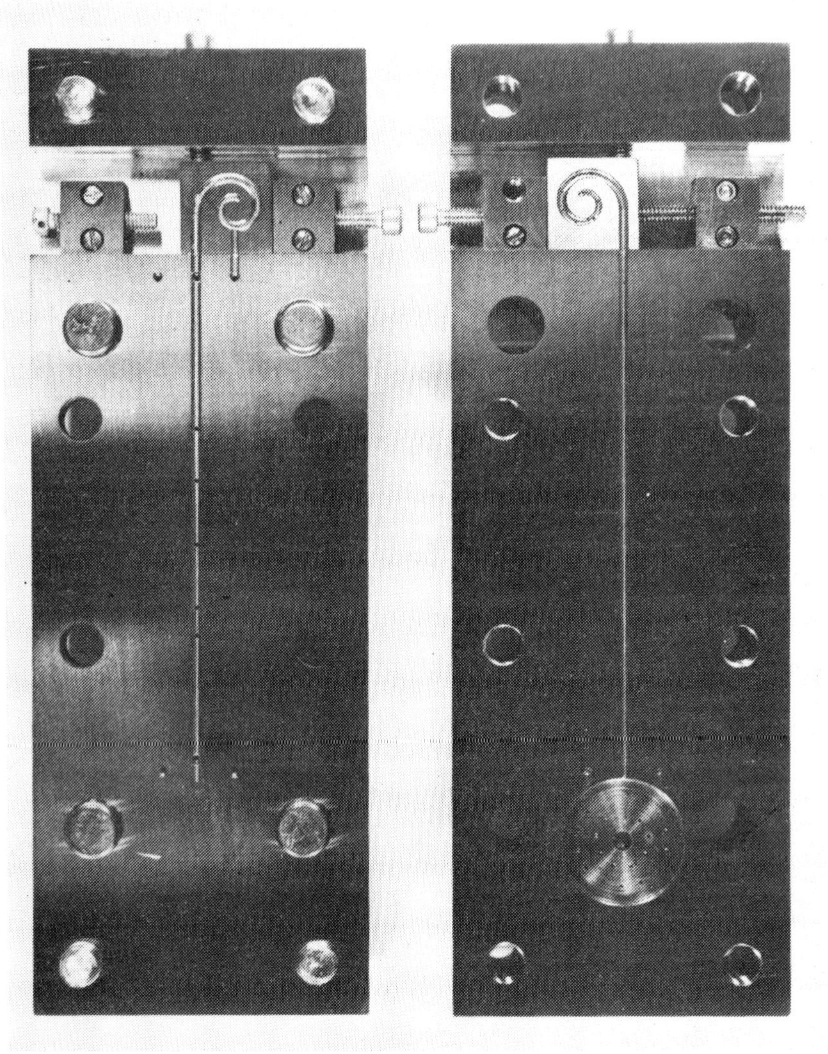

Implant Design and Construction 99

Figure 4.7: UCSF Intracochlear Electrode and Connector Pad. The electrode array, lead segment and connector pad are formed in a single moulding procedure. The 16 connector contacts can be seen on the connector pad (left) reinforced by Dacron mesh.

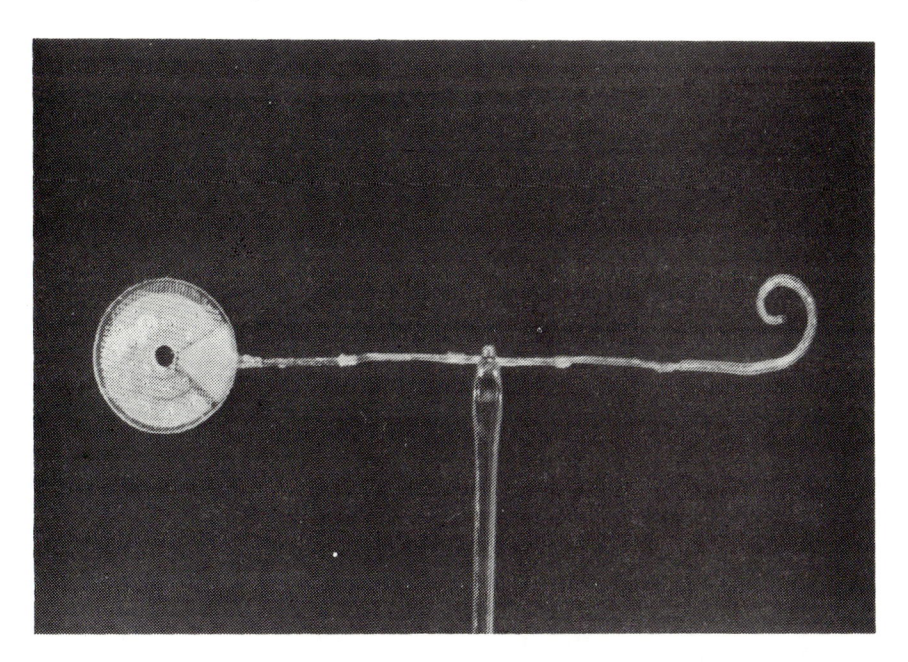

Each electrode contact is 350 μm in diameter at the surface of the carrier and can be addressed in any configuration when used with a percutaneous cable. The edge to edge distance between contacts within each pair is 150 μm with 2 mm separating the centres of each pair. Tests with human temporal bones in which the final orientation of each contact beneath the basilar membrane was measured after insertion have allowed the location of each contact to be correlated with the results obtained from psychophysical testing in experimental patients. Preliminary animal studies have indicated that radial orientation of bipolar stimulating contacts is optimum for efficient, selective stimulation of local groups of residual neurones either in the osseous spiral lamina or spiral ganglion. Psychophysical testing in recent subjects has confirmed that most patients are able to discriminate between the sensations produced by stimulation of adjacent, bipolar electrode pairs with this spacing. It should be noted that when the same electrodes are stimulated in a monopolar fashion (vs. an external or remote ground) there is highly significant interaction between electrodes at different locations and patient failure to discrminate between the sites.

Long-Term Safety of the Intracochlear Electrode

The challenge of developing an electrode array capable of safe stimulation for many

100 *Implant Design and Construction*

Figure 4.8: Cross-section of the Intracochlear Electrode Array. Each of the contact leads is flattened prior to application of the insulation layers and arranged to form a vertical rib within the Silastic carrier. Two electrode mushroom contacts are seen in this section.

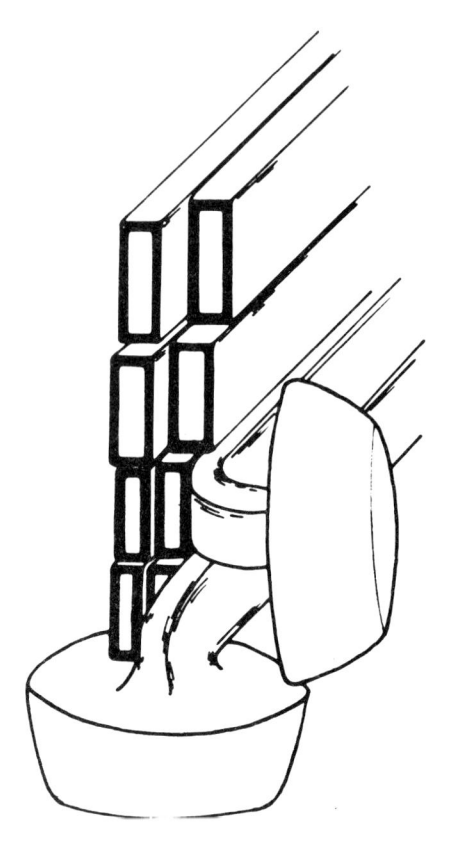

years has prompted many changes in the materials, design and application of these devices. Few data regarding the long-term effects of intracochlear electrical stimulation are available. However, we do know some of the issues of importance. Charge density (the amount of stimulating charge transmitted across the electrode/tissue interface in each phase of a balanced waveform divided by the real contact area through which this charge is passed) appears to be the primary factor. It has been proposed that 300 $\mu C/cm^2$ is a safe upper limit for chronic use. Unfortunately the restricted area stimulated by a bipolar electrode pair also means that fewer neurones will be activated by a given amount of current. Thus discrete multichannel stimulation requires increased current levels to achieve a particular level of loudness. For this reason the surface area of each contact must be as large as possible to decrease the charge density. Either the geometric surface area may be increased or the surface texture may be increased by roughening or sintering materials on to the contact. As shown in Figure 4.9, the contacts used in the UCSF electrode

Figure 4.9: Scanning Electron Micrographs of a Mushroom-shaped Electrode Contact.

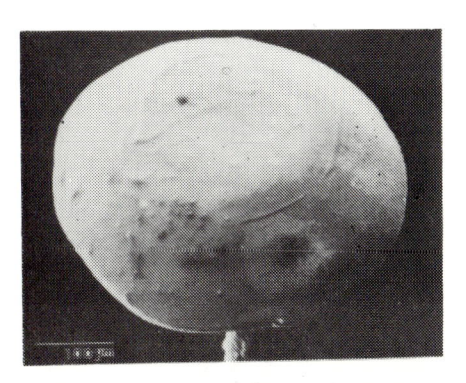

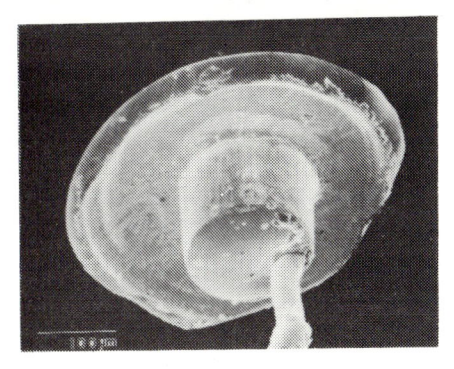

are a mushroom shape to provide maximum surface area with minimum internal volume.

The materials used in the intracochlear electrode have been selected for long life with minimal host reaction. Pt90Ir10 is a stable alloy for electrode contacts and leads. Alloyed in this proportion the platinum provides enough softness to allow forming while the iridium provides protection from dissolution and electrolytic bubble formation at higher current levels. Each contact lead is initially coated with Pyre-ML which provides a mechanically robust adhesion layer for Parylene-C. As described earlier Parylene is an excellent insulating material for implanted devices because of its pin-hole free, consistent deposition and its exceptional biocompatibility. The carrier which forms the body of the electrode array is cast from Dow Silastic MDX 4-4210 which in our experience generates lower levels of tissue response than other types of silicone rubber.

To protect against the possibility of infection the electrode leads are placed in a channel along the ear canal and a plate of bone is used both to hold the leads in place and to prevent the erosion of the canal wall as it passes over the electrode leads (Chapter 6 and Schindler *et al.*, 1981).

102 *Implant Design and Construction*

Figure 4.10: Cross-section of the UCSF Surgical Connector. The surgical disconnect base holds the connector pads (stippled) for the electrode and internal receiver antenna array. The contacts (0.5 mm balls) held in these pads mate with a mirror image set of feedthrough pins on the lower surface of the four-channel receiver capsule, which occupies the majority of the space within the connector, and forms its lid.

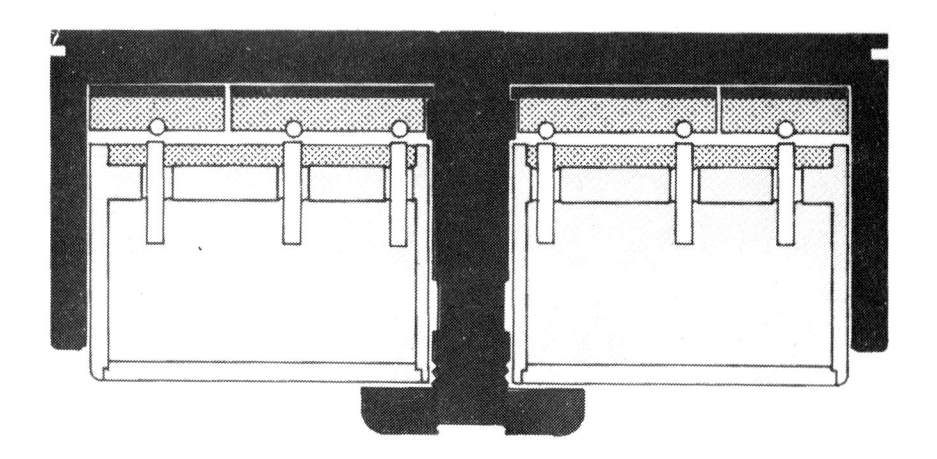

UCSF Surgical Connector

The design requirements for the UCSF surgical connector included the following. (1) The connector must be functional over the expected lifetime of the electrode, i.e. 30 years. (2) The connector must be fabricated from materials which have good performance in the biological environment. (3) The connector must make low impedance connections between the electrode leads and feedthroughs from the implanted receiver but must exhibit high resistance to shorting between adjacent contacts. (4) Surgical application of the connector must be simple ensuring correct orientation and failure-free connection. (5) Repeated opening of the connector must not affect the integrity of the device.

Figure 4.10 shows the present surgical connector. The shell is machined from titanium (Ti6A14V) and acts both to protect and pressurise the Silastic pad within. These pads hold the contacts from the electrode leads and percutaneous cable. The contacts are formed by melting a small ball (0.5 mm) on the end of each lead and the pad is moulded as a part of the electrode. When this pad and a mirror image pad from the percutaneous cable (or receiver feedthroughs) are placed together within the connector the corresponding balls from each pad make contact with each other. To make the orientation of this connection more reliable, the bottom surface of both the cable contact balls and the receiver feedthroughs are flattened to provide greater contact surface and an orientation pin in the lid mates with a slot in the base. When the lid is closed and tightened with a screw, the elasticity of the Silastic maintains a high pressure. This pressure is sufficient to prevent water vapour, which permeates all polymers, from condensing.

The use of balls formed directly on the ends of electrode and cable leads (also Pt90Ir10) and platinum feedthrough pins in the receiver reduces the possibility of galvanic corrosion between the contacts as may occur with solder or weld joints. In all tests the UCSF connector has produced low impedance contact of all appropriate leads while maintaining high isolation (5–20 Mohms) between channels. This strategy is used in the Australian device apparently with excellent results in both *in vitro* tests and clinical use.

The temporary percutaneous cable used in psychophysical testing of experimental patients is constructed of 18 platinum-iridium leads (16 electrode leads and two grounds) in a Silastic tubing sheath. Each lead is formed from seven-stranded wire to prevent breakage with flexing. The cable terminates internally in a Silastic connector pad with each lead ending in a ball contact which is precisely oriented. In use the cable is passed subcutaneously over the scalp and extends 12–14 inches beyond the skin. After the surgery a standard multipin electrical connector is soldered to the distal cable end.

Transcutaneous Receiver

The transcutaneous receiver is incorporated in the lid of the connector. After completion of the three-month experimental test period the four-channel RF receiver is fitted on the connector base and directly stimulates the electrode lead contacts located in the connector pad.

The receiver operates on four RF carrier frequencies (2, 3, 4.5 and 6 MHz). Each channel is independent and electrically isolated from the others, having individual antennae, detecting circuits and bipolar output feedthroughs. The configuration of electrodes to be driven by each channel can be set prior to or during the surgical procedure. The output of each channel is capacitively coupled to prevent the passage of a net direct current charge. An internal array of four antennae receive transmitted signals from a matching external set of coils. A complete UCSF implant system for clinical application is shown assembled in Figure 4.11.

An external speech processor and transmitter is adjustable to adapt the device to patients with varying dynamic range and thresholds (Figure 4.12).

Fabrication of the UCSF Cochlear Implant System

Intracochlear Electrode

Assembly of the intracochlear electrode begins with the formation of mushroom-shaped contacts on each of the 16 lead wires. Two sizes of round PtIr (90:10) wire (0.0015 in. D and 0.002 in. D) are flattened to 0.00075 × 0.0025 in. and 0.001 × 0.003 in. to produce the required flexural characteristics in the finished electrode. This wire is coated with a triple layer of Pyre-ML polyimide (California Fine Wire Co.) and tested to assure insulation. The process of forming the mushroom contact is shown in Figure 4.13. A measured section of wire is melted in a flame to

Figure 4.11: Assembled UCSF Four-channel Cochlear Implant (Implanted Components).

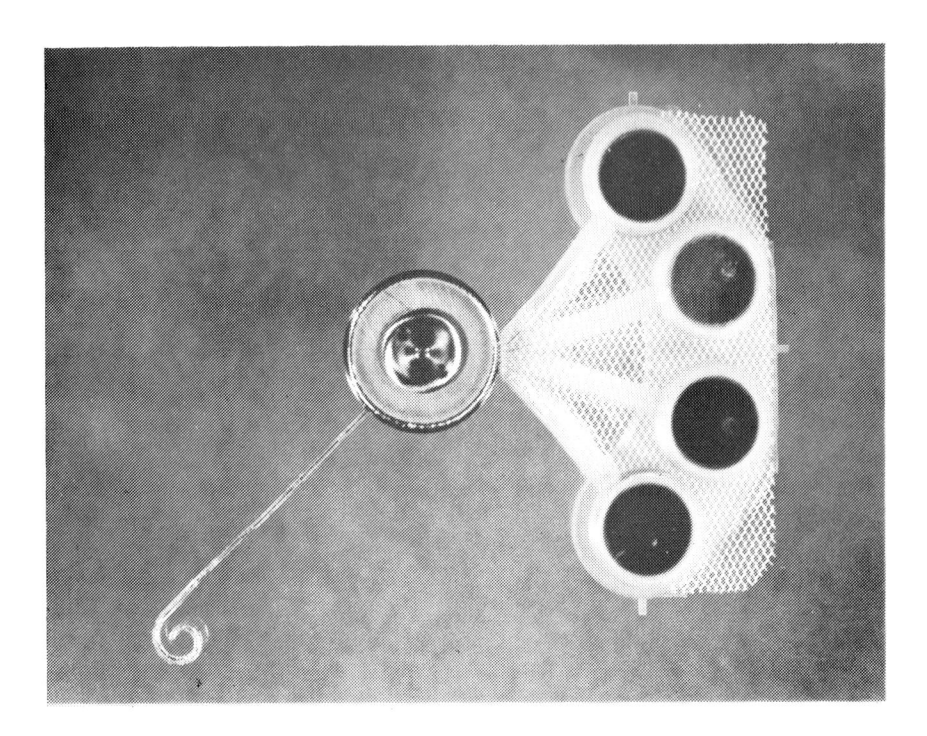

form a ball on the tip of the lead. A pair of forceps is used to heat sink the lead and minimise the insulation burned back during the melting process. The wire is then threaded through a swaging die and the mushroom stamped from the ball. Completed mushrooms are next assembled on to racks for coating with a 2 μm layer of Parylene-C (Viking Technology, Santa Clara, CA).

The electrode mould allows precise placement of the 16 stimulating contacts, their leads and connector balls. Present electrode moulds are computer numerical control (CNC) machined from stainless steel. The advantage to the later method is a much harder mould surface which will not become scratched or release contaminating particles of plating during use. The electrode mould includes the moulding cavity required to form the connector pad so that the electrode, lead cable and pad can be injection moulded in one step.

Ensuring correct placement of the mushroom contacts requires orientation and a method of holding the electrodes during filling of the mould with Silastic. Sixteen locating holes 300 μm in diameter have been drilled into the mould (Figure 4.14). As each successive pair of electrodes is secured the vertical rib of wires grows and is held by guide pins and occasional application of Silastic. The lead for each contact is placed in turn in position on the connector pad and

Implant Design and Construction 105

Figure 4.12: UCSF External Four-channel Speech Processor/Transmitter. The wearable four-channel stimulator allows patient adjustment of individual channel level and overall threshold/level control. The four-coil external antenna array is held in position by four magnets which correspond to matching implanted magnets.

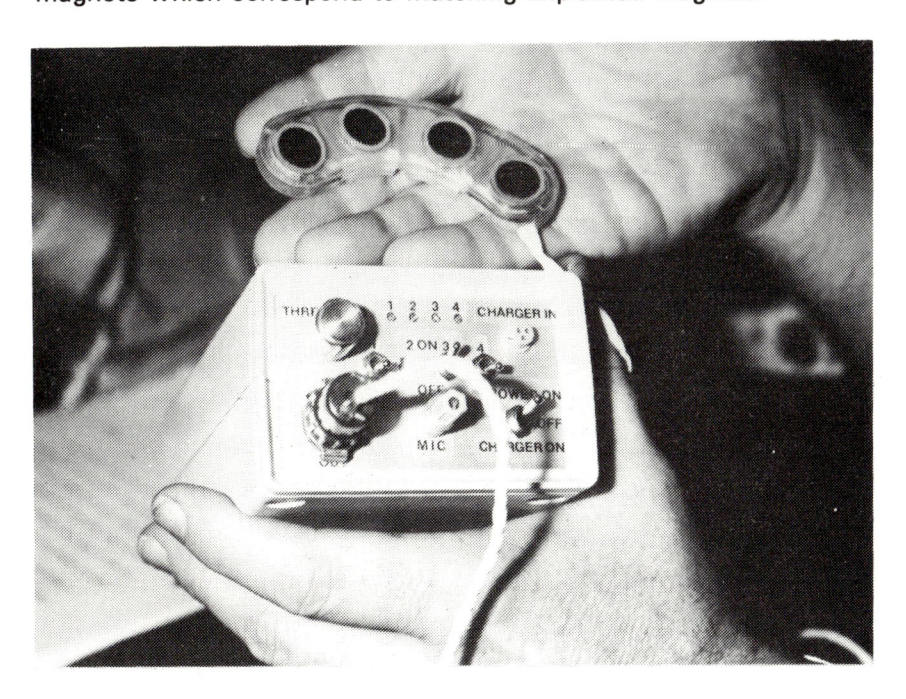

Figure 4.13: Electrode Contact Forming Process. The swage on the left deforms the ball to a mushroom as shown in the four sequential drawings on the right.

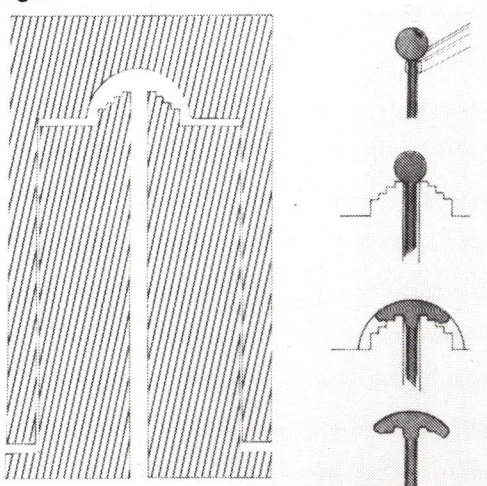

Figure 4.14: Schematic Diagram of the UCSF Electrode Mould. Electrode contacts and leads are oriented in the intracochlear spiral section of the electrode mould with the use of guide pins. The vertical rib can be seen forming between the seven pairs of guide pins.

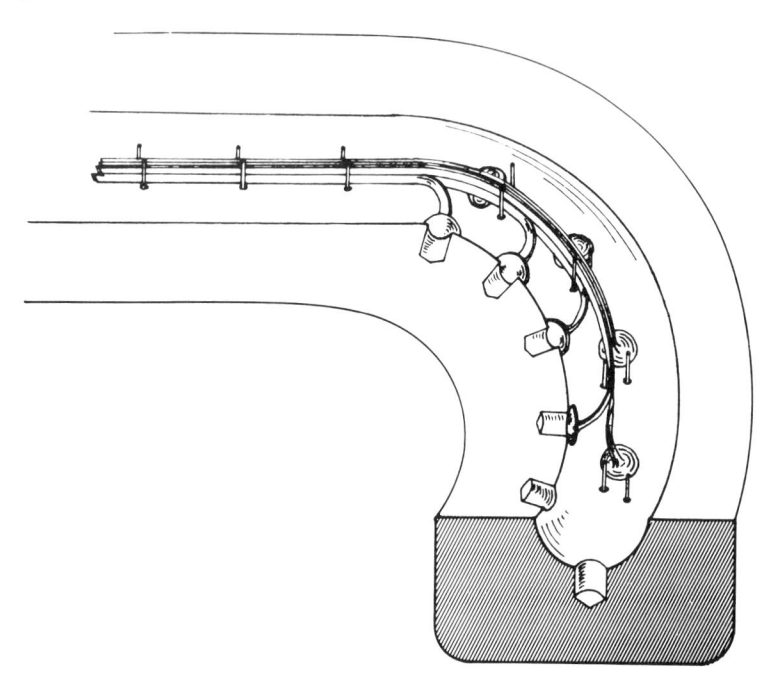

its length adjusted by melting back a 0.5 mm sphere to form the connector contact ball. After positioning the sixteen mushrooms and connector balls a fine layer of Dacron mesh is laid in to act as a backing.

Percutaneous Cable

Seven-stranded PtIr cable (Teflon insulated) is drawn through Silastic tubing to create an 18 wire percutaneous cable. To form the connecting pad, 0.6 mm balls are melted on the ends of the wires and pressed to produce a flat surface 0.5 mm in diameter. These contacts are positioned in a mirror image mould, backed with Dacron mesh and moulded in Silastic. The resulting cable connector pad is held in contact with the electrode by a simple connector lid which is replaced by the four-channel receiver when the cable is removed following the initial testing period. To prevent entry of bacteria at the skin exit site a 10 mm long cuff of Dacron felt (1 mm thick) is attached with Silastic Type A adhesive and positioned below the skin surface during surgery.

Four-Channel Receiver

Titanium (Ti6Al4V) capsules for the RF receiver are produced by AstroSeal Inc,

Figure 4.15: The UCSF Four-channel Implanted Receiver is Shown Before (Left) and After (Right) Electron Beam Welding of the Titanium Lid to Hermetically Seal the Capsule. The hybrid electronic components are attached to the pre-soldered ceramic substrate in a single operation. Each circuit is then tested prior to silicone conformal coating and welding of the lid. The receiver module is 1 inch (25 mm) in diameter.

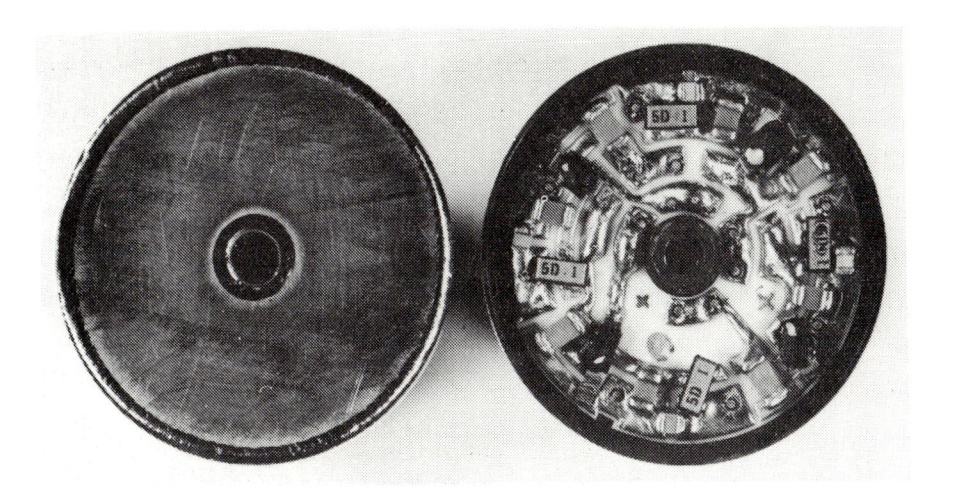

Los Angeles, CA (Figures 4.1 and 4.4). Twenty-four hermetic feedthroughs are required for the four-chanel receiver, 16 for electrode contacts and eight for the four antenna coils. Each feedthrough is made by press forming a cylindrical ceramic collar. The feedthrough pins are cut from 0.5 mm pure platinum stock and roughened with sodium bicarbonate 'sand blasting'. To prepare the titanium cans for sealing each can is heated to 1100°C to form a thick oxide layer which will bind to the ceramic during firing. The 24 platinum pins, preformed ceramic inserts and titanium capsule are aligned in carbon jigs and the assembly is fired at 1700°C to fuse and seal the unit. The sealed feedthrough plane is helium leak tested.

Electronic components are assembled onto a pretinned ceramic hybrid circuit substrate which has been laser drilled to fit over the 24 feedthrough pins (Biomed Concepts Inc., Clarksburg, MD) (Figure 4.15). All components and connecting pins are soldered during a single reflow solder operation. After testing each of the four circuits, a Silastic conformal coating is applied over the substrate and the receiver lid is electron beam welded over the capsule. Each completed receiver is tested in hot freon for gross leaks and in krypton 85 for fine leaks. The four 13 mm diameter antennae provide both power and signal information for each channel of the receiver and are wound from seven-strand PtIr wire and coated with medical grade epoxy, Parylene-C and Silastic. The antenna leads terminate in 0.5

108 *Implant Design and Construction*

Figure 4.16: Four-channel Implanted Receiver Antenna Array. The four independent receiver channels are driven by four, matched antenna coils via the surgical connector. The circular connector pad at the bottom of the photograph holds the leads and eight contacts from the coils which mate with eight input feedthroughs on the lower surface of the receiver. Dacron mesh is moulded into the coil array to provide strength and an anchorage to the skull. A ceramic magnet in the centre of each receiver coil positions and supports each external transmitter coil.

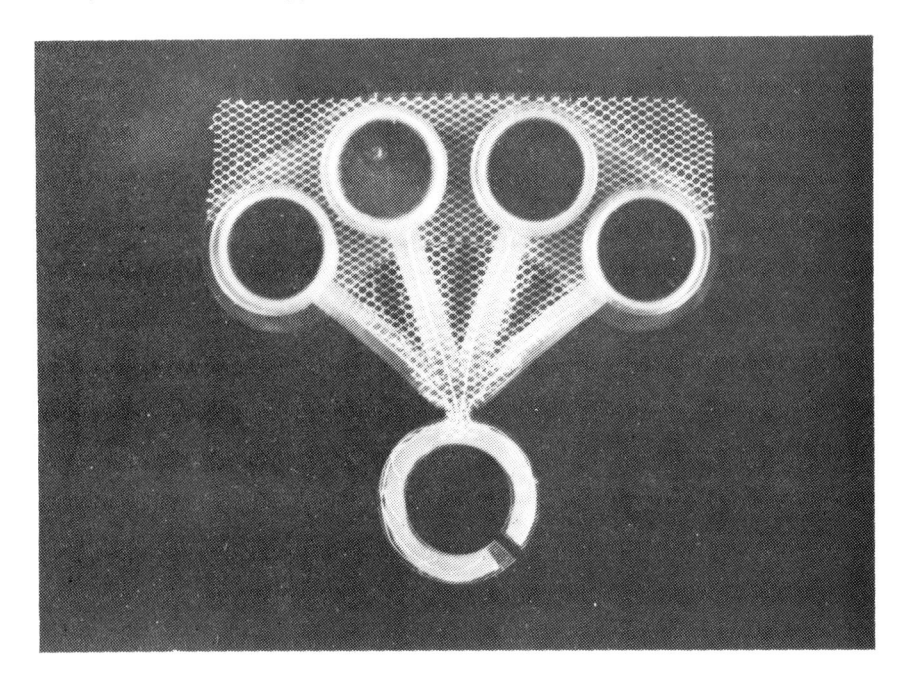

mm balls moulded into a ring-shaped connector pad which fits around the electrode pad (Figure 4.16).

Other Cochlear Implant Designs and Projects

House Ear Institute, Los Angeles

More cochlear prostheses have been implanted at the House Ear Institute, and by their collaborators, than in all other centres combined (see Chapter 1). Beginning in 1961 with a cochlear electrode array consisting of five separate leads and an extracochlear ground they now use a single-channel system manufactured by McGann Surgical Products, a subsidiary of the 3M Corporation. Over 400 patients have received this device, which is currently the only intracochlear device presently under review by the United States Food and Drug Administration for commercial market approval. The House implant programme, as well as details on the implant itself (Danley and Fretz, 1982), are thoroughly described in House *et al.* (1981) and in a special supplement of the *Annals of Otology, Rhinology and Laryngology* (House and Edgerton, 1982).

The internal components of the House single-channel system are extremely simple and have proven to be equally reliable. The device consists of a copper induction coil wound around a delrin bobbin and ferrite pot core to which two platinum leads, an active and ground electrode, are soldered. The receiving coil wire is insulated with Isonel and then impregnated with Epoxylite to reduce further the possibility of fluid shorting between adjacent coil windings. A coating of silicone rubber is applied as a final encapsulation layer. The electrode leads themselves are fabricated from 0.008 in. pure platinum wire. The active (cochlear) lead is 78 mm in length with a 0.5 mm ball formed at the distal end and 15 mm left uninsulated. The ground lead is constructed from the same wire with a total length of 68 mm of which 53 mm is uninsulated. The insulated portions of both leads are passed through Silicone rubber tubing. A matching external coil drives the internal device by direct induction of an amplitude modulated 16 kHz carrier signal (Figure 4.17).

Considerable controversy has surrounded the engineering of the House device in respect to both the safety and efficacy of the signal transmission system. Because the internal coil is directly coupled to the electrodes without filtering or decoding, the 16 kHz carrier signal is continuously transmitted to the cochlea and central nervous system. The effects of such stimulation are not currently understood. It is also clear from studies on a bilaterally implanted patient (Johnsson *et al.*, 1982) who later died of natural causes, that balled electrodes without clearly defined flexural characteristics may penetrate the basilar membrane during insertion leading to cochlear injury and profound effects on the populations of surviving cell bodies and neurons within the osseous spiral lamina (see Chapter 3). Although this pathology does not seem to degrade the percepts of a single channel user with present signal-processing techniques there is clear evidence that this loss of neural population may seriously degrade future multiple-channel, or sophisticated single-channel, perceptions. However, as mentioned earlier, the device is exceptionally reliable and by nature of its simplicity has allowed the implantation of a large group of patients. House and Edgerton (1982) also describe continued studies with a series of electrodes consisting of four active and three ground leads, similar in construction to the single-channel leads, connected to a skin plug for investigation of multichannel stimulation.

Biostim Inc., New Jersey, USA

In the Spring of 1983 Biostim Inc. introduced a single-channel intracochlear electrode system for clinical evaluation and eventual commercial application. The device resembles the House implant in basic configuration, but has several significant improvements. First, the electrode is driven by an RF receiver which is hermetically sealed in titanium. The receiver delivers a demodulated analogue signal from which the RF carrier has been effectively filtered and which has been charge balanced

110 *Implant Design and Construction*

Figure 4.17: The House Single-channel Cochlear Prosthesis Which Has Been Implanted in Over 400 Patients. The implanted portion of the device (left) consists of an induction coil of copper wire wound round a ferrite core, an active intracochlear stimulating lead (longer of the two leads) and a ground lead which is placed outside the cochlea. The induction coil assembly is encapsulated in epoxy and Silastic and the leads pass through Silastic tubing. The external stimulator consists of a microphone, processor and transmitting coil. The House device is produced by a subsidiary of the 3M Corporation.

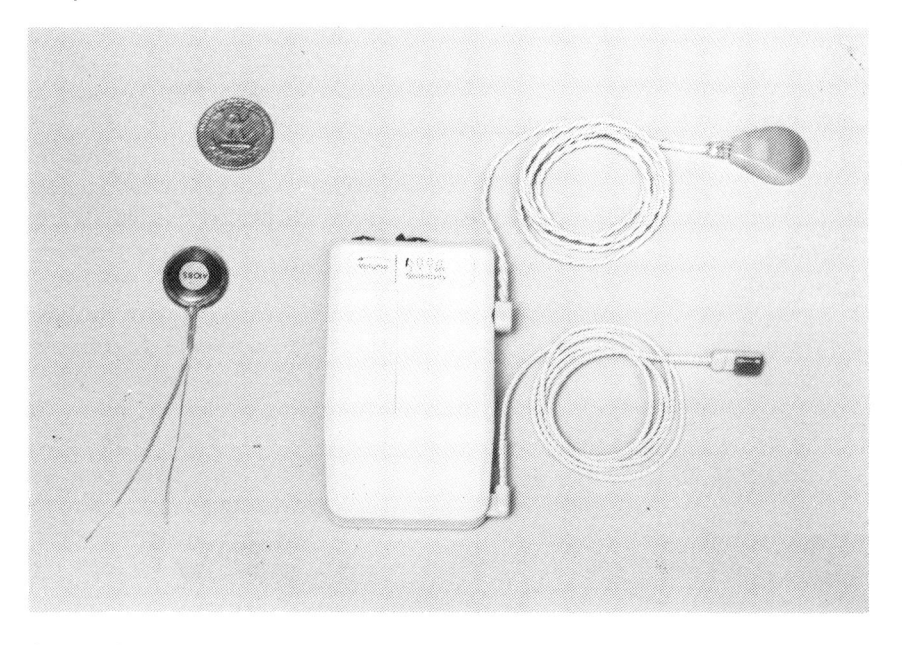

Source: Courtesy House Ear Institute, Los Angeles, California.

by capacitive coupling. These two features are a significant step in improving safety and efficiency of information transfer. The Biostim system also includes a more versatile sound processor unit with greater control over waveform and processing functions in a small, wearable package. With this system the otologist also has the option of positioning the electrode extracochlearly, e.g. in the round window niche.

University of Utah, USA

Dr Eddington has intensively studied several multichannel implant patients at the University of Utah in Salt Lake City. The electrodes used in these studies consist of five or six balled wire leads and two ground leads placed on the promontory and in temporalis muscle. In early devices the electrodes were made with Pyre-ML insulated silver wire whereas the later prostheses were made with Teflon-coated platinum. The leads in the cochlea ended with balls approximately 0.5 mm in diameter. To provide a flexible system within which a wide variety of stimulus strategies could be applied the leads were connected to a plug which exits the skin through a carbon pedestal. This system has recently been approved for clinical investigation and is being produced by the Kolf Medical Corporation of Utah. The ball-tipped wire electrodes used in the device are prone to produce the same type of trauma observed by Johnsson et al. (1982); however the long-term effectiveness of this multichannel strategy has been demonstrated in past patients (Eddington et al., 1978; Eddington, 1983).

Technical University of Vienna, Austria

The cochlear prosthesis team at the Technical University of Vienna has developed a great variety of implantable systems and tested a large group of patients with multichannel devices. A review of the design generations and patients studied during the time from their first clinical application of a prosthesis in 1977 is presented in their summary of these results in the New York Academy of Sciences publication, *Cochlear Prostheses: An International Symposium* (Burian et al., 1980, 1981; Hochmair-Desoyer et al., 1983). During this time they have implanted 19 multichannel intracochlear devices and 15 single-channel extracochlear prostheses. It is interesting to note that this group began by building an extremely sophisticated eight-channel CMOS hybrid receiver and found, as have other groups, that optimising sound processing strategies for even a small number of channels is very complex. For this reason they reduced the number of channels to six and finally to four in the most recently reported generation. This has also allowed use of a more simple, broad bandwidth (20 kHz) analogue receiver.

The intracochlear electrode developed by Drs Hochmair and Hochmair-Desoyer consists of four bipolar pairs of PtIr (90:10) contacts on a tapering 25 mm-long carrier of Silastic 382 as shown in Figure 4.18 (Hochmair-Desoyer and Hochmair, 1980). The stimulating surface is formed by allowing a portion (0.25 mm diameter) of the 0.35 mm contact ball to be exposed at the carrier surfaces. These contacts form a real surface area measured at 0.15 mm(2) to 0.33 mm(2). The electrode wires are Teflon insulated and lead directly into the receiving unit which is encapsulated with epoxy overcoated with Silastic 382. The receiving system allows the electrodes to be stimulated either in a bipolar or monopolar scheme with the use of a magnetic reed switching network (Burian et al., 1981).

The Hochmairs feel their electrodes can be safely inserted 12–22 mm into the human cochlea. To modify the handling characteristics of the electrode, a stiffening wire is placed in the centre of the carrier. The Vienna group has reported three successful revisions of devices which failed electronically. These reports add hope that it may be possible to remove and replace an intracochlear implant should this be required.

Hopitaux de Paris — Hopital Saint-Antoine

Dr Chouard has studied 48 long-term multichannel implant users from 1973 to the present (Chouard, 1980; Chouard et al., 1983). Early patients in this series

112 *Implant Design and Construction*

Figure 4.18: Intracochlear Electrode Developed at the Technical University of Vienna.

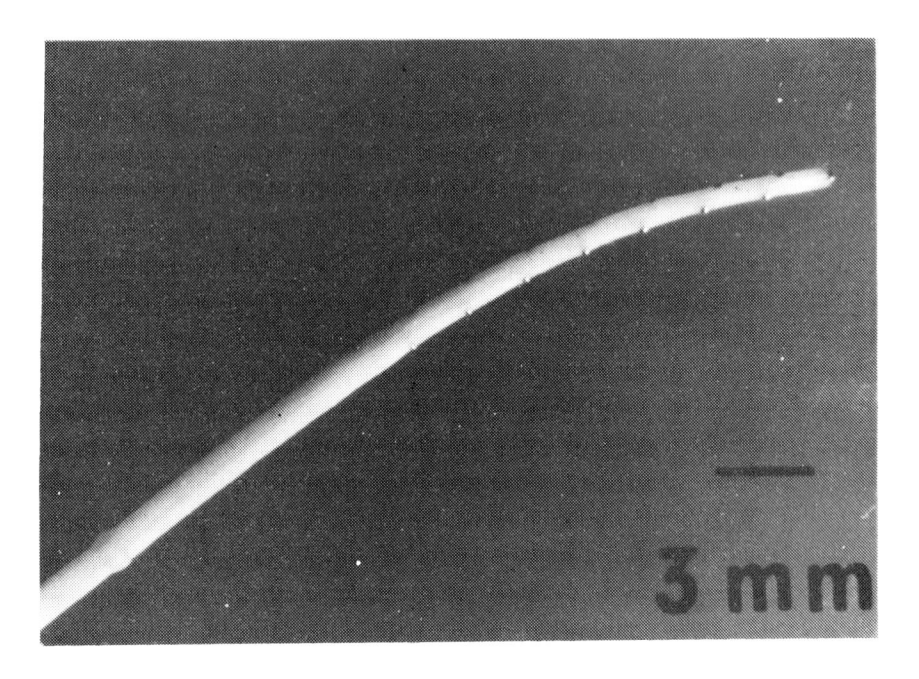

Source: Courtesy Dr E. Hochmair and Dr I. Hochmair-Desoyer, Technical University of Vienna.

were implanted by placing 12 fine wires in the scala tympani via small fenestrations drilled into the cochlear from the middle ear space. Each electrode consisted of a Teflon-coated platinum iridium (90:10) lead (0.005 in. in diameter) with the insulation bared at the tip to expose a contact surface area of 0.2–0.5 mm(2). In order discretely to stimulate specific positions along the cochlea, Dr Chouard creates a partition between each stimulating electrode by placing small wedges of Silastic above and below each contact. Seven of these compartments are placed in the basal turn and five in the middle turn of the cochlea. The first patients in the series received percutaneous cables; these were replaced by a multiplexed receiver which generates non-simultaneous monopolar stimulation by activating one electrode while the remaining eleven are tied to ground.

In later patients an improved electrode system has been implanted with a Silastic carrier inserted through the round window. In an attempt to create isolated stimulation sites as in the previous technique, the newer electrode features deeply recessed contacts. This recess also prevents immediate contact between the stimulating surface and intrascalar structures, a point which Dr Chouard feels is essential in electrode design.

University of Melbourne/Nucleus Ltd, Australia

As early as 1977, Dr Clark (Clark *et al.*, 1977; see also Chapter 11) reported the development of advanced multichannel scala tympani electrodes both in wireform and thin film versions and a complex ten-channel receiver based on CMOS integrated circuitry. The receiver contained three levels of stacked hybrid circuits and was driven by separate power and data coils above the encapsulated electronics. A gold-coated Kovar box was used to hermetically seal the electronics. Feedthroughs from the receiver extended to an attached connector which consisted of moulded conductive and non-conductive silicone rubber. The entire receiver package was finally coated with Silastic to minimise tissue reaction to the unit. Although the design has changed in many respects, the basic concepts of this generation are clearly present in the current system.

The Melbourne/Nucleus electrode consists of a Silastic (MDX 4-4210) carrier with 22 bands of platinum-iridium (90:10) (Clark *et al.*, 1983). The bands are formed from strips of Pt-Ir foil and a lead (also Pt-Ir) is welded to the band. As the 22 bands are assembled in the tapered mould each lead is run back through the growing series of bands. After injection moulding with Silastic the electrode has 22 regularly spaced bands along a longitudinal axis of approximately 25 mm as shown in Figure 4.19. The Melbourne group feels the bands are an advantage to point source contacts because they offer very large surface areas, are relatively easy to fabricate and mould into the Silastic carrier and their performance is not affected by the axial rotation of the electrode after insertion. The bands may be driven in many configurations by the processor circuitry but are usually stimulated in a longitudinal bipolar fashion with one band versus an adjacent band. The leads are helically wound to allow free movement without breakage, a technique used in many pacemaker and nerve stimulator lead designs. The leads are connected to the receiver outputs through a Silastic elastomer pad which holds platinum foil strips in contact with each when the connector is closed. The connector (which is not fixed to the skull) is closed under pressure to exclude fluid and to prevent eventual condensation of water vapour as in the UCSF system.

The current Nucleus receiver is built around a single, custom CMOS chip which digitally selects the level of stimulation and to which pair of bands each signal will pass as directed by the speech processor worn externally. A full description is to be found in Chapter 10. To avoid current summation between electrode pairs only one pair of contacts is stimulated along the array at any given instant. Thus, a sound component characterised by the speech processor as a high pitch signal would be directed to a basal electrode pair whereas a low pitch tone would stimulate a more apical set of bands. The receiver is encapsulated in a titanium (Ti6Al4V) can with a ceramic floor containing the 22 output feedthroughs. The ceramic feedthrough plate is brazed to the titanium can with a copper/silver brazing compound. The Melbourne group feels that galvanic corrosion between the copper, silver and titanium will not be a problem under the seal of compressed Silastic. The receiver operates with a single data and power coil. To minimise the voltage levels at the coil, a single turn is used and the voltage of this input is later stepped up in the

114 *Implant Design and Construction*

Figure 4.19: Nucleus Ltd/Melbourne University Multichannel Implant System. The internal components of the Australian device. The receiver (upper left) is a hermetically sealed titanium capsule containing the electronic circuits to drive 22 electrodes in a non-simultaneous scheme. Twenty-two platinum feedthroughs can be seen on the lower surface of the receiver corresponding to a matching set of contacts terminating the electrode leads (lower sub-assembly). These mirror-image contacts are connected via a Silastic pad (upper, centre) with flexible platinum foil strips on both the upper and lower surface.

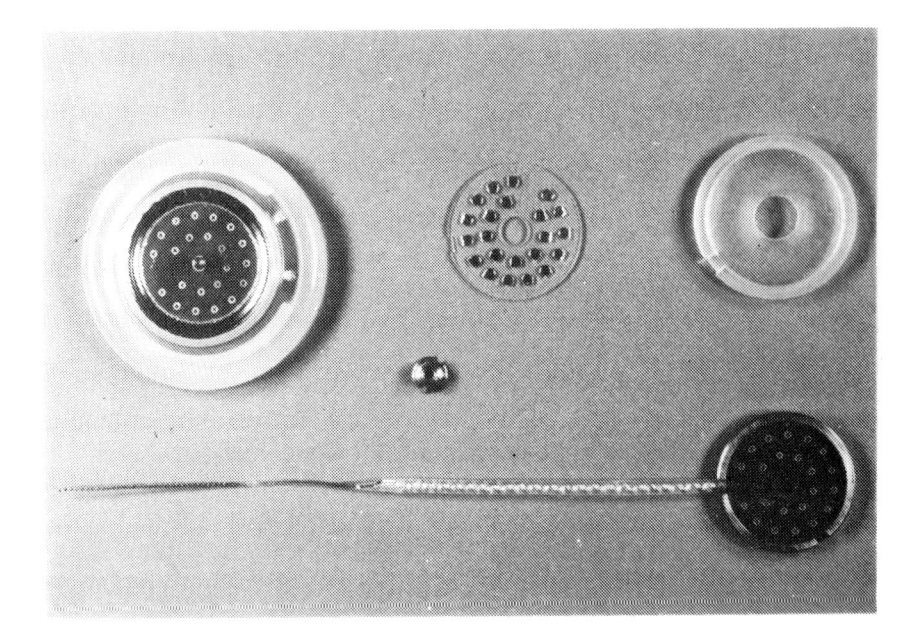

Source: Courtesy Nucleus Ltd, Australia.

receiver. The single antenna coil is moulded in Silastic and surrounds the upper edge of the receiver capsule.

The speech processor/transmitter is also innovative in both design and realisation. The unit is small in size and utilises both analogue and digital circuitry to provide up to 50 hours of battery life with three AA cells. The processor is programmable to allow custom fitting of the device for each patient depending on his or her individual thresholds, dynamic range and place/pitch rankings for the electrode.

Stanford University, Palo Alto, California

Cochlear implant research at Stanford University began in 1964 with the insertion

Figure 4.20: Eight-channel Digital Receiver in Development at Stanford University.

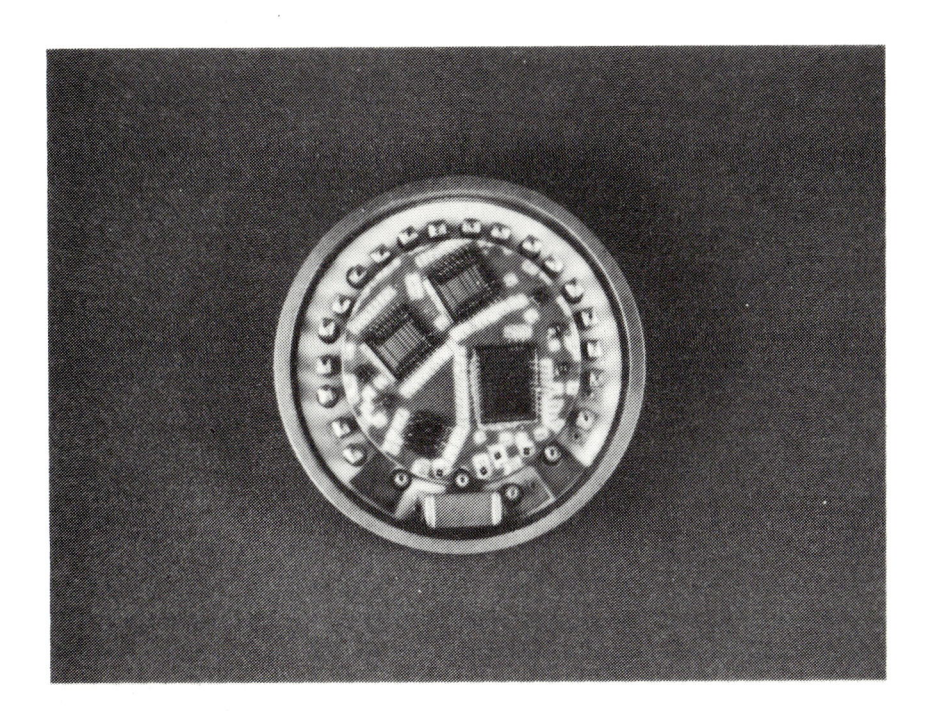

Source: Courtesy Applied Electronics Laboratory, Stanford University.

of a six wire modiolar electrode (Simmons, 1966). Since that time the Stanford group has developed both modiolar and scala tympani electrodes utilising advanced thin-film photolithographic techniques (White, 1982, 1983). They have also developed the electronics and packaging for prototype 8 and 12 channel integrated circuit receivers (Figure 4.20). Due to technical problems with the thin-film electrodes, the Stanford group has chosen to use Hochmair style eight-contact arrays with percutaneous connectors in their current set of patients.

The thin-film techniques developed at Stanford offer promising solutions to the problems of economical production of these complex electrode arrays and of achieving greater contact density. The electrodes are built up in layers by vacuum deposition (sputtering). Alternating layers of conductors and insulators, and photo-etching patterns into these layers allows in principle almost limitless control over the location, size and number of contacts for an electrode array. The modiolar electrode consists of a rigid sapphire support 125 μm thick. Tantalum conductor strips and electrode pads are formed by deposition and etching after which insulation layers of tantalum pentoxide, silicon nitride, silicon dioxide and Parylene are applied. Platinum is deposited over the tantalum contact pads to act as the stimulating contact surface. One of the possibilities for such an electrode is the ability to create a very large number of contacts within a small area. This is possible because photolithographic techniques allow masking and etching of layers to a resolution of 1 μm. Particularly in the case of the modiolar electrode, where the stimulating surfaces are in direct contact with the neural tissue, a dense packing of stimulation sites could conceivably activate a large number of discrete nerve groups. Because a large number of densely packed contacts would create tremendous difficulties in attaching leads and feedthroughs to a receiver future plans include directly building integrated circuits on the sapphire substrate to direct the signals to the electrode. With this technology one can conceive an electrode with hundreds of stimulation channels with only four leads (two for power and two for data). However, significant problems are anticipated in protecting active semiconductor circuits in the absence of conventional hermetic packaging.

The intracochlear thin-film electrode is constructed in the same manner (Figure 4.21). Because this electrode must be flexible the substrate chosen was polyimide. A 6,000 Å layer of platinum is vacuum deposited onto the polyimide and etched to produce the desired pattern of electrode contacts and leads. After this a second layer of polyimide is applied as an insulating layer and partially cured. At this stage openings can be etched through the upper layer to expose the electrode pad sites. Next the electrode is put through a final curing stage after which the polyimide becomes very inert and chemically resistant. It was found that the electrodes produced in this way tended to damage intracochlear structures due to their tall, thin shape. To counter this the group has moulded a Silastic backing on to the electrode.

Delamination of insulating layers and contact metals, as well as problems bonding leads, have plagued thin-film electrode production. Intermediate layers of active metals and new polymers appear to be improving the delamination problems. In the next generation of thin-film scala tympani electrodes the Stanford group plans to incorporate a Silastic-under-pressure connector system in collaboration with UCSF.

As mentioned earlier two patients were recently implanted at Stanford with Hochmair style eight contact electrodes. These electrodes were fabricated with 0.001 in. platinum-iridium wire and Silastic MDX4-4210 (Roberts, 1983). The leads are connected to a pyrolitic carbon percutaneous plug for the current studies.

University of Copenhagen, Denmark

The multichannel array developed at the University of Copenhagen (Lauridsen et al., 1983) incorporates several innovative design concepts. The electrode array has been made utilising thin-film production techniques with 24 contacts capable of providing either 12 channel bipolar or 24 channel monopolar stimulation. The most innovative aspect of the design, as shown in Figure 4.22, are the moveable electrode flaps which are held in a retracted position as the electrode is inserted and released with the removal of a piece of fine suture. Also unique is the overall configuration which consists of two intracochlear segments, one for the basal turn and a second one for the middle turn.

As mentioned earlier the electrode is produced using photolithographic thin-

Implant Design and Construction 117

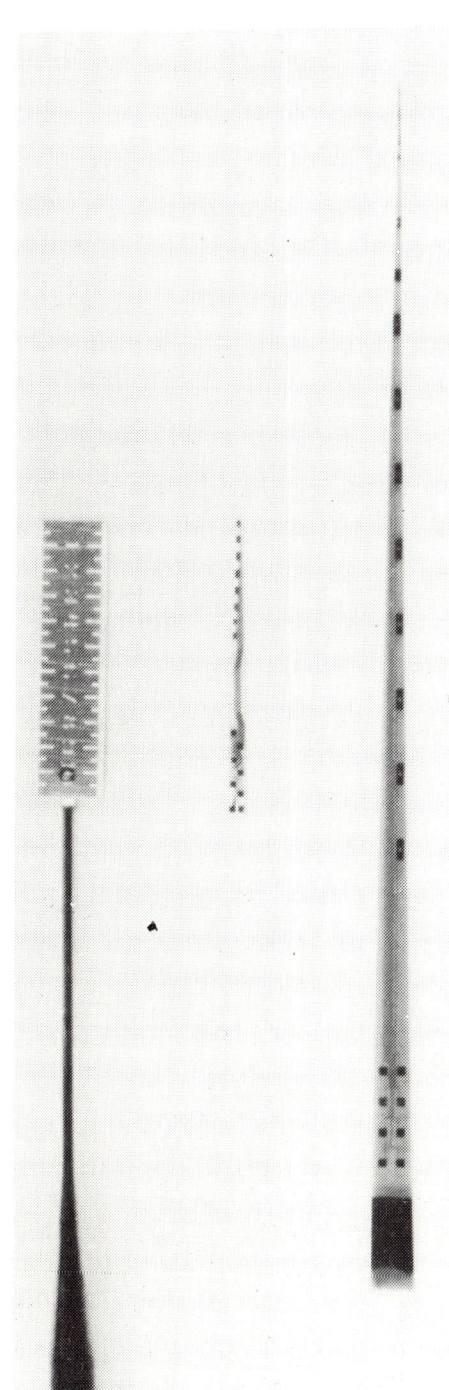

Figure 4.21: Two Thin-film Electrodes Developed at Stanford University Are Shown in This Photograph. The scale is 1 cm in length. The electrode on the right is a flexible scala tympani array fabricated by photolithographic techniques on a polyimide substrate. The left electrode is produced in essentially the same way on a rigid sapphire substrate for implantation in the modiolus.

Source: Applied Electronics Laboratory, Stanford University, Stanford, CA.

film techniques. The carrier consists of Kapton plastic 25 μm thick. A 0.1 μm layer of pure platinum is deposited on the surface of the Kapton substrate. The platinum contact patches and lead traces are defined photolithographically. Finally the intercontact spaces and leads are overcoated with a Kapton-like polymer for insulating leaving only the stimulating surfaces exposed. As with the Stanford thin-film electrodes the leads are run to a larger connector pad which could either be wire bonded to receiver electronics or incorporated in a Silastic pressurised connector. At this time the Denmark group has not reported on the development of any electronics to drive their electrode system.

During surgical insertion two openings are made into the scala tympani. The first fenestra allows access for the basal, curved segment of the electrode which carries 16 contacts while the second allows access to the middle cochlear turn for the smaller, eight contact elements of the electrode. The basal portion of the electrode is inserted until its tip can be seen through the second opening. At this time the suture holding the contacts is withdrawn allowing the flaps to unfold and contact the basilar membrane. Finally the apical segment of the array is inserted into the second turn of the cochlea. Although two openings must be made in the cochlea to perform this technique it permits the electrode to be placed in a region of tonotopically lower pitch than a round window approach. Only *in vivo* testing and psychophysics will reveal whether the benefits of this placement are offset by the increased trauma inherent in the procedure.

At the time of their last publication the Denmark group had not completed testing of the electrode to ascertain the extent to which the array is susceptible to delamination and dissolution. They stress that the present electrode is experimental in design and eventually hope to define a generation suitable for human implantation.

Extracochlear Devices

Two devices for single-channel excitation of the cochlea through active electrodes placed in the middle ear have been developed at the University College of London (Douek *et al.*, 1983; Fourcin *et al.*, 1979, 1983) and the Technical University of Vienna (Hochmair-Desoyer *et al.*, 1983). Preliminary patient results indicate that performance with these systems is equal to that of a single-channel intracochlear implant. This is particularly significant in patients who have some residual hearing in the ear to be implanted and it leaves the cochlea unaltered for possible implantation of a more sophsticated multichannel device in the future.

The two devices currently studied were developed with different applications in mind. The English system is a wholly external device which can be removed at will by the user. The prosthesis consists of an ear mould which supports a spring-loaded stainless-steel ball electrode contacting the promontory during use. The ear mould is given a conductive coating for use as the ground electrode. Signals from a speech processor are delivered to the device via two fine wire leads. Patients with open middle ear cavities have been suitable subjects for this technique. In patients with intact tympanic membranes the membrane has been stretched down to contact the promontory and attached at that point (tympanopexy). Although

Figure 4.22: Diagram of a 24-contact Thin-film Electrode Under Development at the University of Copenhagen. The array has two sections. An apical segment containing eight contacts is designed to be inserted in a window in the middle turn of the cochlea and a second segment with 16 contacts to be inserted through a window in the basal turn. The lower drawing shows how the contact flaps are held flat against the body of the basal segment of the array by a suture. After implantation in the scala tympani the suture is removed and the contact flaps are released to rest gently against the basilar membrane.

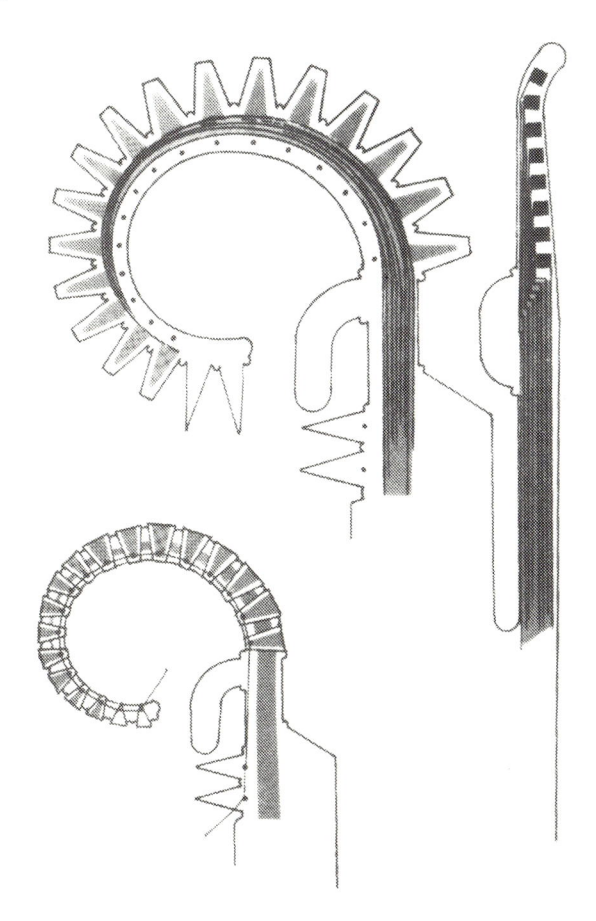

Source: Redrawn from Lauridsen et al., 1983.

extremely straightforward in application these devices suffer from difficulty achieving repeatable, positive contact between the electrode and its stimulating site. For this reason a permanently implanted device may be preferable for most patients.

The extracochlear prosthesis developed in Vienna consists of an implanted AM receiver and two Pt-Ir electrodes. The ball-shaped active electrode lead is wedged into the round window niche or attached to the promontory. To provide maximum contact area the ground electrode is three lobed and placed in adjacent temporalis muscle. The AM receiver demodulates the signal from a transmitter antenna coil behind the ear and assures charge symmetry between the electrodes. Epoxy and Silastic 382 are used to protect the antenna coil and receiver components.

Acknowledgements

The design of the UCSF cochlear implant system has evolved over nearly 20 years with contributions from many members of the project. Principal among these are Dr Michael Merzenich and Dr Gerald Loeb (NIH). Mr Chuck Byers, chief project engineer, and the author have been responsible for the actual designs and fabrication of the intracochlear electrode, surgical connector and hermetic packaging of the implanted electronics. Dr Robin Michelson and Dr Robert Schindler have provided insight to the practical application of these devices in humans. Animal studies conducted by Dr Patricia Leake, in collaboration with Dr Sheila Walsh, were essential in determining *in situ* biological performance of materials chosen for the implant and in evaluating and quantifying the extent of cochlear pathology which can be associated with the prosthesis.

Electronics for the system were developed by Dr David Wilkinson, Dr Gerald Loeb, Mr Lindsay Vurek, Mr Marshall Fong, and Mr Bernard Borenstein. Early circuit prototypes were constructed with the assistance of Mr Lloyd Ferreira (Biostim Inc). During the past six years several visiting surgeons, sponsored by the TWJ Foundation, have made significant contributions to the project. These include: Dr Brian O'Reilly, Dr Roger Gray, Dr Frank Wilson, Dr David Aird, Dr Gerard O'Donoghue and Dr Anthony Jefferis. I also want to thank Dr Robert Jackler for his work in evaluating methods by which cochlear implants could be safely applied in children.

The fabrication of these devices for human implantation is extremely difficult. Mr Peter Zimmerman, and earlier Mr David Casey, have continually generated new ideas and strategies for more efficient and better quality manufacture of the implant system. I want to thank Dr Jerry Loeb for his critique of this manuscript and Mr Joseph Molinari for his help in preparing the manuscript and coordinating the efforts of all of the above. The work was supported by NIH Contract no. NO1-NS-7-2367, NO1-NS-3-2353, NIH Grant no. NS-11804, the Saul and Ida Epstein Endowment Fund, the Coleman Fund, and Hearing Research Inc.

References

Black, J. (1981) *Biological Performance of Materials: Fundamentals of Biocompatibility*. Marcel Dekker, New York, 265 pp.

Blencke, B.A., Bromer, H. and Deutscher, K.K. (1978) Compatibility and long term stability of glass-ceramic implants. *J. Biomed. Mat. Res.*, *12*, 307–16

Boretos, J.W. (1981) The chemistry and biocompatibility of specific polyurethane systems for medical uses, in D.F. Williams (ed.), *Biocompatibility of Clinical Implant Materials*, Vol. II, CRC Press, Boca Raton, Florida, pp. 127–44

Bruck, S. (1973) Polymeric materials: current status of biocompatibility. *Biomat. Med. Dev. Art. Org., 1*, 79–98

Brummer, S.B. and Turner, M.J. (1977a) Electrochemical considerations for safe electrical stimulation of the nervous system with platinum electrodes. *IEEE Trans. Biomed. Eng., 24*, 59–63

―― and ―― (1977b) Electrical stimulation with platinum electrodes. I. A method for determination of 'real' electrode areas. *IEEE Trans. Biomed. Eng., 24*, 436–9

―― and ―― (1977c) Electrical stimulation with platinum electrodes. II. Estimation of maximum surface redox (theoretical non-glassing) limits. *IEEE Trans. Biomed. Eng., BME 24*, 440–3

―― and McHardy, J. (1977) Current problems in electrode development, in F.T. Hambrecht and J.B. Reswick (eds.), *Functional Electrical Stimulation*, Marcel Dekker, New York, pp. 499–514

Burian, K., Hochmair, E., Hochmair-Desoyer, I. and Leseer, M.R. (1980) Electrical stimulation with multichannel electrodes in deaf patients. *Audiology, 19*, 128–36

――, Hochmair-Desoyer, I.J. and Hochmair, E.S. (1981) Cochlear implants: further clinical results. *Acta Otol., 91*, 629–33

Charnley, J. (1970) *Acrylic Cement in Orthopedic Surgery*. E. and S. Livingstone, London, 127 pp.

Chawla, A.S. (1978) *In vitro* interactions between novel filler free silicone rubber and blood. *Biomat. Med. Dev. Art. Org., 6*, 89–102

Chouard, C.H. (1980) The surgical rehabilitation of total deafness with the multichannel cochlear implant. *Audiology, 19*, 137–45

――, Fugain, C., Meyer, B. and Lacombe, H. (1983) Long-term results of the multichannel cochlear implant, in *Cochlear Implants, Ann. NY Acad. Sci., 405*, 187–411

Clark, G.M., Black, R., Denhurst, D.J., Foster, I.C., Patrick, J.F. ad Tong, Y.C. (1977) A multiple-electrode hearing prosthesis for implantation in deaf patients. *Med. Prof. Tech., 5*, 127–40

――, Sheperd, R.K., Patrick, J.F., Black, R.C. and Tong, Y.C. (1983) Design and fabrication of the banded electrode array, in *Cochlear Prostheses, Ann. NY Acad. Sci., 405*, 191–201

Danley, M.J. and Fretz, R.J. (1982) Design and functioning of the single channel cochlear implant. *Ann. Otol. Rhinol. Laryngol., 91* (Suppl. 91), 21–6

deGroot, K. (1981) Degradable ceramics, in D.F. Williams (ed.), *Biocompatibility of Clinical Implant Materials, Vol. I*. CRC Press, Boca Raton, Florida, pp. 200–16

deWijn, J.R. and van Mullen, P.J. (1981) Biocompatibility of acrylic implants, in D.F. Williams (ed.), *Biocompatibility of Clinical Implant Materials, Vol. II*. CRC Press, Boca Raton, Florida, pp. 99–126

Dillier, N., Spillman, T., Fisch, V.P. and Leifer, L.J. (1980) Encoding and decoding of auditory signals in relation to human speech and its application to human cochlear implants. *Audiology, 19*, 146–63

Dillingham, E., Webb, N., Lawrence, W.H. and Autian, J. (1975) Biological evaluation of polymers. I. Poly(methylmethacrylate). *J. Biomed. Mat. Res., 9*, 569–96

Douek, E., Fourcin, A.J., Moore, B.C.J., Rosen, S., Walliker, J.R., Frampton, S.L., Howard, D.M. and Abberton, E. (1983) Clinical aspects of extracochlear electrical stimulation, in *Cochlear Implants, Ann. NY Acad. Sci., 405*, 332–6

Eddington, D.K. (1983) Speech recognition in deaf subjects with multichannel intracochlear electrodes, in *Cochlear Prostheses, Ann. NY Acad. Sci., 405*, 241–58

――, Dobelle, W.H., Brackmann, D.E., Mladejovsky, M.G. and Parkin, J.L. (1978) Auditory prosthesis research with multiple channel intracochlear stimulation in man. *Ann. Otol. Rhinol. Laryngol., 87* (Suppl. 53), 5–39

Eskin, S.G., Trevino, L. and Chimoskey, J.E. (1978) Endothelial cell culture on Dacron fabrics of different configurations. *J. Biomed. Mat. Res., 12*, 517–24

Evans, E.M., Freeman, M.A.R. and Vernon-Roberts, B. (1974) Metal sensitivities as a cause of bone necrosis and loosening of the prosthesis in total joint replacement. *J. Bone. J. Surg., 56B*, 626–42

Fourcin, A.J., Douek, E.E., Moore, B.C.J., Rosen, S., Walliker, J.R., Howard, D.M., Abberton, E. and Frampton, S. (1983) Speech perception with promontory stimulation, in *Cochlear Prostheses, Ann. NY Acad. Sci., 405*, 280–94

――, Rosen, S.M., Moore, B.C.J., Douek, E.E., Clarke, G.P., Dodson, H. and Bannister, L.H. (1979) External electrical stimulation of the cochlea: clinical, psychophysical, speech-perceptual and histological findings. *Br. J. Audio., 13*, 85–107

Griss, P. and Heimke, G. (1981) Biocompatibility of high density alumina and its application in orthopedic surgery, in D.F. Williams (ed.), *Biocompatibility of Clinical Implant Materials, Vol. I*.

CRC Press, Boca Raton, Florida, pp. 156–95

Guidoin, R., Gosselin, G., Domurado, D., Marios, M., Levaillant, P., Awad, J., Rouleau, C. and Levasseur, L. (1977) Dacron as an arterial prosthetic material: nature, properties, brands, facts and perspectives. *Biomat. Med. Dev. Art. Org.*, 5, 177–203

Hahn, A.W., Yasuda, H.K. and James, W.J. (1983) Glow discharge study; materials development and evaluation. Quarterly Progress Reports. National Institutes of Health Contract no. NO1-NS-1-2382

Harms, J. and Mausle, E. (1979) Tissue reaction to ceramic implant material. *J. Biomed. Mat. Res.*, 13, 67–87

Hastings, G.W. (1981) Biocompatibility of polyethylene and polypropylene, in D.F. Williams (ed.), *Biocompatibility of Clinical Implant Materials, Vol. II*. CRC Press, Boca Raton, Florida, pp. 44–55

Haubold, A.D., Shim, H.S. and Bokros, J.C. (1981) Carbon in medical devices, in D.F. Williams (ed.), *Biocompatibility of Clinical Implant Materials, Vol. II*. CRC Press, Boca Raton, Florida, pp. 4–38

Heimke, G., Griss, P., Jentschura, G. and Werner, E. (1978) Direct anchorage of Al2O3 ceramic hip components: three years of clinical experience and results and future animal studies. *J. Biomed. Mat. Res.*, 12, 57–65

Hochmair, E.S., Hochmair-Desoyer, I.J. and Burian, K. (1979) Investigations towards an artificial ear. *Int. J. Art. Org.*, 2, 255–61

Hochmair-Desoyer, I.J. and Hochmair, E.S. (1980) An eight channel scala tympani electrode for auditory prosthesis. *IEEE Biomed. Eng.*, BME 27, 44–50

——, Hochmair, E.S., Burian, K. and Stiglbrunner, H.K. (1983) Percepts from the Vienna cochlear prosthesis, in *Cochlear Prostheses, Ann. NY Acad. Sci.*, 405, 295–306

Homsy, C.A. (1981) Biocompatibility of perfluorinated polymers and composites of these polymers, in D.F. Williams (ed.), *Biocompatibility of Clinical Implant Materials, Vol. II*, CRC Press, Boca Raton, Florida, pp. 59–79

House, W.E. (1982) Cochlear implants: progress and perspectives. *Ann. Otol. Rhinol. Laryngol.*, 91 (Suppl. 91), 1–124

House, W.F., Burliner, K.I., Eisenberg, L.S., Edgerton, B.J. and Thielemeir, M.A. (1981) The cochlear implant: 1980 update. *Acta Otol.*, 91, 457–62

—— and Edgerton, B.J. (1982) A multiple electrode cochlear implant. *Ann. Otol. Rhinol. Laryngol.*, 91 (Suppl. 91), 104–15

Johnsson, L., House, W.F. and Linthicum, F.H. (1982) Otopathologic findings in a patient with bilateral cochlear implants. *Ann. Otol. Rhinol. Laryngol.*, 91 (Suppl. 91), 74–89

King, M., Blais, P., Guidoin, R., Prowse, E., Marcois, M., Gosselin, G. and Noel, H. (1981) Polyethylene terephthalate (Dacron) vascular prostheses — material and fabric construction aspects, in D.F. Williams (ed.), *Biocompatibility of Clinical Implant Materials*, Vol. II, CRC Press, Boca Raton, Florida, pp. 178–25

Krainess, F.E. and Krapp, W.W. (1978) Strength of a dense alumina ceramic after aging *in vitro*. *J. Biomed. Mat. Res.*, 12, 241–6

Lauridsen, O., Gunthersen, C., Bonding, P. and Tos, M. (1983) Experiments with a thinfilm multichannel electrode for cochlear implantation. *Acta Otol.*, 95, 219–26

Leake-Jones, P.A. and Rebscher, S.J. (1983) Cochlear pathology with chronically implanted scala tympani electrodes, in *Cochlear Prostheses, Ann. NY Acad. Sci.*, 405, 203–23

Loeb, G., Bak, M.J., Salcman, M. and Schmidt, E.M. (1977) Parylene as a chronically stable, reproducible microelectrode insulator. *IEEE Trans. Biomed. Eng.* BME 24, 121–8

——, Byers, C.L., Rebscher, S.J., Casey, D., Fong, M. and Merzenich, M.M. (1983) Design and construction of an experimental cochlear prosthesis. *Med. Biol. Eng. Comput.*, 21, 241–54

McHardy, J., Robblee, L.S., Martin, J.M. and Brummer, S.B. (1980) Electrical stimulation with platinum electrodes. IV. Factors influencing platinum dissolution in organic saline. *Biomaterials*, 1, 129–34

Merritt, K., Shafer, J. and Brown, S. (1979) Implant site infection rates with porous and dense materials. *J. Biomed. Mat. Res.*, 13, 101–8

Merzenich, M.M., Rebscher, S.J., Loeb, G.E., Byers, C.L. and Schindler, P.A. (1984) The U.C.S.F. cochlear implant project: state of development. *Adv. Audiol.*, 2, 119–44

Michelson, R.P. and Schindler, R.A. (1981) Multichannel cochlear implant, preliminary results in man. *Laryngoscope*, XCI, 38–42

Myojin, K. and von Recum, A.F. (1978) Experimental infections along subcutaneous conduits. *J. Biomed. Mat. Res.*, 12, 557–70

O'Reilly, B.F. (1981) Trauma and reliability of placement of a 20 mm long model human scala tympani electrode array. *Ann. Otol. Rhinol. Laryngol.*, *90* (Suppl. 82), 11–12

Osterholm, H.H. and Day, D.E. (1981) Dense alumina aged *in vivo*. *J. Biomed. Mat. Res.*, *15*, 279–88

Robblee, L.S., McHardy, J., Marston, J.M. and Brummer, S.B. (1980) Electrical stimulation with platinum electrodes. V. The effect of protein on platinum dissolution. *Biomaterials*, *1*, 135–9

Roberts, L.A. (1983) Development of multichannel electrodes for an auditory prosthesis. Quarterly Progress Reports. National Institutes of Health Contract no. N01-NS-0-2336

Sawyer, P.N., Stanczewski, B., Hoskin, G.P., Sophie, Z., Stillman, P.M., Turner, R.J. and Hoffman, H.L. (1979) *In vitro* and *in vivo* evaluations of Dacron velour and knit prostheses. *J. Biomed. Mat. Res.*, *13*, 937–56

Schindler, R.,A., Gray, R.F., Rebscher, S.J. and Byers, C.L. (1981) Multichannel cochlear implants: electrode design and surgical considerations. *Art. Org.*, *5* (Suppl.), 258–60

Simmons, F.B. (1966) Electrical stimulation of the auditory nerve in man. *Arch. Otol.*, *84*, 24–76

Sutow, E.J. and Pollack, S.R. (1981) The biocompatibility of certain stainless steels, in D.F. Williams (ed.), *Biocompatibility of Clinical Implant Materials, Vol. I*, CRC Press, Boca Raton, Florida, pp. 46–90

Thompson, N.F., Buchanan, R.A. and Lemons, J.E. (1979) *In vitro* corrosion of Ti-6Al-4V and Type 316 stainless steel when galvanically coupled with carbon. *J. Biomed. Mat. Res.*, *13*, 35–44

van Noort, R. and Black, M.M. (1981) Silicone rubbers for medical applications in D.F. Williams (ed.), *Biocompatibility of Clinical Implant Materials, Vol. II*, CRC Press, Boca Raton, Florida, pp. 79–98

White, R.L. (1982) Review of current status of cochlear prostheses. *IEEE Trans. Biomed. Eng.*, *BME 29*, 233–8

—— (1983) Thin film electrode fabrication techniques, in *Cochlear Prostheses. Ann. NY Acad. Sci.*, *405*, 183–90

Williams, D.F. (1981a) *Biocompatibility of Clinical Implant Materials*, Vols I and II, CRC Press, Boca Raton, Florida, 262–72

—— (1981b) Titanium and titanium alloys, in D.F. Williams (ed.), *Biocompatibility of Clinical Implant Materials, Vol. I*, CRC Press, Boca Raton, Florida, pp. 9–44

—— (1981c) The properties and clinical uses of Co-Cr alloys in D.F. Williams (ed.), *Biocompatibility of Clinical Implant Materials, Vol. I*. CRC Press, Boca Raton, Florida, pp. 100–23

5 SELECTION OF PATIENTS

J. Graham Fraser

Any centre starting a cochlear implant programme must take a decision early on as to the main group of patients that it intends to treat. The implantation of patients with congenital deafness is controversial. Centres which now regard cochlear implantation as a routine therapeutic procedure, such as the House Ear Institute and Otological Group in Los Angeles, feel that it is unreasonable to withhold implants from the congenitally deaf. On the other hand those who still regard cochlear implantation as experimental feel that the value of the procedure must be proven first with those who have acquired deafness so that we have a clear understanding of what the patient can gain from the procedure. These patients are able to describe clearly the sensation they are receiving by referring back to their memory of sound before they were deafened.

Once the decision has been taken as to which group of patients is to be implanted, an efficient and logical protocol is needed to select those patients who are suitable. Any centre offering implants will be approached by a large number of potential patients and there is a danger of being overwhelmed by unsuitable cases. The selection process therefore is really a question of excluding those who are unsuitable for implantation. Various stages in this process can be recognised.

Stages in Patient Selection

(1) Postal questionnaire
(2) Initial medical assessment
   (a) Aetiology
      (i) Acquired Deafness
      (ii) Congenital Deafness
   (b) Age
   (c) General health
   (d) Personality
   (e) Availability
   (f) Language
   (g) Otological examination
(3) Special audiometric investigations
   (a) Pure tone audiometry
   (b) Electrical response audiometry
   (c) Tests of auditory discrimination
(4) Radiological examination of the cochlea
(5) Hearing aid trial
(6) Electrical stimulation of the cochlea

(7) Tinnitus evaluation
(8) Vestibular testing
(9) Psychological assessment
(10) Informed consent to operation
    (a) Explanatory literature
    (b) Meeting with implanted patient
    (c) Counselling
(11) Voice production

Postal Questionnaire

Many initial enquiries come by post, but the letters seldom contain the information needed. It is most useful, therefore, to send out a questionnaire to see whether it is worth bringing the patient to the clinic. The questionnaire used by University College Hospital/Royal National Institute for the Deaf (UCH/RNID) in London is given as an example:

Postal Questionnaire for Potential Cochlear Implant Patients.

> Do you have any hearing in either ear?
> If yes, which ear?
> Name or type of hearing aid used?
> What can you hear with the hearing aid?
> Can you hear speech?
> Can you hear loud noises? doors banging etc?
> At what age did you lose your hearing?
> What was the cause of hearing loss? (if known)
>
> Can other people easily understand when you speak?
> (a) Everything you say
> (b) Some words only
> (c) Very little
>
> How much can you understand by lip-reading?
> (a) A member of your family 100% 75% 50% 25%
> (b) A stranger 100% 75% 50% 25%
> (please tick)
>
> Have your ears ever discharged or run?
> If yes, which ear?
>
> Have you a perforation of the eardrum?
> If yes, which ear?

126   Selection of Patients

Have you ever had surgery performed on the ears?
If so, what operation?
(a) Mastoid operation   What age?
(b) Middle ear surgery
(c) Other

Have you any medical complaints?

Are you on any treatment from your doctor or specialist?
Please give names of drugs

Do you suffer from severe anxiety or depression?

Could you spend some time living near the hospital?

When the questionnaire is mailed, information about the nature of cochlear implants should be sent as well since most patients have a very poor understanding of what to expect. Many imagine that hearing can be restored to normal by a cochlear implant and it is vital at every stage to emphasise that this is not the case, so that their expectations are realistic.

Replies to the questionnaire will enable patients who are hearing aid users and those who have middle ear infections to be excluded, neither condition being suitable for implantation. If the answers to the questionnaire indicate that further investigation is justified, the patient is brought to the clinic for an initial medical assessment.

Initial Medical Assessment

Aetiology of Deafness

Acquired Deafness. Most centres will be looking for patients in this group. The work of Otte, Schuknecht and Kerr (1978) shows that certain causes of acquired deafness are more likely to leave a useful neuronal survival pattern than others. Initially they counted the ganglion cells of 100 post mortem ears, the hearing of which had been tested two days to eight years before death; 65 had predominantly sensorineural hearing loss and eight had normal hearing. The ganglion cell populations were determined for each of four segments and for the cochlea as a whole.

Tone threshold (average 500, 1,000 and 2,000 Hz) showed that ears with normal or near normal thresholds had at least 20,000 cells. Threshold losses of up to 50 to 60 dB generally had at least 10,000 cells. The correlation of spiral ganglion cell populations with speech discrimination scores showed that some speech discrimination is possible with total counts as low as 10,000 cells.

In the second part of the study Otte *et al.* examined 62 deaf ears from 43 subjects who had been profoundly deaf. In acquired lesions the loss of ganglion cells was found to parallel the extent of the injury to the supporting cells (Deiter's cells and pillar cells) rather than the hair cells. Addressing the problem of which ears might have been theoretically suitable for implantation with some hope of speech recognition, they looked to see which ears had a total of at least 10,000 spiral ganglion cells with at least 3,000 in the apical 10 mm of the organ of Corti.

Viral Labyrinthitis and Sudden Deafness. Overall nine of 17 had more than 10,000 cells. The eight cases of measles had poor cell survival on the whole whereas the single case of mumps deafness had an excellent population of cells. Cell survival in the cases of sudden deafness was very variable.

Bacterial Labyrinthitis may be secondary to middle ear infection or meningitis. Of 17 ears 12 had poor ganglion survival throughout and of the remaining five, with more than 10,000 surviving cells, all had poor counts in the basal turn.

Congenital Syphilis. Of the four ears deafened by congenital syphilis, two had poor ganglion survival throughout and one had surviving cells in the middle and apical turns only. Only one case had more than 10,000 surviving ganglion cells.

Otosclerosis. Of the three individuals with profound deafness from otosclerosis, two had good neuronal survival and one had poor survival. Of the four involved ears, two had more than 10,000 surviving cells.

Ototoxic Drugs. The one case of bilateral deafness from Kanamycin therapy had excellent ganglion survival.

Traumatic. The two individuals with fractures of the petrous bone showed ganglion survival commensurate with the degree of injury.

Meniere's Disease. Three of the four ears had more than 10,000 surviving cells and in two there were surviving ganglia in the basal turn.

Vascular. There were two ears from an individual who suffered sudden hearing loss believed to be of vascular origin and both showed poor ganglia survival.

Perilymph Fistula. No cases were available for examination.

It is evident from this work that some causes of profound deafness are more likely to leave a good population of surviving neurons than others. There is, however, great variability even within the groups. Furthermore the assumption that a ganglion population of at least 10,000 is necessary for speech recognition is derived from acoustic stimulation and it does not necessarily follow that the same will apply with electrical stimulation. Thus a clinical method of determining ganglion populations in patients is still badly needed.

Central causes of acquired deafness such as bilateral acoustic neuroma or fractures of the petrous bone are unsuitable for cochlear implantation.

Congenital Deafness. Otte *et al.* (1978) also counted the ganglion population in nine cases of cochlear dysplasias. Overall three of them had more than 10,000 spiral ganglion cells. Two out of three with Scheibe type (cochleosaccular) dysplasia had excellent ganglia in all three turns. Of the four ears with Mundini dysplasia (abnormalities of the bony and membranous labyrinths) the overall nerve survival was poor although two had more than a third of the ganglia surviving in the basal turn.

It has been found in Vienna (Hochmair-Desoyer, personal communication) and Los Angeles (Berliner, personal commuication) that teenagers with congenital deafness who have been persuaded by their parents to have implants do badly. Deaf teenagers have already adjusted to living in the deaf world and to communicate with their friends by signing. Many find the sensations from their implants mysterious and unpleasant and they do not have the patience to persist until the signals become meaningful. Congenitally deaf adults also have a very difficult period initially when they do not recognise the sensations as sounds. Sometimes they feel as if the feelings are arising in other parts of the body initially, such as the chest. If they are prepared to continue using the implant they come to associate the electrical signal as sounds in the head and they may ultimately derive benefit from it if they are motivated to persist with prolonged training.

The implantation of congenitally deaf children is an area of controversy. The team at the House Ear Institute is now concentrating entirely on the implantation of children and so far they have implanted about 60 between the ages of two years four months and eighteen. They have developed special intensive conditioning tests to ensure that the diagnosis of deafness is as certain as possible and they carry out brainstem evoked response audiometry preoperatively to reduce the chance of error to a minimum. No other group thinks it is appropriate to implant children because of the difficulty in being sure that there is no residual hearing, which would be destroyed by the insertion of an implant. The view of the team at the House Institute is that they now have enough experience through their work with adults to be confident that the implant they are offering is of proven clinical value. They have been able to compare its performance with that of hearing aids in the same individual. They feel that it is unreasonable to withhold this technique of proven value from children, since childhood is the time most benefit should be derived from an implant. Furthermore, there is always the possibility of using the child's second ear should hearing aid technology advance.

This ethical problem does not arise if an extracochlear electrode is used. In the next few years it should be possible to decide whether the results of using an extracochlear round window electrode are as good as a single-channel electrode inserted 6 mm into the cochlea.

Age

There need be no upper or lower limit to the age at implantation as long as the patient is generally fit. The ethical problems associated with implanting children have been discussed above. Since children are more liable to acquire middle ear infections, the chances of developing labyrinthitis or meningitis must be higher in children. Once again this problem should not arise with extracochlear electrodes.

General Health

The patient must be fit enough to withstand an operation under general anaesthesia but there are other conditions which would make implantation impractical because rehabilitation would be so complicated and time consuming as to be unrealistic. Such conditions would include degenerative neurological disease, cerebrovascular accident or associated blindness.

Personality

The physician who first sees the patient at the initial medical assessment must judge whether the patient is intelligent and motivated enough to cooperate fully with the operation and rehabilitation. More detailed psychological tests will be carried out on those who appear suitable.

Availability

The patient must be prepared to give up enough time to attend the postoperative sessions of instruction and rehabilitation, otherwise he is unlikely to become a successful implant user. A minimum requirement would be a week to carry out the selection procedure, two weeks to cover the hospitalisation and recovery from surgery and a further period of two weeks for special training once the implant has been switched on. This makes a total of five weeks initially which includes about one week in hospital. Because implants are still experimental, time is also needed for special follow-up testing in the hope of advancing knowledge. Most implantees feel that it takes about six months to derive the maximum benefit from the devices and so two further test sessions may be best arranged three months and nine months postoperatively.

Language

Good understanding of language is essential if a patient is to understand the nature of the operation and what is expected of him. It is also necessary in order to ensure that his expectations are realistic.

Otological Examination

A full otological examination must be done to exclude middle ear disease.

Special Audiometric Investigations

There is no area more controversial in cochlear implant surgery than the question of residual hearing. It must be assumed that if an intracochlear electrode is inserted it will destroy any remaining hearing. Even if the patient cannot use a hearing aid effectively at present, this is highly undesirable because hearing aids are advancing rapidly and signal processing aids may become available in the near future which could help the patient. If the patient has had an intracochlear electrode, this opportunity will be lost to them. For this reason most centres using an intracochlear electrode will insist on there being no residual hearing.

A different view is put forward by Berliner (1983). She comments that in any new medical or surgical treatment the nature of the selection process and the criteria for including patients changes from one of obtaining good experimental subjects to one of acceptable clinical practice. Since clinical trials of their single-channel intracochlear electrode have now been continuing for 18 years at the House Ear Institute, the selection process has evolved into a clinically efficient procedure. They now feel that they have sufficient experience of cochlear implants, with more than 300 patients implanted, to be able to assess accurately whether patients can do better with the implant than with their residual hearing and a hearing aid. They acknowledge that hearing aids may advance but their view is that many patients have not got time to wait for possible hearing aid development and in any case they have a second ear.

The position can best be summarised by saying that anyone starting a cochlear implant programme with an intracochlear electrode should concentrate initially on patients with no residual hearing. When they gain more experience and can compare the results they are achieving with a cochlear implant with the patients' success with a hearing aid, then they may be able to justify operating on patients with minimal residual hearing. Fortunately, with an extracochlear electrode, this dilemma does not arise. The Austrian group have found that in using a round window electrode the residual hearing is undamaged. This also has the great advantage that hearing aid performance can be compared with electrical stimulation of the cochlea in the same ear in the same patient. If it is found that patients with round window electrodes do just as well as those with a single-channel electrode inserted a short distance into the cochlea, then there will be no justification for implanting a single-channel intracochlear electrode where there is residual hearing. The insertion of a multichannel intracochlear electrode might still be justified if it can be shown to lead to better speech discrimination.

Pure Tone Audiometry

Martin (in preparation) addresses the problem of defining the term 'total deafness'. The term is being used around the world to describe people whose hearing loss varies considerably. It is very important to produce an agreed definition now that electrical stimulation of the cochlea is being widely used. Many patients are labelled as having total deafness merely because they have not responded to the maximum output of the available audiometer. The audiometer and headphones used for potential implantees should have a maximum output of 130 dB HL. The Telephonics TDH 39 headphones are capable of delivering this sound pressure level but many audiometers currently in use are not designed to give more than 110 dB HL.

When putting in such a powerful stimulus it is essential to differentiate between hearing and tactile sensation. Martin suggests that, to be sure of an acoustic response, at least one of the following criteria should be satisifed:

(1) The patient should exhibit marked tone decay.

Selection of Patients

(2) There should be an unambiguous loudness discomfort level.
(3) The hearing threshold should be better in one ear than the other.
(4) The patient should indicate positively that the sensation is hearing rather than tactile.

It was hoped that reaction times would also show a difference between tactile and auditory stimulation but this has not proved to be a useful test for this purpose.

Using such techniques Martin (1983) recognised two groups of patients in those referred to the UCH/RNID group as potential cochlear implant candidates. Only those patients who have no sensation of hearing at 130 dB HL or who show only one or two points at the maximum output of an audiometer capable of giving that output can be considered totally deaf. A second group who show some response over a range of frequencies do have potentially usable hearing and are therefore not candidates for intracochlear electrodes. Against this view must be set the views of Owens et al. (1981). This San Francisco group emphasise that the mere awareness of sound is not important if there is no discrimination ability. They emphasise that the ability to distinguish a voice from noise is of unique importance as it appears to play a role in whether or not a hearing aid will prove useful. When a voice is heard as merely another noise patients tend to find hearing aids unsatisfactory.

Electrical Response Audiometry

All candidates for cochlear implantation should have electrical response audiometry (ERA) to exclude a functional deafness. One patient presenting to us for implantation satisfied all the other criteria but was found to have normal thresholds on electrocochleography and normal cortical responses. She was a teacher of lip-reading!

When children are evaluated for possible implantation, ERA is quite mandatory since subjective testing may be impossible. A negative test does not exclude some low frequency hearing and so further special tests will be needed for children (see below).

Tests of Auditory Discrimination

The Minimum Auditory Capabilities (MAC) battery of tests was designed in the University of California in San Francisco in the department of otolaryngology (Owens et al., 1981, 1982; Owens and Telleen, 1981). The object was to design a battery of tests which would lend consistency to the evaluation of implant patients at different centres. Full details of the test and tapes are available commercially.

The MAC battery consists of 13 auditory tests and one lip-reading test. Twelve consist primarily of spoken materials and the tests are of graduated difficulty. In the first group of tests the simplest is designed to see whether the patient can differentiate a rising pitch from a falling pitch. Another test asks which word in a sentence is accented. The most important part of this first group of tests shows whether a patient can distinguish between a voice and speech-modulated noise. The tests take the form of multiple choice responses where the patient is given a list of the possible answers and has to choose the correct one (closed list).

A second group of tests requires identification of phonemes and also takes the form of multiple choice responses. The consonant items are designed to test whether nasality, voicing and glide features of speech may be detected. The spondee recognition test is a relatively easy speech recognition test because the patient only has to make a selection from a closed list of four choices.

The remaining tests in the battery are open response (open list) tests in which the patient is required to describe the sound, word or sentence he has been given. Fifteen environmental sounds are delivered for identification such as a car horn or a dog barking. A spondee recognition tests uses 25 two-syllable words for the patient to identify. An everyday sentence test employs sentences from a series developed at the Central Institute for the Deaf at St Louis, Missouri, USA. The two most difficult tests in the battery involve repetition of single words and identification of words in context.

The final test involves a single speaker presenting the subject with sentences while sitting one metre in front of the patient. Scores are compared with the amplification device turned on and off. This test is designed to test how much the device aids lip-reading.

The total time of the recorded material of the MAC battery is 67 minutes and the test takes about two hours with a good subject. It may take much longer if a lot of explanation is needed. One of the problems of using this test in practice is that even though one is looking for minimum auditory capabilities most patients do not have even this and so one is asking them to continue for at least two hours without the encouragement of getting answers right. Edgerton et al. (1983) describe their experience administering the MAC battery to nine post-lingually deafened adults using cochlear implants. The subjects did very poorly on the open response tests. The tests which were within the subjects' capabilities were: question/statement, vowel, noise/voice, accent, initial consonant, spondee same/different, everyday sounds, four choice spondee, final consonant and visual enhancement (lip-reading).

Despite these problems there is no doubt that if the MAC battery were used in all centres carrying out cochlear implants it would be much easier to compare results between different centres.

In the same paper (Edgerton et al., 1983) the authors summarise the assessment strategy used at the House Ear Institute. The protocol used for auditory assessment at the House Ear Institute has grown simpler with experience. During the early stages of evaluation the only tests of discrimination they recommend are the Environmental Sounds test and the MTS test (monosyllable, trochee and spondee). The more elaborate protocol that they used previously was much more time consuming and they did not find this justified in helping to make the decision between a hearing aid and an implant.

More basic tests are being devised at the Royal National Institute for the Deaf in London to assess the ability to discriminate the sort of acoustic information that is needed for speech discrimination. The tests being tried include the ability to detect changes of pitch, gap detection in an acoustic signal, change of amplitude in the middle of a signal and periodicity to see whether a patient is able to distinguish between a crackle and a hum. Synthetic speech is used to test perception of formant spacing. When these tests have been fully developed it should be possible to automate and standardise them.

Only the House Ear Institute has as yet faced the special problems of selecting young children for implantation. Edgerton *et al.* detail the techniques they use. Negative respones to ERA do not exclude usable low frequency hearing so it was essential to find tests that assessed discrimination of simple speech or speech components through a hearing aid. They found existing tests unhelpful and devised the Discrimination after Training Test (DAT). The DAT test is based on the MTS test but is broken down into much simpler discriminations using non-speech and speech discriminations. If the child cannot initially perform a task, training is initiated. If the child is progressing better with a hearing aid than would be expected with an implant then cochlear implantation would not be recommended.

Equally important is observation over time. They strongly believe that children be given an adequate trial with hearing aids. However if no progress is seen in awareness of sound or speech development then cochlear implantation would be considered.

Radiological Examination of the Cochlea

Good visualisation of the cochlea can be achieved either with polytomography or with high-definition computed tomography. If a multichannel electrode is to be used it is essential to know whether it will be possible to insert it into the cochlea. Many cases of acquired deafness have scar tissue or new bone growth in the cochlea which would make implantation impossible. Figure 5.1 shows the image of the cochlea that can be achieved with a Philips Tomoscan 310; the cochlea is shown to be clear and suitable for an intracochlear electrode. If the patient has suffered from meningitis it is a wise precaution to do a brain scan at the same time to exclude damage to the auditory cortex.

Hearing Aid Trial

Many of the patients presenting themselves as cochlear implant candidates have not seen an otologist or audiologist for many years because they had been told that 'nothing can be done'. They may have tried a hearing aid unsuccessfully in the past but they have not tried modern high-powered hearing aids. In the UCH/RNID study about half the patients who seemed suitable for implantation from the postal questionnaire had sufficient residual hearing to benefit from a hearing aid. Because their hearing is minimal the quality of sound perceived will be poor and they will need persuasion to try the hearing aid over a period of at least a month before they can be said to have failed the hearing aid trial. It must be remembered that most patients who receive a cochlear implant do not really

134 *Selection of Patients*

Figure 5.1: CT Scan of Cochlea Showing Patent Scala Tympani.

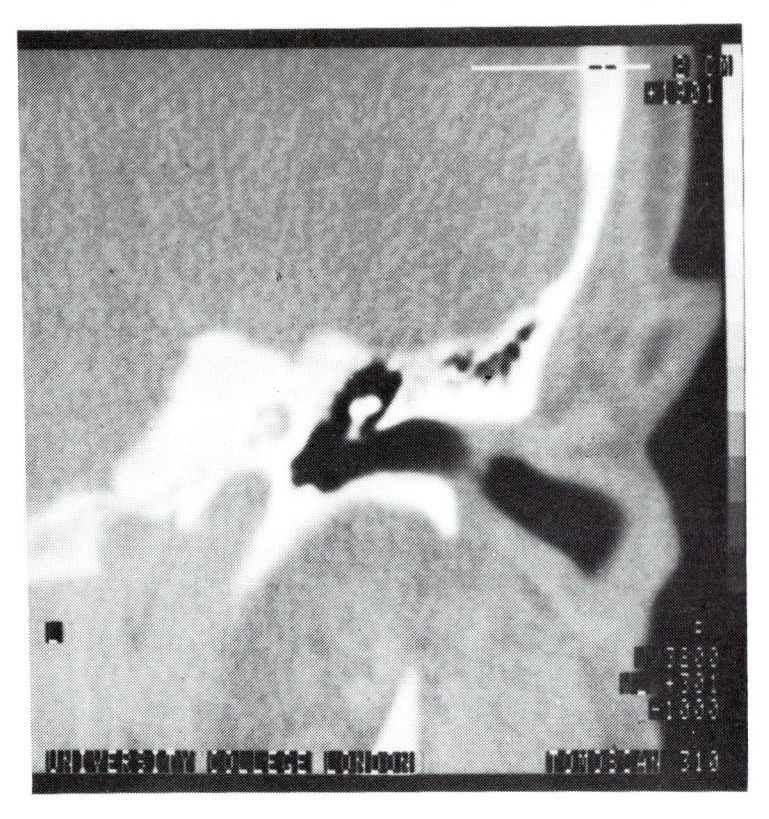

Source: Courtesy Dr D. Edwards, FRCR and Miss C. Munro.

appreciate its full advantages for about six months. On receiving an acoustic signal for the first time after many years of silence a learning period is needed in exactly the same way. It is essential to make sure that the best possible aid is fitted and then to give rehabilitative support and encouragement. A systematic protocol is needed for the hearing aid trial just as it is for the implant.

Electrical Stimulation of the Cochlea

Stimulating the cochlea electrically preoperatively has two advantages. First, if the patient has a sensation of sound, then there is clearly some neuronal survival. Secondly it gives the patient an idea of what type of sensation they can expect from the cochlear implant so avoiding unrealistic expectations. Although used initially in the House Ear Institute, it has now been given up as a test there because they found that some patients who had no perception of sound on promontory stimulation still did well with an implant.

Most other centres are using promontory stimulation, although they are using it in different ways. Only in Vienna is the decision to implant decided by the results of promontory stimulation. They use the transtympanic needle which is used for electrocochleography and have developed a simple test which they call the stimulus identification test. It has the advantage that it can be done in the congenitally and prelingually deaf as well as those with acquired deafness. Three different stimuli are presented to the patient; these are bursts which have different frequencies, namely 62.5, 125 and 255 Hz. The patient has to remember that these are stimuli 1, 2 and 3 and, after some training, the test consists of asking the patient to identify these stimuli. Some patients are unable to do this task. At the moment these patients are excluded from implantation.

The UCH/RNID group (Brightwell et al., 1983) is testing threshold and discomfort level by promontory stimulation and also the ability to appreciate pitch change. These tests are carried out using a stainless-steel needle electrode placed on the promontory of the middle ear for the purpose of transtympanic electrocochleography. The reference electrode is a silver chorlide disc on the ear lobe. The following parameters are then measured:

(1) The smallest current that produces a sensation of sound.
(2) The current that produces a sound level that the patient finds uncomfortable, or
(3) The current level that produces pain or discomfort from somatosensory stimulation.

It seems likely that the patients who have the widest dynamic range and the greatest ability to perceive pitch change will be the best candidates for implantation but as yet there are too few for evaluation.

At Stanford University (Simmons, 1983) a tympanomeatal flap is turned forward and an electrode is placed in the round window. Once again threshold and loudness discomfort levels are tested.

Electrically induced brainstem responses have also been recorded (Brightwell et al., 1983; Meyer, 1983; Simmons and Smith, 1983). If the technique for eliciting these responses becomes reliable it will be a crucial pre-implantation test in children since it will give objective evidence of neuronal survival. Similarly it is to be hoped that using different stimuli it might be possible to decide whether a patient was better suited to a single-channel or multichannel electrode.

A completely different approach is used by the Guy's Hospital Cambridge Group (Douek et al., 1983; Fourcin et al., 1983). Under a general anaesthetic a tympanomeatal flap is turned forward and an electrode is inserted into the round window. It is then kept in position for a few days. They have concluded that threshold tests are of limited value. Particularly helpful has been the ability of patients to distinguish between a periodic and aperiodic random sound (scratch versus buzz). They then proceed with speech tests using not only speech but speech pattern components. The temporary electrode is left in position for several days so that the patient hears a considerable amount of speech and so really does have

136 *Selection of Patients*

an understanding of what they are likely to hear if they have an implant. It does meant that the patient makes a decision on implantation, and is very well informed about what to expect. One of the problems that may be encountered with this approach is that many implant subjects at other centres do not like their implant for the first few weeks and frequently report that it takes about six months before they found they perceive sounds in any way natural.

Tinnitus Evaluation

It is evident from the recent survey carried out by the Institute of Hearing Research (MRC Inst. Hearing Research, 1981) and the British census (UK Govn. Stat. Survey, 1981) that between 0.5 per cent and 2 per cent of the population suffer from severely disabling tinnitus. It is thus a much commoner symptom than profound deafness and yet little attention has been given to it so far in cochlear implant programmes. It is reported that about 30 per cent of patients get relief of their tinnitus from the implant as used in the House Ear Institute (Edgerton, 1982). It may well be that in the long run more patients will receive cochlear implants for tinnitus than for profound hearing loss but it is vital to collect information on the subject now. Because it is a subjective symptom the only way of obtaining information about it is to administer a questionnaire. It is very important that this should be done pre- and postoperatively.

Where promontory stimulation is being done as part of the preoperative protocol the effect of stimulation on the tinnitus should be noted. Much work has been done by Aran and his colleagues in Bordeaux on tinnitus suppression using a promontory electrode and a ball electrode in the round window (Aran and Cazals, 1981). Their results of electrical stimulation for tinnitus suppression were not encouraging because they found that a train of positive pulses was a more effective suppressor of tinnitus than sinusoidal signals. Such suppression is probably due to a DC shift (Cazals, 1982) which causes cochlear damage in animals if used long term. Hazell *et al.* (1983), however, did show tinnitus suppression using low-frequency sinusoidal promontory stimulation. They achieved tinnitus suppression in seven out of twelve patients being assessed for cochlear implantation and in some there was a period of post-stimulus inhibition. They also tried short-term DC stimulation and found that it had no advantage over sinusoidal stimulation. The reason for these contradictory results could be that although silence may be obtained by DC stimulation, there may be a worthwhile masking effect from AC stimulation of the cochlea (Hazell, personal communication). The authors propose that, where the clinical facilities allow, a comprehensive pre- and post-implant assessment of tinnitus should be carried out. So far this has not been done.

Vestibular Testing

Thorough vestibular testing should be carried out before using an intracochlear electrode because it is important not to destroy the only functioning labyrinth. Routine caloric tests may be adequate to demonstrate labyrinthine function, although if there is no response, ice-cold water may be needed together with the abolition of optic fixation, using Frenzel's glasses or electronystagmography.

Psychological Assessment

It is important to have a thorough psychological assessment prior to implantation especially while cochlear implantation remains an experimental procedure. The psychological assessments should take the form of standardised tests and structured interviews. One of the difficulties with standardised tests is that many of them are geared to patients' verbal ability which is likely to be impaired in profound deafness. It is also more difficult to administer the tests to a deaf person and it is important in the assessment of a deaf person's intellectual functioning that the problems of test administration should not bias the final result. It is best therefore to use self-administered tests with written instructions.

In the UCH/RNID protocol the psychological testing procedure is as follows.

The Mill Hill vocabulary scale is used as a simple untimed test of verbal ability. Standard progressive matrices test non-verbal intelligence.

The Eysenck personality questionnaire is used as a personality test which gives three scores:

(1) Extraversion/intraversion.
(2) Neuroticism.
(3) Psychoticism.

The second test is the Spielberger State Trait Anxiety Inventory, which is a useful test of anxiety. Thirdly the Crown Crisp Experiential Inventory is a brief self-rating questionnaire devised to pick up psychiatric symptomatology. It provides scores on the following six scales:

(1) Obsessional
(2) Somatic
(3) Phobic
(4) Hysterical
(5) Depressive
(6) Free floating anxiety

This test battery has been selected by Dr Philip Richardson who also conducts a brief semi-structured interview which is designed to supplement the test data and focus on the following areas: educational/occupational background, social functioning and social adjustment, adjustment to deafness, knowledge about expectations of the implant, including attitudes to the rehabilitation programme.

The object of this rather elaborate psychological testing is firstly to make sure that unsuitable candidates are not subjected to surgery but also to assess whether they have some improvement in their psychological state as a result of the implant.

Informed Consent to Operation

Explanatory Literature

Because of problems in communicating with the deaf, it is absolutely essential that detailed literature is provided for the patient to explain the nature of the operation and what benefits can be expected from an implant.

Meeting with Implanted Patients

In centres with an on-going implant programme it is possible to introduce candidates for implantation to patients who have already had one. There is no doubt that this is very valuable in showing the potential implantee what it is really like to have an implant and wear the speech processor.

Counselling

Time must be found for a member of the rehabilitation team to sit down with the patient and explain in detail what the timetable for operation, recovery and rehabilitation will be. This interview can also be used for checking that the patient does really have a proper understanding of what can and cannot be achieved by a cochlear implant.

In the House Ear Institute in Los Angeles, they actually submit the patient to a small written test to see how much of the information he has absorbed. This is such a valuable contribution to patient understanding that I reproduce it below.

Cochlear Implant Questionnaire: Part 2. (as devised and used at the House Ear Institute)

The following are some questions about your expectations regarding the cochlear implant. Please circle the answer you feel will most likely be true if you have the cochlear implant surgery and use the cochlear implant unit.

1. I will hear people talking and be able to understand speech without watching the speaker's lips.

   yes   maybe   no

2. I will have normal hearing when I use the complete cochlear implant stimulator.

   yes   maybe   no

3. I will eventually be able to carry on a telephone conversation, as I did before I lost my hearing, with people I know well.

   yes   maybe   no

4. I will eventually learn to use the sounds I hear to help me recognise the number of syllables in a word.

   yes   maybe   no

5. The cochlear implant will make a big change in the life of a deaf person.
    yes   maybe   no
6. I will be able to hear many of the sounds around me, such as a phone ring, a dog bark, and so on.
    yes   maybe   no
7. I will be able to understand everything a person says when I lip read them.
    yes   maybe   no
8. I will be able to hear my voice and the voices of people around me.
    yes   maybe   no
9. Music will sound the same as I remember before I lost my hearing.
    yes   maybe   no
10. It will take time to learn to recognise all the sounds.
    yes   maybe   no

After the test has been done the counsellor can go through each question with the patient pointing out whether their answers were correct or incorrect and supplementing their knowledge where necessary with further instruction.

Voice Production

Surprisingly little information has been collected on the improvement in voice production which cochlear implantation provides. Voice recordings should be made before and after implantation. Such recordings can be analysed by a speech therapist to assess improvements in loudness modulation and intonation. Segmental features can also be studied.

At the end of this detailed assessment some patients will emerge as suitable candidates for cochlear implantation. When insertion of an implant becomes a routine clinical procedure the selection process may well be simplified. For the time being, while implantation is still at an experimental stage, it is most important that a proper protocol is devised and adhered to so that results can be compared between patients and between centres. It would clearly be advantageous if standardised tests were used and a first step has already been taken along this road with the MAC test. It is also important that the testing should become more efficient since it is very time consuming; many of the tests as they become established will lend themselves to automation.

References

Aran, J.M. and Cazals, Y. (1981) Electrical suppression of tinnitus. *CIBA Found. Symp.*, 85, 217–31
Berliner, K. (1983) Implant patient selection, pp; 395–403. In, Schindler, R.A. and Merzenich, M.M. (eds), *Cochlear Implants*, Raven Press, New York (1985), pp. 343–9.
Brightwell, A., Rothera, M.P., Conway, M. and Graham, J.M. (1983) Evaluation of the status of the auditory nerve psychophysical tests and ABR. In, Schindler, R.A. and Merzenich, M.M. (eds), *Cochlear Implants*, Raven Press, New York (1985), pp. 343–9

Cazals, Y. (1982) Round table discussion on electrical stimulation and tinnitus. *Symposium on Artificial Auditory Stimulation*, Erlangen, Sept. 29

Douek, E.E., Fourcin, A.J., Moore, B.C.J., Rosen, S., Walliker, J.R., Frampton, S.L., Howard, D.M. and Abberton, E. (1983) Clinical aspects of extra cochlear electrical stimulation. *Ann. NY Acad. Sci.*, *405*, 332-6

Edgerton, B.J. (1982) Round table discussion on electrical stimulation and tinnitus. *Symposium on Artificial Auditory Stimulation*, Erlangen, Sept. 29

Edgerton, B.J., Eisenberg, L.S. and Thielemeir, M.A. (1983) Auditory assessment strategy and materials for adult and child candidates for cochlear implantation. *Ann. NY Acad. Sci.*, *405*, 435-42

Fourcin, A.J., Douek, E.E., Moore, B.C.J., Rosen, S., Walliker, J.R., Howard, D.M., Abberton, E. and Frampton, S.L. (1983) Speech perception and promontory stimulation. *Ann. NY Acad. Sci.*, *405*, 280-4

Hazell, J.W.P., Graham, J.M. and Rothera, M.P. (1983) Electrical stimulation of the cochlea and tinnitus. *10th Anniversary Conference on Cochlear Implants*, San Francisco, June 22-4 (in press)

Martin, M.C. (1983) Alternatives to cochlear implants. In, Schindler, R.A. and Merzenich, M.M. (eds) *Cochlear Implants*, Raven Press, New York, 1985, pp. 549-61

—— (in preparation) Total deafness for acoustic stimulation

Meyer, B. (1983) Implant patient selection. In Schindler, R.A. and Merzenich, M.M. (eds) *Cochlear Implants*, Raven Press, New York, 1985, pp. 387-95

MRC Institute of Hearing Research, Nottingham, UK (1981) *Epidemiology of Tinnitus*, Ciba Foundation 85, Pitman Books, London, pp. 16-34

Otte, J., Schuknecht, H.E. and Kerr, A.G. (1978) Ganglion cell population in normal and pathological human cochleae — implications for cochlear implantation. *Laryngoscope, 38*, 1231-46

Owens, E. and Telleen, C. (1981) Speech perception with hearing aids and cochlear implants. *Arch. Otolaryngol.*, *107*, 160-3

Owens, E., Kessler, D.K., Telleen, C.C. and Schubert, E.D. (1981) The minimal auditory capabilities (MAC) battery. *Hearing Aid Journal*, Sept. 9, p. 34

——, ——, Kessler, D. and Schubert, E.D. (1982) Interim assessment of candidates for cochlear implants. *Arch. Otolaryngol.*, *108*, 478-83

Simmons, F.B. (1983) Implant patient selection. In Schindler, R.A. and Merzenich, M.M. (eds) *Cochlear Implants*, Raven Press, New York, 1985, pp. 383-7

—— and Smith, L. (1983) Estimating nerve survival by electrical ABR. *Ann. NY Acad. Sci.*, *405*, 422-3

UK Government Statistical Service (1983) *General Household Survery: The Prevalence of Tinnitus 1981*. OPCS Monitor GHS 83/1. Dept. M, Office of Population Censuses and Surveys, Kingsway, London WC2

6 SURGICAL IMPLANTATION

Robert A. Schindler and Roger F. Gray

The majority of electrodes are placed on or through the round window of the cochlea and two approaches are used.

(1) External Auditory Canal Groove
(For the type of electrode shown in Figure 6.1)
(2) Posterior Tympanotomy or Facial Recess Approach
(For the type shown in Figure 6.2)

Preoperative (Figure 6.3)

The patient is prepared as for any major ear operation except that the hair is shaved from the scalp a hand's breadth from the ear. A thermostatically controlled heating pad beneath the patient is required as the surgery may take four to seven hours. A supine position on the operating table with the head turned 40° away from the surgeon is best. A head up–foot tilt down of 30° aids venous hypotension; the head is individually levelled by adjusting that part of the table separately. Equipment to test the implanted device is made ready in a corner of the operating room. Brainstem-evoked responses may be measured to electrical stimulation if care is taken to exclude the stimulus artefact. If these can be elicited in the operating room, proof of function of the device *in situ* is certain but such tests are often unduly lengthy. A spare implant for use should the first be faulty is essential.

Anaesthesia

The operation is performed under general anaesthesia; if the systemic arterial and venous blood pressure are reduced by posture and the use of hypotensive agents the surgery is easier. Infiltration of the area with a vasoconstrictor agent acceptable to the anaesthetist also reduces scalp bleeding. Phenylephrine 1 in 10,000 up to 10 ml is recommended.

External Auditory Canal Groove

Instruments (Figures 6.4 and 6.5)

In order safely to insert the San Francisco multichannel sheathed electrode without tearing the silastic covering special instruments had to be designed. The two most important at the moment of insertion are, a microsurgical crutch which has a curved

142 *Surgical Implantation*

Figure 6.1: Electrode Developed in San Francisco. Eight pairs of platinum-iridium mushroom contacts are joined to a circular pad to which the rest of the device may be connected.

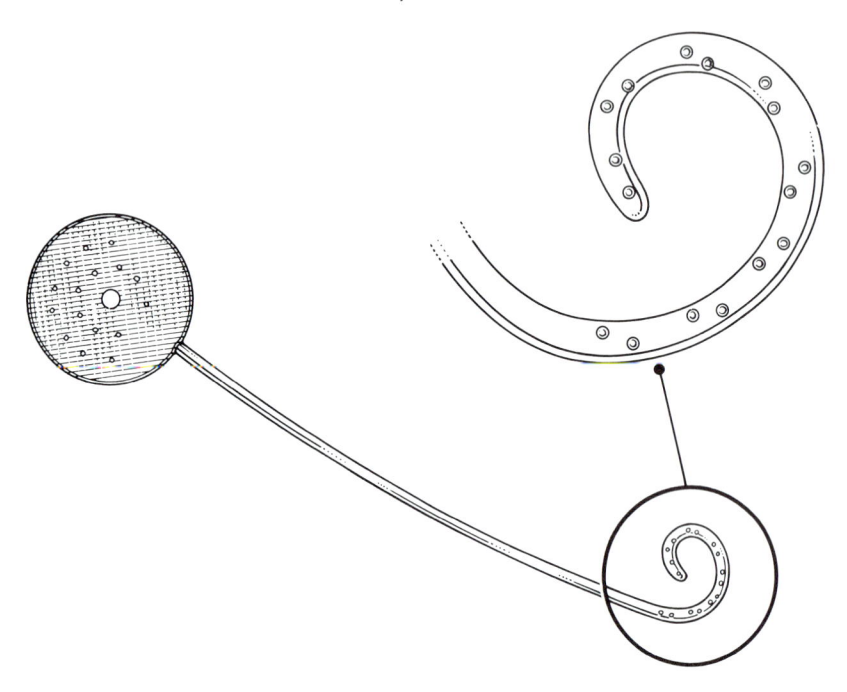

Figure 6.2: Round Window Electrode with Indifferent Electrode and Receiver Coil.

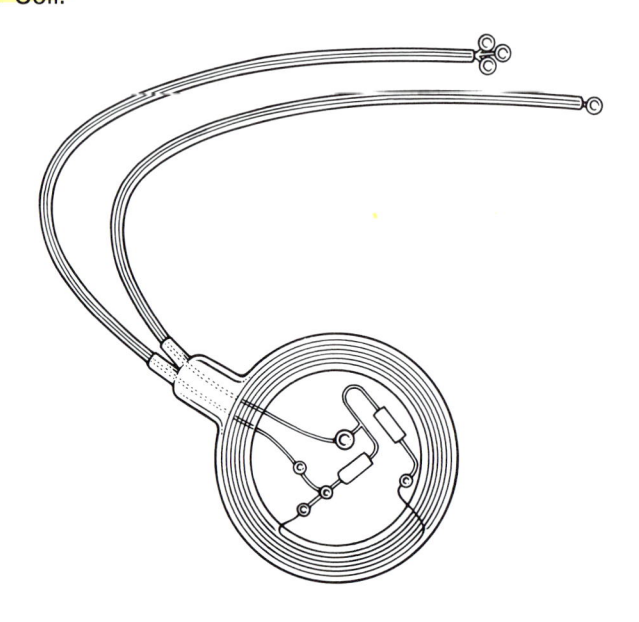

Surgical Implantation 143

Figure 6.3: Patient Positioned and Shaved for Operation.

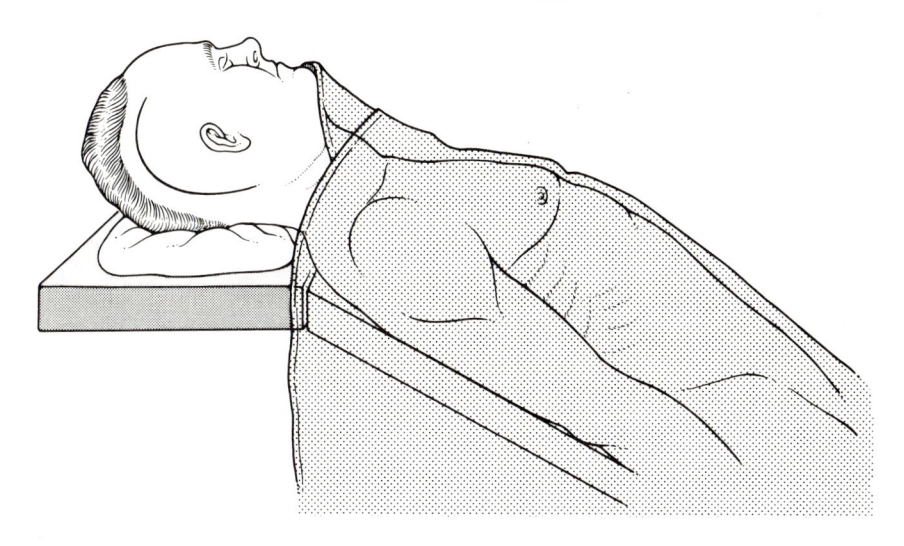

Figure 6.4: Modified Forceps.

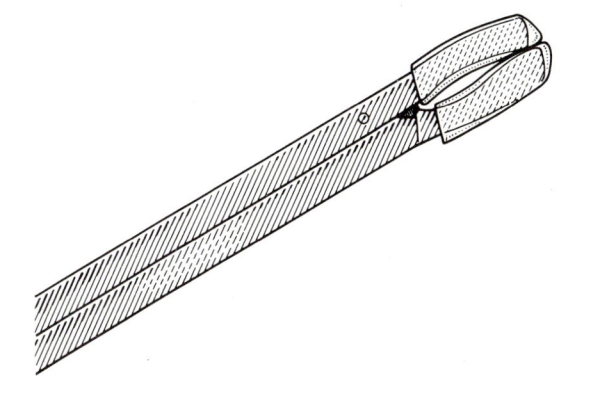

Figure 6.5: Microsurgical Crutch.

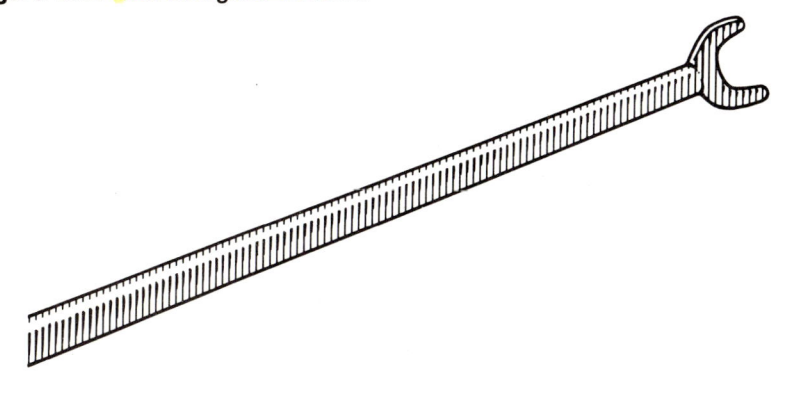

144 Surgical Implantation

end allowing control of the electrode tip around the first turn of the scala tympani (Figure 6.5), and a modified angled cupped forceps with silastic covered jaws which allow the electrode to be gripped and advanced into the scala without injuring the delicate electrode contact surfaces (Figure 6.4). This pair of instruments make it possible to insert the long UCSF multi-electrode array the required distance.

This electrode (Figure 6.1) has been designed with an 'elastic' memory which allows the tip to be straightened and yet retain its ability to adopt the curve of the modiolus.

Incision (Figure 6.6)

Figure 6.6 shows a large postauricular scalp flap. This is raised in continuity with the skin of the posterior ear canal wall and the ear drum. The edges of the flap are secured with Michel clips to stop bleeding. Periosteum is raised on an anteriorly based pedicle and turned forward to uncover bone.

Figure 6.6: Incision.

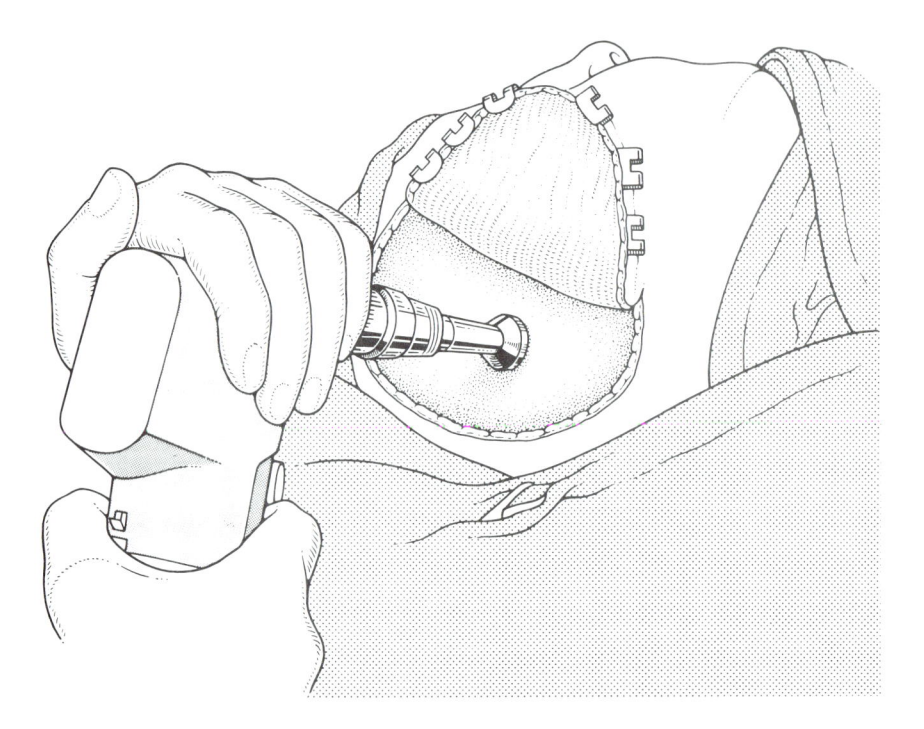

Mastoid Cortex (Figure 6.6)

An electrically powered trephine with a spring-loaded centrepin following a small pilot hole in the bone is used to excavate a 'socket' several millimetres deep in the cortex into which the circular disconnection unit will fit. When this item sits down nicely in its pit it is lifted out and the walls of the pit undercut to provide

Figure 6.7: Grooving the Ear Canal.

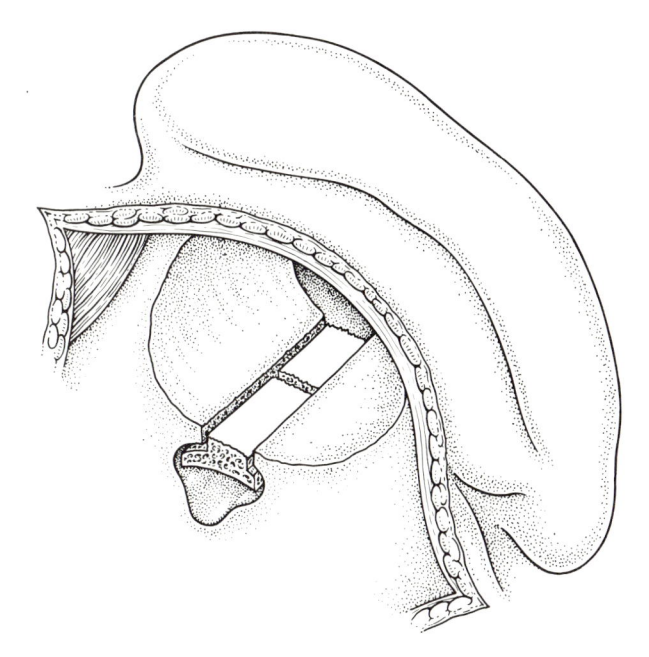

a key for acrylic cement later. The bone from the centre of the depression is removed with a chisel as a small slab and preserved for use in the ear canal.

Grooving the Ear Canal (Figure 6.7)

The soft tissues of the ear are displaced anteriorly exposing the bony meatus. Care is taken not to injure or tear canal skin. Extensive dissection has to be made in the inferior portion of the basal scala tympani, and as this requires large exposure of the hypotympanum it has been found most convenient to place the electrode leads directly in a groove in the posterior canal wall. The groove serves two purposes, providing access to a narrow area at the right angle for the surgeon's line of view and a secure place to lodge the cable.

The groove is created in the posterior canal wall extending from the region of the round window to the outer margin of the mastoid cortex. The descending portion of the facial nerve lies 2 mm deep to the bony tympanic annulus at the medial end of the groove. The sheath of the nerve may become visible at this point and care is needed to prevent heating or laceration.

The edges of the groove are undercut to permit the insertion of bone wedges over the electrode leads. Cortical bone taken from the prepared site of the disconnection unit is shaped with a drill to fit the undercut groove like the lid of a school pencil box. The lid is then covered with a temporalis fascia graft. This technique prevents the vulnerable canal skin dipping into the bony groove or coming into contact with the electrode lead.

146 *Surgical Implantation*

Figure 6.8: Opening the Scala Tympani.

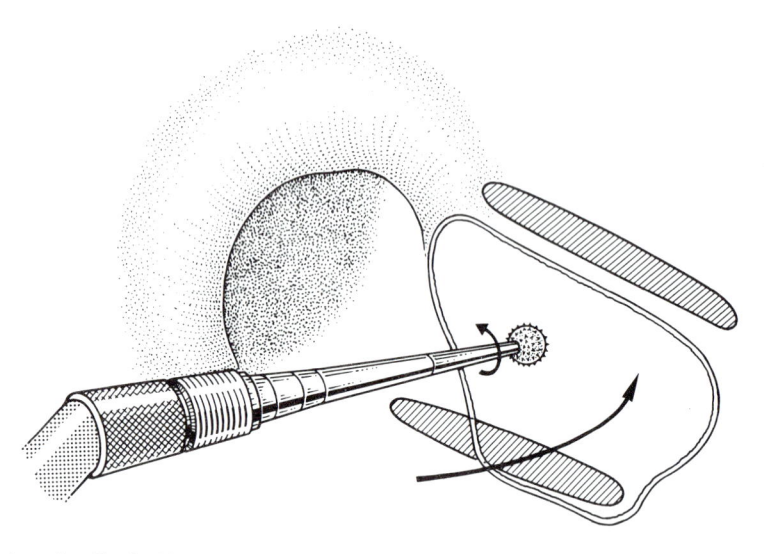

Opening the Scala Tympani (Figure 6.8)

Insertion of the UCSF electrode requires exposure of the basal scala tympani. Bone is removed from the lateral wall of the scala for a distance of approximately 3–4 mm from the round window. This exposure allows the surgeon to negotiate the electrode tip safely around the first turn of the cochlea without perforating the basilar membrane.

A 2 mm diamond paste burr mounted on an angled handpiece is plied just beyond the anterior rim of the round window niche until the endosteum of the scala is visible. Entering the scala too low is almost impossible because the floor of the hypotympanum limits the dissection. Too high and a shelf appears across the field of view: this is the limbus of the cochlear partition and should be treated with the greatest respect for fear of dislocating the basilar membrane of which it is the outer rim.

Final Electrical Tests

The electrode is unwrapped from its sterile covers and tested with a transmitter. A bold copy of the signal seen on an oscilloscope connected to the apical contact electrodes is taken as good evidence that the device has survived transport and sterilisation. Sterile leads and covers are used.

Electrode Insertion (Figure 6.9)

When tested and ready, when a hole in the scala as far round the first turn of the cochlea as is practicable is open at the end of the groove, the electrode may be inserted.

Held uncoiled and presented to the opening in the scala tympani the inbuilt tendency of the electrode to re-coil helps draw it into the cochlea. The two pronged

Surgical Implantation 147

Figure 6.9: Electrode Insertion.

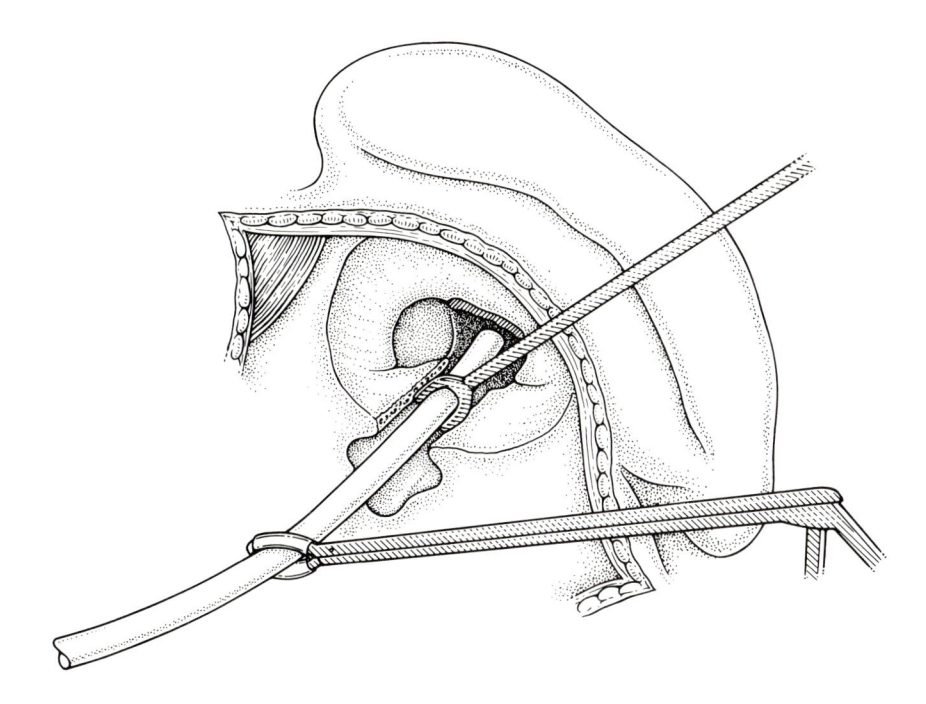

blunt fork and the soft faced crocodile micro-forceps alternately hold and advance the electrode to its optimum position along the basilar membrane which has a total length of 36 mm.

Penetration of 24–26 mm is readily achieved without undue thrust in this way. Excessive force shows itself as buckling of that portion of the electrode still visible and is best avoided by a gentleness of touch born of practice on cadaver temporal bones.

Securing the Lead (Figure 6.10)

The electrode lead is laid in the undercut groove prepared for it and held there by the bone wedges prepared for the groove. No glue or cement is needed if the carpentry has been good!

Securing the Disconnection Unit

The bone is carefully dried, acrylic cement sparingly applied to the prepared bone 'socket' in the mastoid cortex and the hardware pressed home. The remainder of the device, receiver coils or percutaneous temporary cable are secured to dry bone using the minimum of acrylic cement.

Grafting the Canal

A temporalis fascia graft is placed over the bony groove and wedged to further

148 *Surgical Implantation*

Figure 6.10: Securing the Lead.

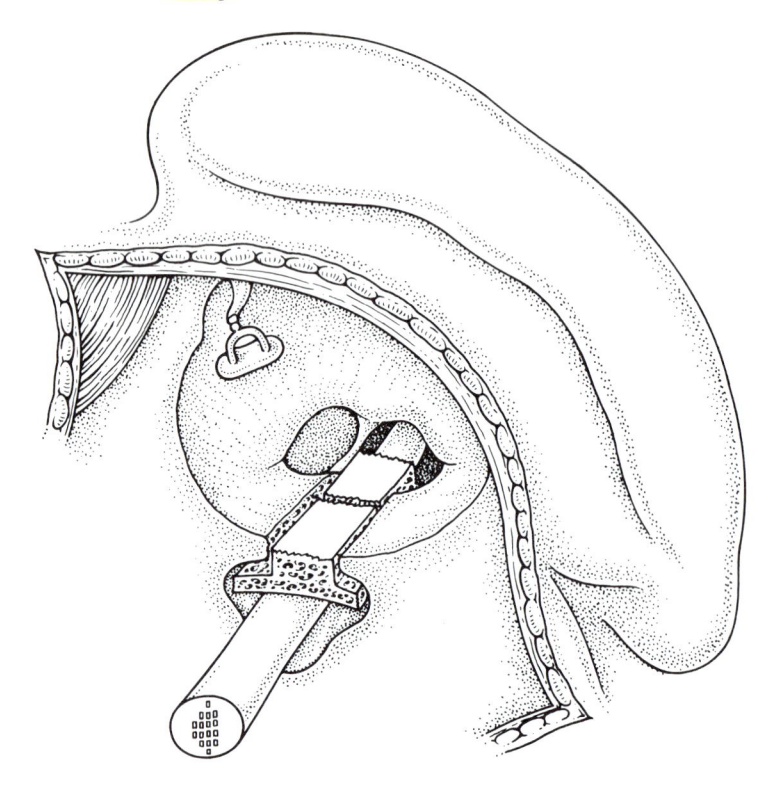

protect canal skin from the possibility of invagination, ulceration and infection.

Closure

The scalp flap is sutured back into place and an antiseptic pack placed in the ear canal to maintain its shape. A mastoid pressure bandage is generally applied over a small open tube drain. Both are removed at 48 hours.

Posterior Tympanotomy Approach (Facial recess route, Figure 6.11)

Single-channel electrodes whether intended to pass into the cochlea or to stop at the round window are often slim, floppy and require support across the middle ear. For this reason and also because ulceration over a subcutaneous wire has been a leading cause of infection of the ear canal in the past, such electrodes are usually passed through the mastoid bone and posterior tympanotomy slot at the site of the facial nerve recess.

The incision is the same as described in the meatal approach above and an identical flap is raised. The mastoid bone is excavated with cutting burrs until an entrance can be made into the middle ear beneath the posterior canal wall at

Figure 6.11: Securing the Receiver.

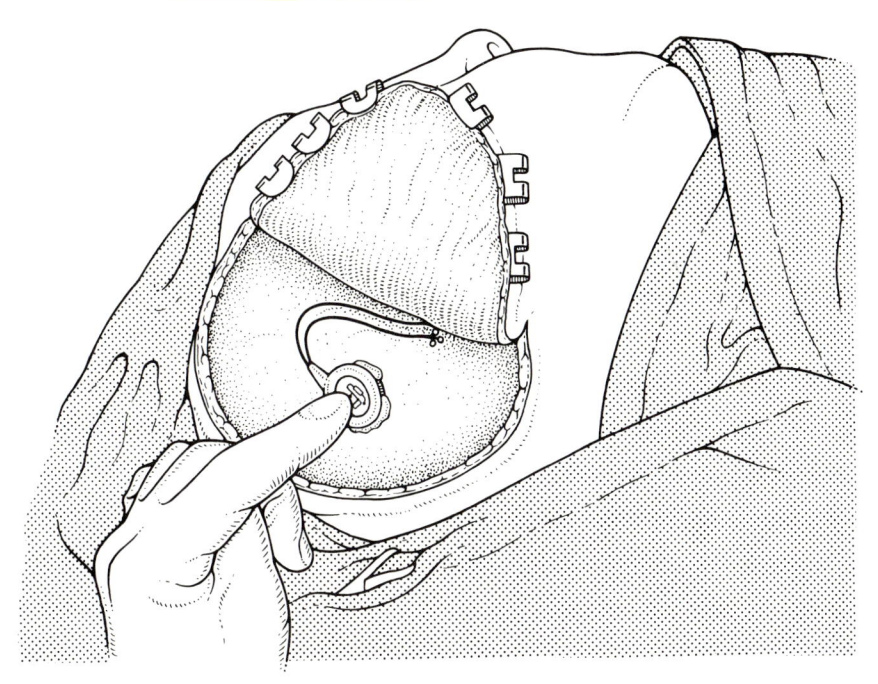

the site of the facial recess. This entrance becomes, as it enlarges, a slot bounded by the short process of the incus (preserved) laterally and the facial nerve (also preserved!) medially. Twisting the patient's head away from the surgeon and looking through the 'slot' at an oblique angle brings the round window into view. If desired, raising a flap of so far undisturbed ear canal skin affords a second view of the scene in the middle ear. This is useful when manipulating a electrode through the 'slot'.

Securing the Receiver (Figures 6.11 and 6.12)

The solid portion of the implant, receiver coils, tuned circuit and junctions all encapsulated in a non-porous material are cemented to hollows in the bone near the mastoid cortex. Non-absorbable sutures may be used in drillings in the bone to hold the device in place instead of acrylic cement. Closure is as described above.

In both approaches it is unwise to secure the solid portion of the implant before positioning the cochlear end of the electrode as twists or a 'bad lie' cannot be corrected easily without imposing a permanent orientation change upon the lead. Stress fractures and insulation breakdown are the likely result of such abuse.

Postoperative Care

For the first few hours the patient may be cold and prone to falls in blood pressure;

150 *Surgical Implantation*

Figure 6.12: The Receiver may be Secured with Acrylic Bone Cement (1) or Monofilament Nylon Tied through Holes in Bone (2).

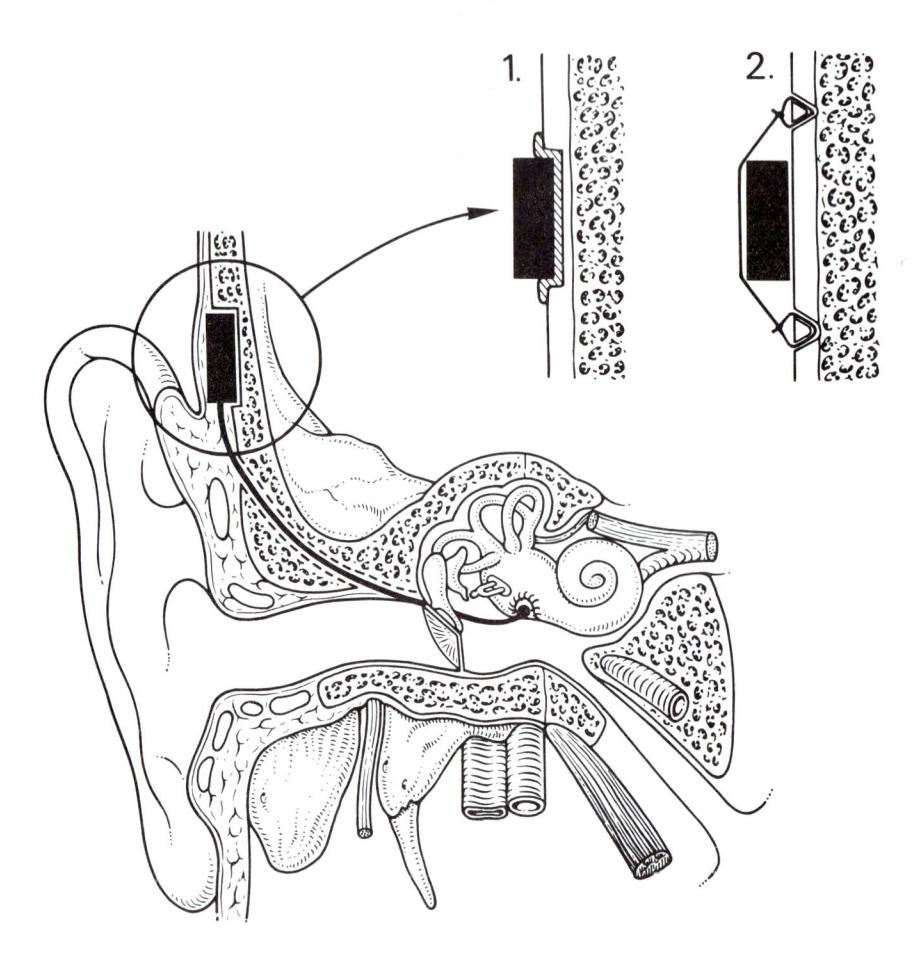

the intravenous infusion used during surgery should be maintained until blood pressure is stable. The patient may then be nursed in a 30° head up position which is both comfortable and minimises scalp bleeding. Leg movements are encouraged as unlike most otological procedures there is a real risk of pulmonary embolism from deep venous thrombosis.

Antibiotic therapy is a wide precaution against infection. The mastoid pressure dressing is removed with the drain at 48 hours and the patient allowed out of bed.

First Stimulation (Figure 6.13)

Few surgeons can resist the temptation to try stimulating the ear when the dressings

Figure 6.13: First Stimulation.

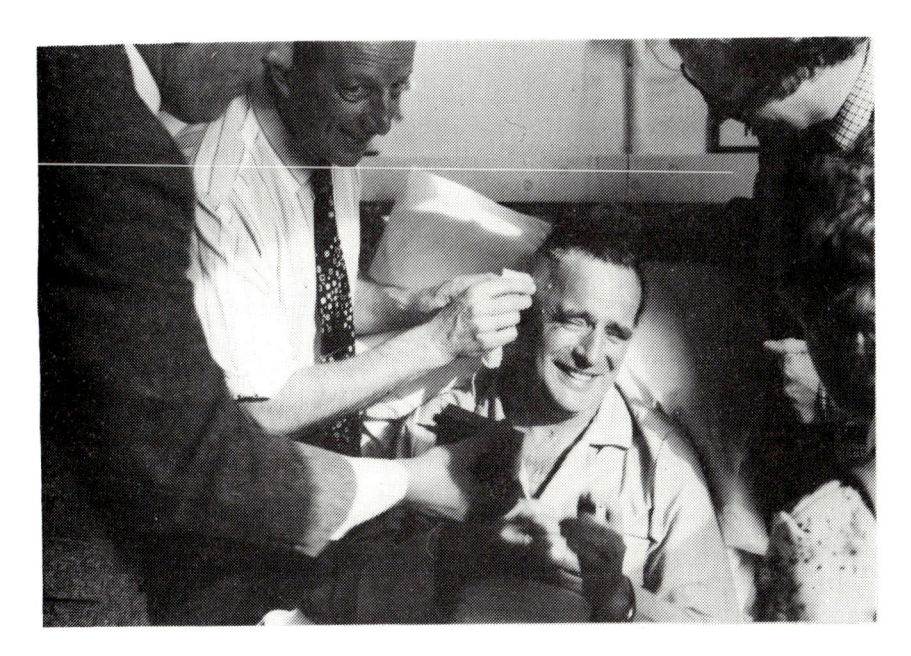

come off. The transmitter placed in a sterile bag is held against the scalp over the receiver and turned on. This is not the time to measure thresholds, frequency responses or tinnitus suppression but a simple reassurance to patient and implant team that the device is 'live' is needed. Oedema in the scalp may hold the transmitter away and give a faint response. If a percutaneous cable is used electrode impedances may be checked objectively without tiring the patient unduly.

Modiolar and Multiple Electrodes

These are inserted from above via the middle cranial fossa. Some multichannel electrodes are placed by making two or several openings into the bony cochlea via the middle ear or middle cranial fossa. Chapter 4 describes and illustrates such prostheses.

References: see Chapter 7 (p. 162).

7 COMPLICATIONS AND FAILURES OF COCHLEAR IMPLANTS

Roger F. Gray and Robert A. Schindler

For purposes of definition, we have chosen the term complications to describe undesirable events associated with the surgical implantation and presence of the cochlear implant. The term failure describes malfunction of the cochlear implant or inability of the patient to use the device.

Early Complications

The hazards of a long anaesthetic and operation are well known and will not be discussed here in detail. The most common early complication is a wound haematoma which can arise from the scalp and galeal incisions. Evacuation of the haematoma is essential to prevent infection. The complication can best be prevented by employing closed suction drainage, such as that offered by a Hemovac or Jackson-Pratt closed drains.

Allergic reactions may occur as a result of medications, suture material, antiseptic agents and adhesive dressings. These may cause serious anaphylactic reactions or may predispose the patient to secondary infection. A stitch abscess may be the result of an allergic reaction to suture material or contamination by organisms. The reaction can be severe enough to require surgical debridement and drainage. If the incision is well away from the implanted device, these stitch abscesses can be controlled without contamination of the entire wound.

The most serious complications of cochlear implantation are associated with infection of the implant site itself. Since all cochlear implants are bio-compatible but not bio-degradable, once they become involved with infection they react like a foreign body. Control and eradication of the infection usually requires removal of the entire implant device in addition to standard modes of therapy.

Opening the inner ear creates a pathway for cerebrospinal fluid (CSF) to flow from the area around the brainstem through the cochlea aqueduct and out around an intracochlear electrode. This complication carries the risk of meningitis if bacteria follow the fluid to its source. However, such leaks occur very rarely and do not seem to be a problem. Perhaps this is because the electrode becomes surrounded by a fibrous sheath (Johnsson et al., 1982) which obstructs the mouth of the narrow aqueduct of the cochlea.

Loss of labyrinthine function may become obvious a few days after surgery. The patient complains of vertigo, is only comfortable with the operated ear uppermost, holds the head askew and has to be supported to the bathroom. Nystagmus made worse by looking away from the implanted ear may be present.

Complications and Failures 153

Life-long poor balance results if the balance organ which has been damaged by opening the cochlea was the only functioning organ but a slow recovery will be made if the contralateral organ is in good condition. Loss of balance after intracochlear implantation is rare. The author knows of only one case where the ear had to be reopened soon after surgery to stop a CSF leak (Ballantyne, personal communication). There are three reasons for this. First, it is possible to open the cochlea without necessarily destroying balance function; successful stapedectomy is a good example. Secondly, most otologists perform caloric tests on potential implant patients to avoid such a disaster and thirdly many patients have such poor caloric responses and inner ear balance function that the loss would not be noticed. Such patients have accommodated to the loss of function over many years and rely upon visual references, muscle tension and joint position sense for their balance.

Tinnitus — noise generated in the ear and apparent to the sufferer as a high pitched whistle or the sound of escaping steam which never stops and which may be very loud — is a common complication of deafness. Any operation on the middle or inner ear may cause or worsen tinnitus and the more invasive the surgery the greater the chance of tinnitus. Electrical stimulation reduces or abolishes tinnitus in a proportion of cases (Aran and Cazals, 1981).

Minor complications at this stage are persistent oedema of the scalp over the receiver coils causing a faint signal and regrowth of hair at the same place. Depilation may be necessary.

Late Complications

Cables routed down or near the external auditory meatus have been the Achilles heel of many implants. Months after a successful operation when the patient is well advanced with auditory rehabilitation the otologist finds a crust in the ear canal and removes it. At the next visit a pink patch of bone cement is visible in the base of a small ulcer on the canal floor. By the third visit granulation tissue has formed and the ear is discharging. Nothing will now stop the ulceration and micro-organisms have a pathway to the cochlea inwards and a pathway to the seat of the electronics outwards. The situation may be endured while the device continues to function but sooner or later all foreign material will have to be removed.

Cables routed through the facial recess are spared the problems of chronic otitis externa but are equally at risk of harbouring organisms from an attack of otitis media perpetuating such an infection and propagating it into the cochlea and out to the lodgement of the receiver electronics. Fortunately adults with normal Eustachian tube function very rarely suffer otitis media but it may present a considerable problem with children.

Mastoiditis occurs at the site of lodgement of foreign material when micro-organisms reach the area via a cable entering the skin or an ulcerated electrode

154 *Complications and Failures*

site. It smoulders despite antibiotic therapy and may lead to the next complication.

Degeneration of residual supporting cells in the organ of Corti and residual cochlear neurones is a late complication particularly of intracochlear electrodes. Ball electrodes and the tips of long stiff electrode arrays have a tendency to penetrate the basilar membrane and fracture the spinal lamina where the nerve fibres are to be found. A detailed discussion of this subject can be found in the second half of Chapter 3.

Failures

Failures Due to Injury

Cochlear implants are delicate; the more complicated the device the more possibilities exist for failure. It should be true that the device left the laboratory or workshop in working order, but what hazards does it face before being safely installed in a suitable patient?

Implants travel long distances. Those made in Austria are installed in London, those made in Minnesota are installed in Los Angeles. Micro-electronics are moved safely all over the world but special packaging techniques are employed, particularly expanded polystyrene, thick-walled boxes tailored to the shape of the item. Water, great heat and violent shocks must be guarded against and in some devices decompression at altitude may cause damage if bubbles exist in silastic-bound electrode arrays.

Sterilisation is a testing event for a composite structure of polymers and metal. Hand the package to the Operating Department Sister and she will put it in a steam autoclave. Not all implants and their packaging are suitable for this method. Figure 7.1 shows an Austrian device half fused to its package by excessive heat and an unsuitable synthetic sterilising bag. Fortunately a spare was immediately available as the operation was far advanced.

Handling prior to use requires care. Opening the final wrappings has resulted in partial avulsion of cables and cutting the top of the bag should not be delegated to the most junior nurse, since the electrode may be snipped clean away from the receiver. The main risk of injury is at the time of insertion when surgical enthusiasm is at its height. Figure 7.2 shows a result one author has witnessd on two occasions.

Loosening of any part of the device from its attachments is eventually fatal to function. If the electrode moves due to repeated stresses like the force reversals due to chewing or true growth as in a child's ear, requirements for current go up, electrode impedances go up and auditory perception goes down. If the receiver in its bony pit comes adrift it may migrate to an unsuitable position for stimulation. It will be restrained in its journey by the cable but this will soon give way by actually parting or being dragged out of the round window.

Even if the intracochlear portion of electrode and receiver stay firmly lodged in their appointed places but the intervening stretch of cable is unsupported and free to move trouble will result. Repeated movements associated with any normal body activity produce stress fractures of fine wires or breakdown of insulation.

Complications and Failures 155

Figure 7.1: Device Half-fused to Package by Excessive Heat and Unsuitable Synthetic Sterilising Bag.

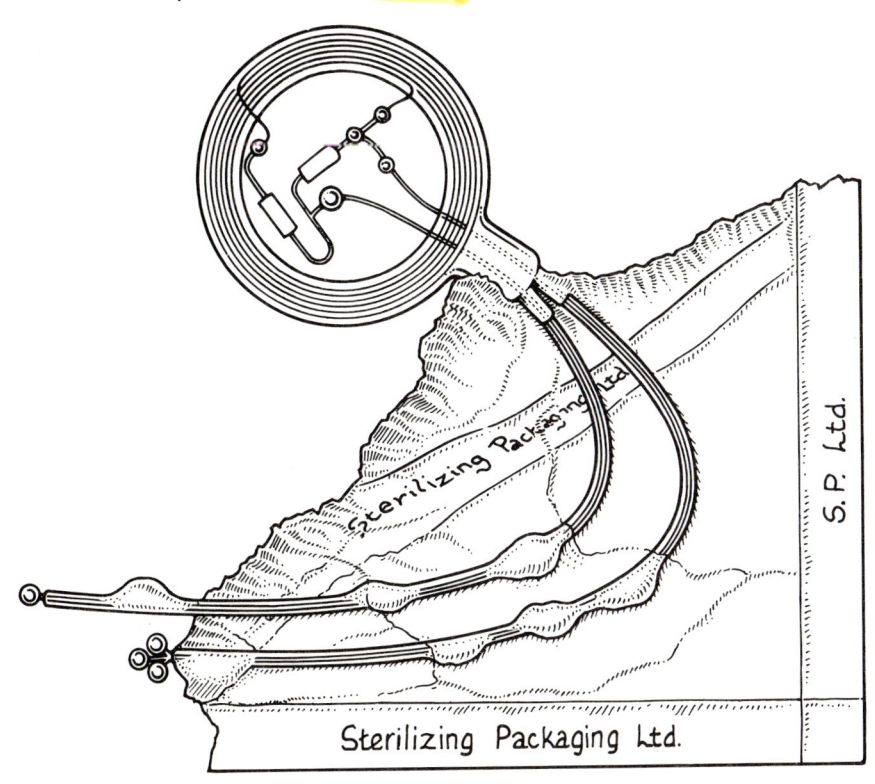

Cables routed through or under muscles are to be avoided. Intermittent failure due to cable stress fracture can often be diagnosed by finger pressure behind the ear. If the right spot is found function will be restored for a few seconds. Figure 7.3 shows a stress fracture 6 mm below the receiver coil.

Failures of Electrical Insulation

Penetration of a neural prosthesis by extracellular body fluid generally stops the prosthesis functioning. The smaller the electrode surfaces the higher the density of current must be for the same biological effect. That current will cheerfully leak away through an ion-rich fluid or to an adjacent uninsulated cable. Implant engineers have put much thought and energy into this aspect of the subject and a detailed study is to be found in Chapter 4. Two substances deserve special mention because their properties are not as expected. Medical-grade silicone rubber absorbs water rendering its insulation properties poor. This may be overcome by enclosing it under a hydrostatic pressure equal to or greater than the vapour pressure of water vapour at body temperature. This keeps it quite dry. Teflon (PTFE) has as its main drawback that it fails to bond to metals and allows creeping fluid penetration along a wire. Figure 7.4 shows a disruption of the insulation of a multichannel

156 *Complications and Failures*

Figure 7.2: Electrode Damaged at Insertion.

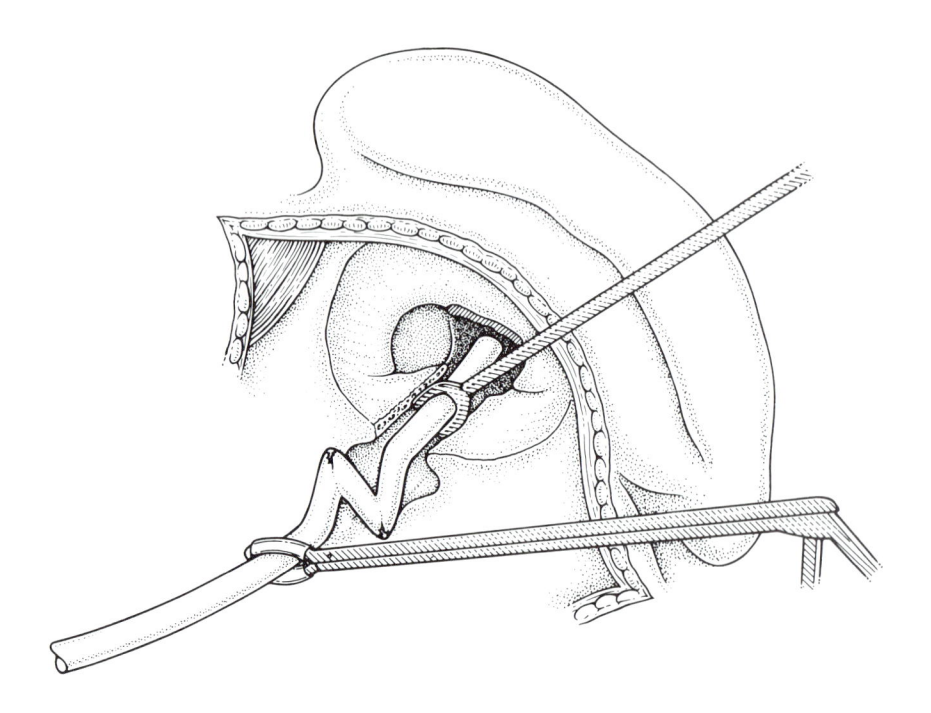

electrode bundle. Short circuits between adjacent wires with loss of 'channels' are to be expected. When a cable is free to move tens of thousands of 'reversals' may occur without wire fracture but the device may fail because of loss of insulation. Epoxy and varnish coats are often more rigid and prone to fracture than the wire itself.

Electrolysis

Dissimilar metal junctions, especially if bathed in a fluid through which ions may pass, can cause spontaneous generation of an electromotive force. Where a current is made to flow for a larger purpose electrolysis occurs in solutions containing ions even if only a single metal is present. Figure 7.5 shows a brazed joint between a platinum electrode and the end of a copper coil into which body fluids have penetrated. The fluffy deposit the artist has drawn at the junction is a chloride of copper.

Intrinsic Component Failure

Five species of component failure are well recognised. Two describe the mode of failure and are called degradation failure and catastrophic failure. Three describe the cause of failure and are titled misuse failure, inherent weakness failure and wear-out failure.

Complications and Failures 157

Figure 7.3: Stress Fracture. This occurs where a movable cable joins a fixed structure; in this case a notch can be seen 6 mm below the rigidly fixed receiver coil.

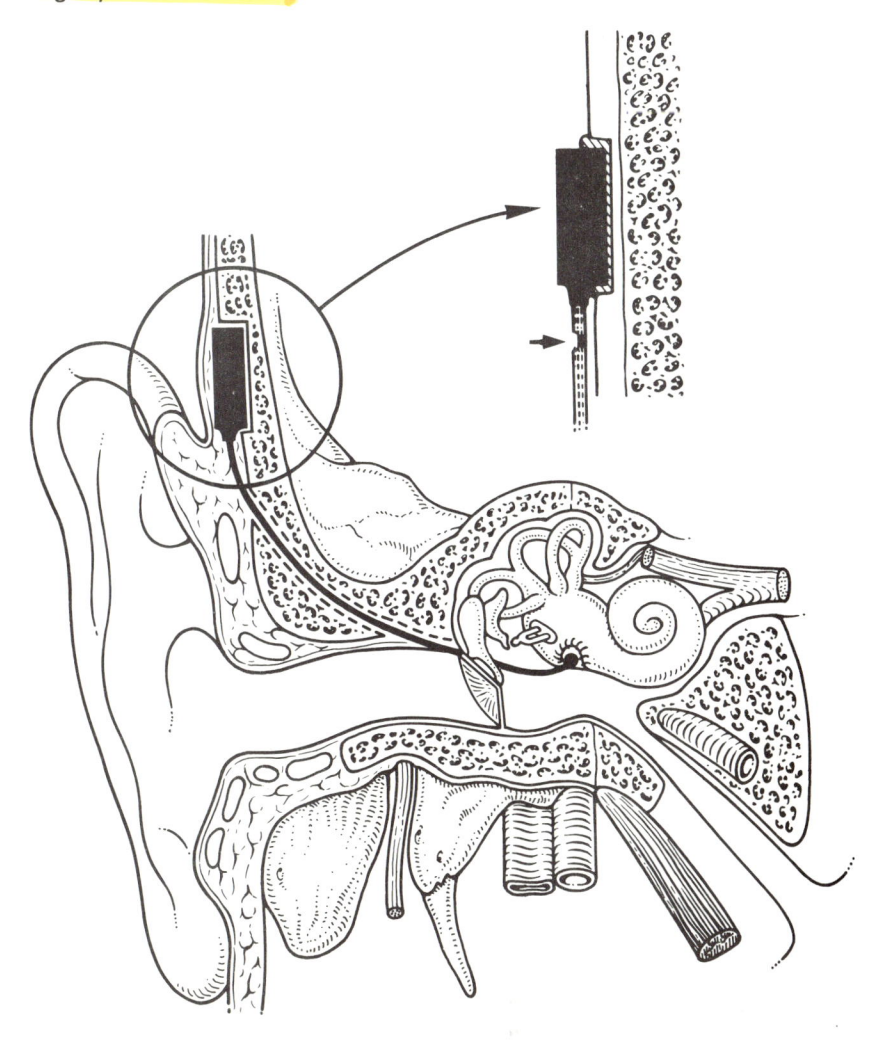

Electronic components are supplied untested, tested by a single demonstration of function, and tested by repeated use for a specified period. This last is what is required for implanted components, is called 'burning in' and should ensure that the item is in the plateau phase of its life. Figure 7.6 shows component failure rate plotted against time. The curve has three segments, initial high failure rate (a) due to inherent weakness, middle plateau phase (b) with minimal failures and terminal phase (c) when wear-out failure begins and progresses (Young, 1981).

Components found in cochlear implants are resistors, capacitors, coils and diodes. Integrated circuits are rare in the surgically implanted portion of prostheses

Figure 7.4: Disruption of Insulation of a Multichannel Electrode Bundle.

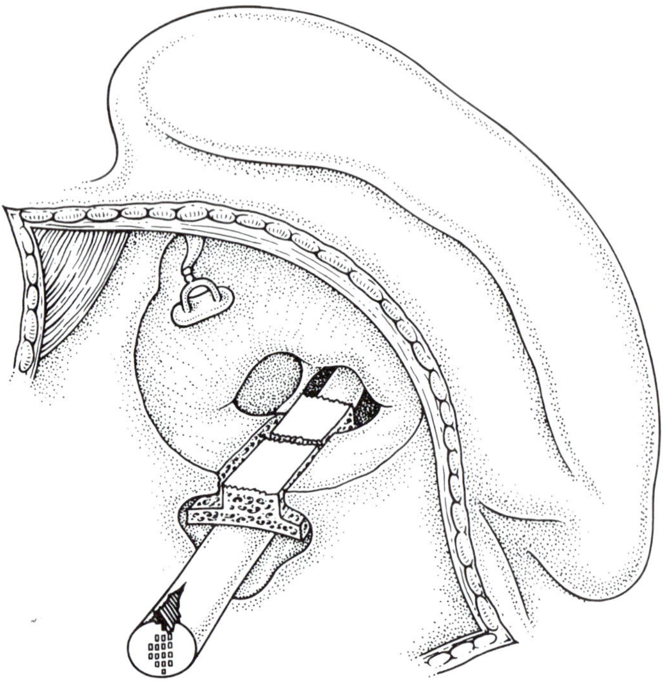

because they generally require an intrinsic power source. This means cells or batteries of limited life inaccessible without surgery. Diode failure is the commonest event in the authors' experience, resulting in loss of a channel in a multichannel device in one case and this would have been the loss of all input in a single-channel device.

Failure of Selection

Implantation may completely fail to improve the hearing and quality of life if an inappropriate choice has been made. Chapter 5 is devoted to this subject, but two striking examples of misjudgement and one of sheer misfortune will be included here. Consider a teenage boy, victim of a severe sensory neural deafness which occurred before the age of one year, from maternal rubella, for example. Brought up to think and communicate by sign language, supplemented by a limited vocabulary of mispronounced monotonic words for essential situations, such a person is likely to be happiest signing fluently among teenagers with the same language. Sudden introduction of the rhythmic skeleton of a strange tongue would probably be rejected as meaningless. Even normal auditory input would fall on unprepared neurological ground at a age less adept at learning than infancy. Where groups of congenitally deaf people have discussed implants their reaction has often been one of scornful rejection.

Complications and Failures 159

Figure 7.5: Brazed Joint between a Platinum Electrode and the End of a Copper Coil into which Body Fluids Have Penetrated.

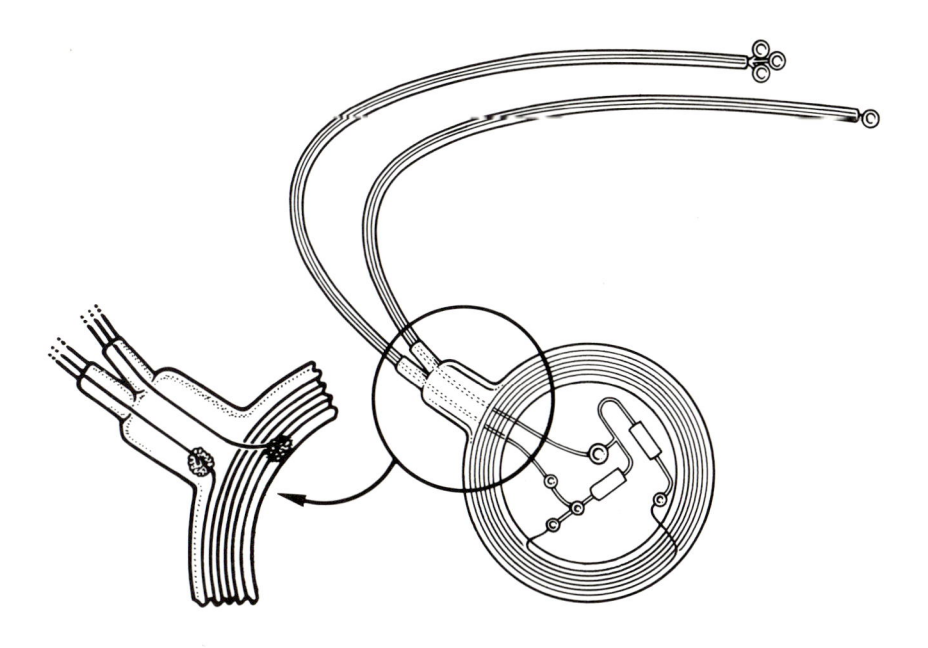

Figure 7.6: Component Failure Rates, Showing Three Phases. See text for explanation.

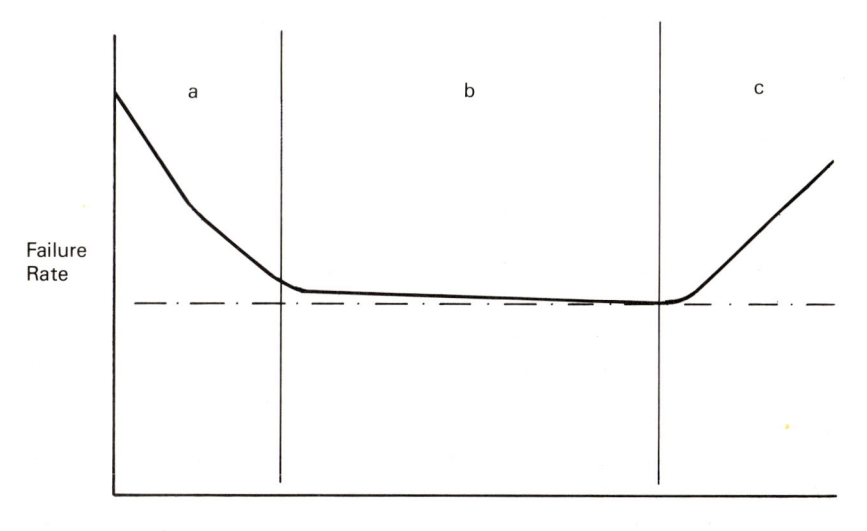

160 *Complications and Failures*

Figure 7.7: A CT Scan Performed Long after Implantation Showing a Large Temporal Lobe Deficit on One Side.

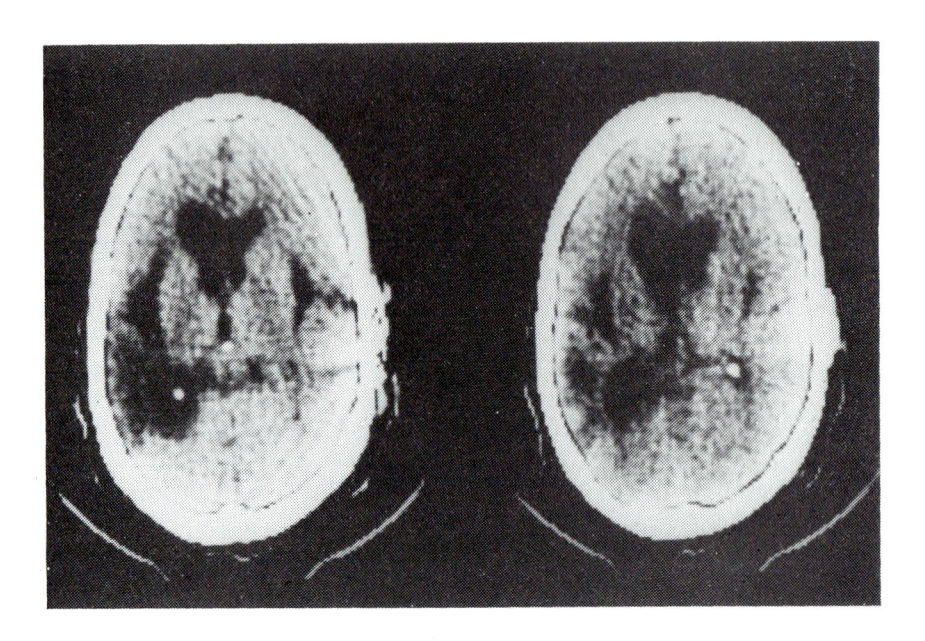

The second example is the resentful and lazy patient who welcomes the attention and fuss associated with preparation for surgery but after the operation complains bitterly of discomfort and inconvenience. The sounds perceived are declared to be far short of expectations despite careful preoperative counselling and the patient refuses to co-operate with any programme of training or rehabilitation. It seems likely that, unless there are large numbers of electrically accessible cochlear neurones remaining in an implanted ear, the success of any individual patient in rehabilitation depends mostly upon his or her willingness and capacity to learn to use the new auditory input. The difference in such a case between multi-channel or single channel is overshadowed by the differences in personality between one patient and the next.

The third case is drawn from the authors' experience of one particular patient. Mr C.H. was chosen carefully for an intracochlear electrode. A willing and likeable fellow he had been deafened at the age of twenty by streptomycin given in good faith twenty years ago for tuberculous meningitis. A radiological examination of the bony cochleas showed that both were free of labyrinthitis ossificans and that insertion of an electrode was possible. Two radiological techniques are available for this, hypocycloidal tomograms of the temporal bone and a high definition CT head scan. Implantation went ahead on the results of the tomograms. Figure 7.7 is a CT scan performed long after implantation and shows a large temporal lobe deficit on one side. Despite this C.H. is pleased with the device, uses it daily,

Complications and Failures 161

and undoubtedly derives considerable prosodic or rhythmical information from it. Had the CT scan been chosen preoperatively the view of the bony cochleas might have been poor, but the cerebral damage would have been considered an example of central deafness unsuitable for a cochlear implant.

Children and Implants

Young children with severe congenital deafness have problems which are not addressed formally in this book. Whether an input through the auditory nerve, such as is described in Chapter 8 or Chapter 10, would be helpful in the learning of a spoken language at the age of three or four is not yet known. The only way to find out is to try and this is certainly happening in Los Angeles. Most hearing people believe that it should be tried, but not at any price. Repeated hospitalisation, raised and dashed hopes, painful or repeated surgical procedures and irrevocable changes in the inner ear which might make a future device useless are all prices considered too high for a small child's welfare. Most people born deaf believe it is quite wrong to do it at all and that the money involved could be much better spent. Anyone declaring in 1920 that electronic amplifiers would never be any use in ameliorating deafness or in assisting the severely deaf child to speak, however, would now have to eat his words. Compromise might be the answer. An extracochlear electrode placed with such care that the ossicular chain was untouched and an appropriate hearing aid could still be worn might satisfy the need. The prosodic information from such a simple implant might be as much use to the 'totally deaf' child as similar information from an aid is when the residual hearing is limited to a corner of the audiogram, the so called 'island of low frequency hearing'. Where doubt exists as to which is the best 'aid' to hearing, the answer would be provided by the child as he or she grew and abandoned the electronic device in favour of the hearing aid or vice-versa. It is hard to imagine a cochlear implant being so successful that the teaching of sign language would not be needed. To be 'bilingual' like the hearing children of deaf parents would be the aim.

Zero Nerve Survival

Unfortunately there is no way of predicting the proportion of cochlear neurones which survive in a deaf ear. A useful proportion is 5 to 10 per cent of the 32,000 or so that populate a normal modiolus (Spoendlin, 1974). These, if present at the time of a cochlear implant, are reduced by progression of the disease which occasioned the deafness, by ageing and by implants that destroy supporting structures in Corti's organ by fracture of the spiral lamina or penetration of the basilar membrane. Chapter 3 gives details on this point.

Promontory stimulation, temporarily arranged in the conscious patient under consideration for an implant, does not provide a reliable answer to the question 'are there surviving neurones'. If the patient reports a strong sensation of sound on stimulation with ability to distinguish frequency differences then nerve survival of some degree is certain. If pain only is reported the converse is not true, as reports of good results from intracochlear electrodes have been made in patients who failed to respond to promontory stimulation. If an extracochlear electrode is planned then a favourable response to promontory stimulation is an essential prerequisite (Douek *et al.*, 1983).

References

Aran, J.M. and Cazals, Y. (1981) Electrical suppression of tinnitus. *CIBA Found. Symp.*, 85, 217–31.
Douek, E.E., Fourcin, A.J., Moore, B.C.J., Rosen, S., Walliker, J.R., Frampton, S.L., Howard, D.M. and Abberton, E. (1983) Clinical aspects of extra cochlea electrical stimulation. *Ann. NY Acad. Sci.*, 405, 332–6
Johnsson, L-G., House, W.F. and Linthicum, F.H. (1982) Otopathological findings in a patient with bilateral cochlear implants. *Ann. Otol. Rhinol. Laryngol.* Suppl. 91(2), Pt 3, 74–89
Loeb, G.E., Byers, C.L., Rebscher, S.J., Casey, D.E., Fong, M.M., Schindler, R.A., Gray, R.F. and Merzenich, M.M. (1983) Design and fabrication of an experimental cochlear prosthesis. *Med. Biol. Eng. Comput.*, 21, 241–54
Merzenich, M.M., Rebscher, S.J., Loeb, G.E., Byers, C.L. and Schindler, R.A. (1984) The UCSF cochlear implant project. *Adv. Audiol.*, 2, 119–44
Schindler, R.A., Gray, R.F., Rebscher, S.J. and Byers, C.L. (1981) Multichannel cochlear implants: electrode design and surgical considerations. *Artificial Organs* (Suppl.), 5, 258–60
Spoendlin, H. (1974) in M.M. Merzenich, R.A. Schindler and F.A. Sooy (eds.), *Proceedings of the First International Conference on Electrical Stimulation of the Acoustic Nerve as a Treatment for Profound Sensory Neural Deafness in Man*, University of California, San Francisco, pp. 7–24
Young, E.C. (1979) *New Penguin Dictionary of Electronics*

8 SPEECH CODING FOR COCHLEAR IMPLANTS

Brian C.J. Moore

Introduction

One of the most critical and difficult processes in producing a cochlear implant is the design of a speech processor and coder. The purpose of such a device is to detect speech sounds, usually via a microphone worn by the implant user, and to process and transform those sounds to electrical signals suitable for driving an implanted electrode system. Several research groups have aimed to produce a speech processor which will allow patients using the device to understand connected discourse using sound alone. Other groups, including my own (the External Pattern Input or EPI group — see later for an explanation of the name) have assumed that the device will not allow unaided speech comprehension, and have designed their speech processor specifically as an aid to *lip-reading*. As we shall see, the design of speech processors can vary considerably depending upon what they are intended to achieve.

Speech-coding strategies can be classified into three main categories. In the first, the aim is to produce in the auditory nerve of the patient patterns of activity which resemble as closely as possible those which would occur in a normally hearing person in response to the same external sounds. This approach has been adopted particularly by those using multichannel implants (see, for example, Merzenich, 1983). The speech is passed through a bank of bandpass filters intended roughly to approximate the filtering which takes place on the basilar membrane (see Chapter 2). The output from each filter is then used to derive a signal which is fed to the appropriate electrode in the multi-electrode array.

In the second strategy, which has been used particularly with single-channel implants, a signal derived more-or-less directly from the analogue waveform of the speech is used to drive the implanted electrode. The idea is to squeeze as much information as possible into the single channel, hoping that the patient will somehow learn to make sense of the information, even if at first the sensation is highly unnatural. This approach has been adopted by the Vienna group (e.g. Hochmair and Hochmair-Desoyer, 1983) and by the House group (House, 1976).

The third approach, which has been adopted by the EPI group and by Clark and his colleagues in Australia, is to simplify the input to the patient by extracting simple patterns from speech and presenting only those simplified patterns to the implanted electrode(s). These patterns are designed to be matched to the discriminative abilities of the patients (as measured psychophysically) and to their needs. In the approach of the EPI group the patterns supplied are primarily designed to be of use as a supplement to lip-reading and to help self-monitoring of voice production.

Later in this chapter each of these approaches will be considered in more detail.

However, before doing this I will outline briefly some of the basic characteristics of speech sounds, and how those sounds are represented in the normal auditory nerve. I will also give a brief summary of the psychophysics of electrical stimulation, since this is important for understanding the limitations of what can be achieved by electrical stimulation.

Basic Characteristics of Speech Sounds

The normal ear is capable of a limited-resolution spectral analysis of complex sounds (see Chapter 2). Each frequency component in a complex sound gives rise to activity at a particular place on the basilar membrane, and hence in neurones with particular characteristic frequencies (CF). Speech sounds such as vowels are distinguished primarily on the basis of differences in the distribution of amount of sound (the energy of amplitude) as a function of frequency. This distribution is known as the energy spectrum or amplitude spectrum, or sometimes simply as the spectrum. However, in running speech the spectrum rarely stays constant for more than a few tens of milliseconds. Thus, in order to display the dynamic characteristics of speech sounds in a way which is comparable with the way that the ear works, it is necessary to show how the spectrum varies as a function of time. This is done by using the speech spectrogram; an example is shown in the middle of Figure 8.1 (taken from Stevens and Blumstein, 1981). Frequency is plotted on the vertical axis, time is plotted horizontally, and amplitude is represented by the darkness of shading. The spectrogram is of the utterance 'the big rabbits'.

The vowel sounds are characterised by high sound energy at particular frequencies, known as formant frequencies and shown as dark bands in the middle of Figure 8.1. The formants can be seen more clearly in the spectra shown in the top part of the figure, which were obtained by sampling at different points in time during the utterance. The patterning of the formants across frequency is different for each vowel sound, and is thought to be the main feature distinguishing one vowel from another. The formants are numbered, the one with the lowest frequency being labelled F1, the next F2 and so on. The first two or three formants seem to be the most important for vowel identification. Notice, however, that the formant frequencies rarely remain constant for any length of time; rather they glide from one value to another.

The situation for consonant sounds is rather more complex. Some consonants, such as the fricatives /s/ or /f/, are stable for fairly long periods of time, and are characterised by a relatively broad distribution of energy across frequency. This is shown in Figure 8.1 for the /s/ sound at the end of the utterance. Other sounds, such as the stop consonants /b/, /t/ and /g/, are characterised by rapid changes as a function of time.

The presence or absence of low-frequency periodicity, associated with vibration of the vocal cords, serves to distinguish voiced from unvoiced sounds. This periodicity is seen in the speech spectrogram as vertical striations, each striation corresponding to a single period of vibration of the vocal cords. For stop consonants

Figure 8.1: Speech Spectrogram of the Utterance 'The Big Rabbits'.

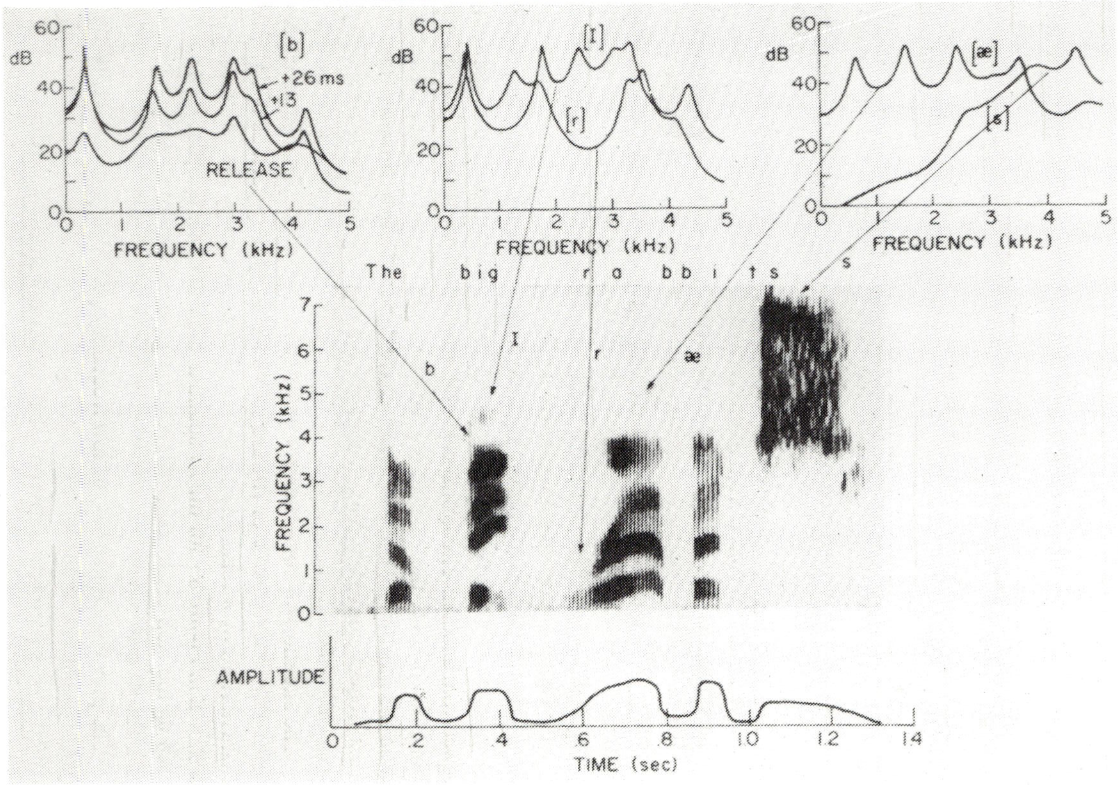

at the beginning of words, the delay between the onset of the sound and the onset of voicing (known as the voice onset time, or VOT) is an important cue. For example, in the English word 'bat' the voicing starts almost at the same time as the sound is released, whereas in the word 'pat' the voicing may start about 50 ms after the onset of the sound.

The stop consonants are produced by a complete closure of the vocal tract at some point along its length, followed by an abrupt release. Hence they are characterised by an abrupt change in amplitude, as may be seen in the bottom part of the figure for the /t/ and /b/ sounds. For other sounds, known as continuants, there may be only a partial closure of the vocal tract, so that the increase in amplitude is more gradual; see, for example the gradual rise in amplitude associated with the /r/ sound. Thus the rate of rise of amplitude can serve to distinguish these classes of sounds. The duration of a certain part of the sound can also be important. For example, the duration of the noise-like part of the sound can distinguish /s/ from /t/.

Certain classes of consonants are distinguished by the properties of the sound in the vicinity of points in time where there is a rapid change in spectrum. An example of such a change is shown in the top left of Figure 8.1; the spectrum close to the onset of /b/ is shown for three points in time 13 ms apart. The consonants /k/ and /g/ (not illustrated) show a prominent mid-frequency peak, whereas /b/ and /d/ show a more diffuse spread of energy without a prominent peak. The spectrum for /b/ tends to be flat or sloping downwards with increasing frequency, while the spectrum for /d/ tends to slope upwards.

The properties listed above are not the only ones which serve to distinguish different speech sounds; for a more comprehensive review see Fourcin (1979) and Stevens (1983). For all speech sounds no single acoustic feature seems necessary or sufficient for the listener to hear the appropriate speech sound. Rather, we can use more than one acoustic property to signal a phonetic distinction, and the combination of properties which is employed may depend upon the context in which a particular sound segment appears. To extract these properties the listener must be able to follow rapid changes of the sound spectrum, to discriminate between rapid and gradual changes in amplitude and between differences in duration, and to distinguish periodic from aperiodic sounds, even when those sounds last only a few tens of milliseconds.

So far I have described some of the acoustic features which are used to make phonetic distinctions, i.e. which allow the identification of particular speech sounds. However, acoustic patterns varying over longer periods of time are important for conveying the *suprasegmental* features of speech such as intonation patterns. Intonation is primarily conveyed by variations in the rate of vibration of the vocal folds, or equivalently in the fundamental frequency of voiced sounds, often labelled F_o. The corresponding subjective variations in voice pitch convey to the listener information about the overall structure of sentences, indicating phrase boundaries, and marking important words.

The Representation of Speech Sounds in the Normal Auditory Nerve

Chapter 2 has described how simple sounds, such as pure tones, are represented in the auditory nerve. To recap: the frequency of a single sinusoid is represented both by the distribution of activity across the nerve-fibre array (place coding) and by the detailed temporal patterns of discharge within nerve fibres (temporal coding). To a *first approximation* the responses of the auditory nerve to complex stimuli, such as speech, can be predicted from the responses to simple sinusoids, but some exceptions do occur.

Several research groups (e.g. Delgutte, 1982; Sachs *et al.*, 1983) have measured responses of single neurones in the auditory nerve to speech, or speech-like stimuli. Many neurones from the same animal have been sampled, so that the distribution of responses across the array of nerve fibres could be determined. In response to a speech sound a complex pattern of responses is evoked in which some neurones are responding more vigorously than others. The more sound energy falls close to the characteristic frequency (CF) of a neurone, the higher the firing rate of that neurone. We will call the distribution of firing rate as a function of CF the rate-place pattern. It is possible that the properties of speech sounds are coded in this pattern. At low sound levels the major features of the spectrum, such as the frequencies of the lower formants, are preserved in the rate-place pattern. However, at moderate-to-high sound levels, the majority of neurones show saturation; they are responding at their maximum firing rates. When this happens the rate-place pattern becomes considerably flatter, and the representation of the formant frequencies is no longer preserved. This may indicate that the rate-place pattern is not of crucial importance for conveying the features of the sound spectrum.

A second way in which features of the sound spectrum are coded is in terms of the temporal patterns of discharge at different CFs. Neural spikes tend to occur at a particular point in time (a particular phase) of the stimulating waveform. This is known as phase locking, and it occurs over a wide range of sound levels, being unaffected by saturation of firing rate at high levels. Thus the timing of the nerve impulses, and particularly the time-intervals between successive impulses, give information about the frequencies in the sound which are most effective in stimulating a given neurone (see Chapter 2 for more details of phase locking). For neurones with CFs close to a formant frequency, the temporal patterns of discharge tend to be synchronised to the formant frequency, provided that the frequency is below about 5 kHz. We may think of the formant as 'capturing' the phase-locking of the neurones over a certain range of CFs. Thus if we sample the patterns of phase-locking as a function of CF, we find that most neurones tend to be synchronised to a formant frequency which lies close to their own CF, and the pattern of phase locking jumps rather abruptly from one formant frequency to another as CF increases. This temporal-place code is much more robust as a function of sound level than the rate-place code. In particular, it is largely unaffected by neural saturation effects.

The coding of the periodicity of voiced sounds, which is related to subjective pitch, is also still a matter of debate. Modern theories of pitch perception suggest that the pitch of a complex tone is extracted in a two-stage process: first the tone is analysed to determine the frequencies of its sinusoidal components, and then the pitch is calculated by some sort of central pattern recogniser (see Moore, 1982, for a review). In principle, the frequencies of the components could be extracted from the rate-place pattern evoked by the complex tone, but Moore, Glasberg and Shailer (1984) have argued that such a code would be inadequate, and that a temporal-place code is probably used. Thus is seems likely that the detailed temporal patterns of discharge as a function of CF are important both for determining timbre (associated with spectral patterns such as formants) and for determining pitch (associated with the periodicity of the sound).

Basic Psychophysics of Electrical Stimulation

One of the most important characteristics of the normal ear is its ability to carry out frequency analysis. When a single implanted electrode is excited, essentially no frequency analysis appears to take place (Shannon, 1983); the different frequency components of the input electrical waveform are not resolved, and hence waveforms can only be distinguished on the basis of differences in their temporal patterning. For low stimulating frequencies, below about 300–500 Hz, changes in frequency can be detected, and are heard as changes in pitch. Presumably this happens because the pitch can be extracted from the pattern of phase locking evoked by the electrical stimulation. However, the ability to detect changes in frequency is much reduced compared to normal hearing; the smallest detectable change in electrical frequency is typically between 5 and 30 per cent for frequencies between 100 and 200 Hz, whereas normally hearing subjects can detect changes of less than one per cent at these frequencies. Furthermore, electrically stimulated patients are relatively insensitive to the exact waveform of the stimulation. For example, if sinusoidal and squarewave stimuli are matched in fundamental frequency, and the magnitude of current is adjusted so that they appear equally loud, then the patient will perceive little or no difference between them. Such stimuli would appear very different from each other if presented in acoustic form to a normal listener.

Although different waveforms can evoke similar percepts, the threshold for detection, and the current at which stimuli become uncomfortably loud, may differ considerably for different types of waveforms. For sinusoidal stimulation the threshold tends to be lowest for very low frequencies, increasing sharply between 100 and 300 Hz, and then flattening off again (Fourcin et al., 1979; Shannon, 1983). The threshold of discomfort varies more slowly with frequency, so that the dynamic range between threshold and discomfort is largest at low frequencies (being typically between 15 and 30 dB) and may be only a few decibels at higher frequencies. When brief current pulses are used as stimuli, the threshold varies only slowly with repetition rate of the pulses. However, the dynamic range tends to be small (between three and six dB) at all repetition rates. Roughly speaking, the threshold for detection seems to be determined by the total charge per cycle

Speech Coding   169

Figure 8.2: Two Patients Tested by the EPI Group with Squarewave Stimuli. See text for explanation.

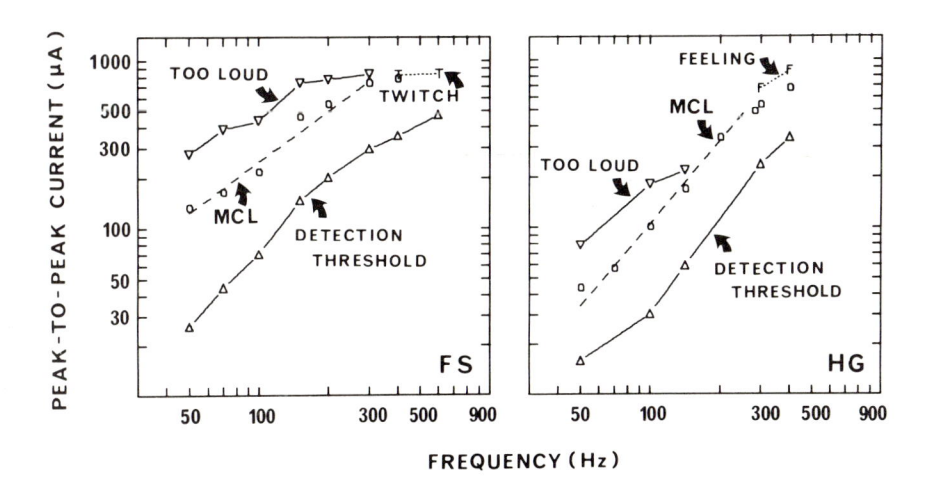

of the stimulus whereas the discomfort level is more related to the peak value of the current. The dynamic range can be maximised by using squarewaves as stimuli. Results for two patients tested by the EPI group with squarewave stimuli are shown in Figure 8.2. Thresholds for detection and discomfort are shown (solid lines) together with the most comfortable level (MCL, broken lines). Each patient was stimulated with an electrode placed on the promontory, outside the cochlea.

The ability to follow changes in the temporal pattern of stimulation is rather good for the majority of patients. For example, temporal gaps only 10 ms in duration can be detected by some patients, and regular periodic stimulation is readily distinguished from aperiodic noise-like stimulation (Fourcin et al., 1979). However, some patients show much reduced temporal acuity, which means that the potential usefulness of an implant will be markedly reduced for them (Hochmair-Desoyer et al., 1984).

Several groups have investigated the percepts associated with the stimulation of individual electrodes in a multi-electrode array within the cochlea. Most have found that different electrodes evoke different percepts, but it is not clear whether the differences should be described as timbre differences (such as differences in 'sharpness') or differences in pitch. Tong et al. (1983) have presented evidence that the percept associated with varying repetition rate on one electrode ('rate-pitch') is different from the percept associated with changing electrodes using a fixed repetition rate ('place-pitch'). The results overall do not fit in with simple conceptions of place and time coding. For example, Shannon (1983) found that the range of pitch sensation associated with changing rate on a single electrode (from 100 to 400 Hz) could be very large (equivalent to a change of over four octaves in an acoustic stimulus according to one patient with previous musical experience) compared with the change in sensation associated with changing electrodes. Furthermore, the pitches perceived did not always vary monotonically with position of the electrodes within the cochlea. Also, the change in pitch associated with change in position within the cochlea was sometimes larger for monopolar stimulation than for bipolar stimulation, even though bipolar stimulation should give a more restricted electrical field within the cochlea.

The experiments with multi-electrode arrays have also shown that there can be interactions between the electrodes; in other words, the electrodes do not act entirely independently. In practice it appears difficult to achieve more than six to eight reasonably independent channels, even for electrodes spaced as widely as possible within the cochlea.

Speech Coding by Multichannel Stimulation to Simulate Normal Auditory-Nerve Activity

Several research groups have implanted multi-electrode arrays with the aim of producing patterns of activity in the auditory nerve which resemble as closely as possible the patterns which would occur in a normal auditory nerve in response to acoustic stimulation (e.g. Banfai et al., 1984; Chouard et al., 1984; Eddington, 1980; Merzenich, 1983). In principle the schemes used by the various groups are similar, but they vary considerably in their implementation. All include a bank of bandpass filters, which split the incoming speech into a number of frequency bands (varying from four to twelve). Either before or after the filter bank there is some means for compressing the dynamic range of speech into the narrow range usable by the implanted patient. The output from each filter determines the electrical signal which will be delivered to a single electrode. In some schemes the analogue waveform at the filter output, or some simple transformation of it, is used to drive the electrode (Eddington, 1980; Merzenich et al., 1984). In other schemes the waveform at the output of the filter is used to trigger current pulses or groups of pulses which are then delivered to the electrode (Banfai et al., 1984; Chouard et al., 1984). A simple example of this type of speech processor, taken from White (1983) is shown in Figure 8.3.

Although in principle these schemes are capable of conveying more information about speech than schemes using single electrodes, in practice they have proved somewhat disappointing. Patients have generally found the devices useful in recognising environmental sounds, and as an aid to lip-reading. However, in most cases the devices have not allowed patients to understand normal conversational speech. It is worth considering some of the reasons for this limited performance. First, in the majority of patients the auditory nerve will have degenerated to a considerable extent. The schemes assume that there are some surviving nerve fibres at each electrode position, but often this will not be the case; there may be only patchy survival of neurones. Unfortunately, there seems to be no reliable test for determining in advance the degree of survival of the auditory nerve.

Secondly, the number of independent channels which can be achieved by multi-

Figure 8.3: One Type of Speech Processor.

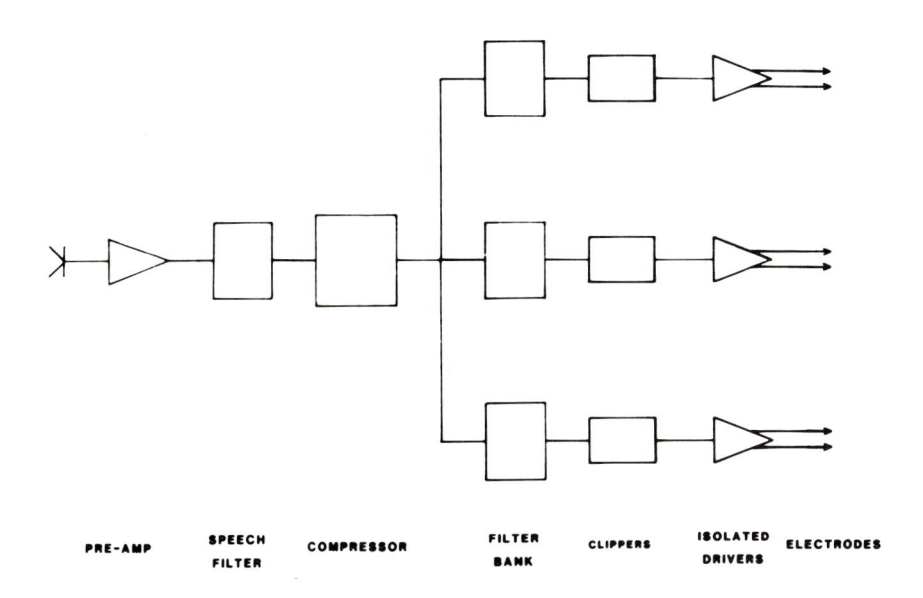

| PRE-AMP | SPEECH FILTER | COMPRESSOR | FILTER BANK | CLIPPERS | ISOLATED DRIVERS | ELECTRODES |

electrode arrays may be insufficient to allow speech comprehension. It appears that a minimum of about eight channels is required for adequate understanding of speech (Flanagan, 1972). While the number of implanted electrodes may be as high as twelve, there are usually significant interactions between channels, so that the number of independent channels is considerably less than eight.

Finally, the temporal patterns of neural firing evoked by electrical stimulation are generally very different from the patterns which would be evoked by acoustic stimulation in the normal ear. This is true of all the schemes, although the degree of the disparity will vary depending upon the exact scheme employed. I have already reviewed evidence suggesting that temporal information is of crucial importance both for the coding of timbre and of pitch. Hence the fact that the temporal patterns evoked by electrical stimulation are grossly abormal may limit the usefulness of the devices. It is not at present clear whether patients can learn to make effective use of the abnormal temporal patterns evoked by electrical stimulation.

In summary, schemes using multichannel electrode systems to simulate normal auditory nerve activity have so far had only limited success. Considerably more research is needed before we can determine the extent to which this limited success reflects inadequacies in the particular devices used as opposed to fundamental limitations imposed by degeneration of the auditory nerve, current spread between channels and inadequate temporal coding. Even if the performance of these devices is improved, it seems likely that only a limited proportion of patients will be able to benefit from them.

172 *Speech Coding*

Figure 8.4: Block Diagram of Sound Processor of House Group.

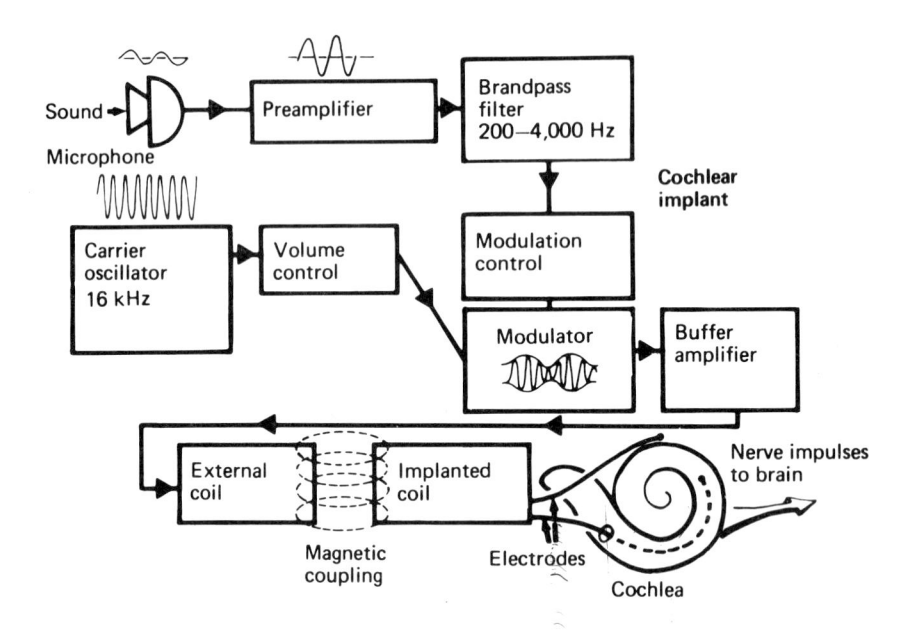

Speech Coding by Analogue Transformations of the Speech Waveform

In this method of coding, the speech waveform itself, or some relatively direct transformation of it, is used to drive the implanted electrode. Usually the method has been used with a single implanted electrode, although sometimes several electrodes have been implanted, and they have either been driven in parallel or the 'best' one has been selected.

The House group (House, 1976) has developed a sound processor based on amplitude modulation of a high-frequency sinusoid. A block diagram of the device is shown in Figure 8.4, taken from Edgerton *et al.* (1984). Sound picked up by a microphone is amplified and passed through a filter which attenuates frequencies outside the range 200–4,000 Hz. This filtered speech is then used to modulate the amplitude of a 16 kHz sinusoidal carrier wave, and this modulated signal is transmitted to the implanted electrode. The modulation device behaves in a nonlinear way, and at sound levels above about 70 dB SPL the modulator produces only a series of rectangular bursts of the 16 kHz carrier, with 'silent' intervals between. There seems to be no particular theoretical rationale for this system; it has simply been found empirically to work reasonably well for the majority of patients. The principal benefits are that the device is useful as an aid to lip-reading, and it allows the identification of certain environmental sounds; it does not allow speech comprehension without lip-reading. This device has been used with more patients than any other system; over 200 deaf adults and 27 children

Figure 8.5: Block Diagram of Speech Processor of Vienna Group.

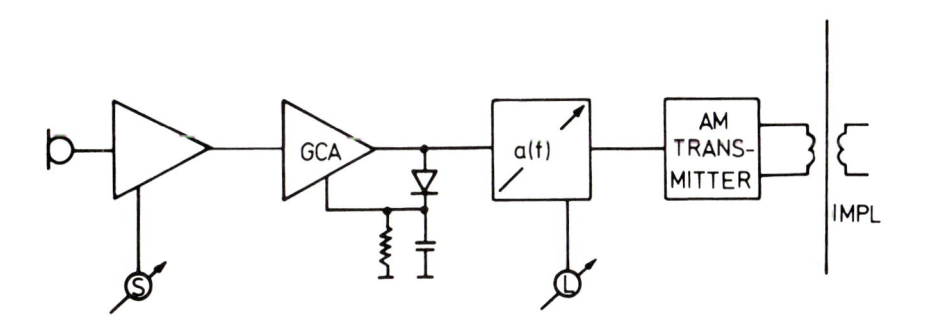

have been implanted with it (Edgerton *et al.*, 1984).

The Vienna group has also used a method of analogue stimulation (Hochmair-Desoyer *et al.*, 1980). A block diagram of their speech processor is shown in Figure 8.5, taken from Hochmair and Hochmair-Desoyer (1983). The signal picked up by a microphone is amplified, and compression of dynamic range is achieved by a gain-controlled amplifier. The compressed signal is then passed through an equalisation network which adjusts the frequency response so that equal loudness at the most comfortable level is achieved with a constant voltage output from the microphone, for frequencies between 100 and 4,000 Hz. This network is adjusted individually for each patient, and the adjustment is reported to be critical for achieving good results (Hochmair and Hochmair-Desoyer, 1983). Finally, the output of the equalisation network is transmitted to an implanted electrode, which may be either within the cochlea, or placed externally to the cochlea, on the round window. More details are given in Chapter 10.

As with most cochlear implants, the majority of patients find the device useful for the recognition of environmental sounds and as an aid to lip-reading. However, some patients have been reported to achieve significant levels of speech understanding without lip-reading (Burian *et al.*, 1984). It is not at present clear why some patients do so much better than others; there is no obvious relationship between benefit and factors such as number of years of deafness, aetiology, age, or electrode position. However, speech discrimination scores do show a correlation with temporal resolution as measured psychophysically (Hochmair-Desoyer *et al.*, 1984).

There are two principal difficulties with schemes based on analogue stimulation. First, it is difficult to determine exactly what information about speech the patient is getting. As discussed earlier, there are generally multiple acoustic cues associated with any given speech sound. The analogue stimulation schemes attempt to 'squeeze' all of the acoustic cues (i.e. the whole of the speech) into a single channel, in the hope that the brain will somehow be able to disentangle the information. It seems likely that in fact the patient will only be able to extract a very limited proportion of the information available in the electrical signal, but it is difficult to determine exactly what sort of information is extracted. This means that there is no well-defined procedure for changing the device to produce further improvements. The approach has to be 'suck it and see'!

The second difficulty is a practical one. In everyday life the patient will often be trying to understand speech in the presence of background noise. In a normal ear the frequency selectivity of the cochlea plays a major role in separating desired signals from background noise. With a single electrode there is essentially no frequency selectivity; signals can be discriminated only on the basis of their time pattern. In schemes using analogue stimulation, any background noise will be processed along with the desired speech, and presented to the implanted electrode. This will severely limit the usefulness of the device in noisy situations, since the patient cannot separate the speech from the background noise.

In summary, schemes based on analogue stimulation seem to give comparable, and, in exceptional cases, possibly superior performance to schemes using multiple electrodes to simulate normal auditory nerve activity. However, the schemes do not have a clear theoretical basis, which makes it difficult to plan future improvements, or to understand individual differences. The effectiveness of the devices is severely reduced by moderate levels of background noise.

Speech Coding by Extraction and Presentation of Speech Patterns

The approach adopted by my own research group, the EPI group, is based on the extraction of simple features or patterns from speech, thus considerably simplifying the information in the speech. The extracted patterns can be transformed in various ways, so that when presented in electrical form they are matched to the patient's perceptual abilities. The electrical signal is applied to a single electrode placed on the surface of the cochlea; hence the name of our group — External Pattern Input (Douek *et al.*, 1977; Fourcin *et al.*, 1979, 1983).

We have worked on the assumption that the electrical stimulation is to be used primarily as an aid to lip-reading, and the speech processor is designed with that goal in mind; the information supplied by the processor is *complementary* to that visible on the face. The acoustical features of the spectrum of speech in the middle-to-high frequency region are quite well correlated with the visible positioning and movements of the tongue, lips and jaw. Hence there is little point in trying to convey those features via electrical stimulation. However, visible information about the activity of the vocal cords is almost completely lacking. Thus the feature of voicing, which as we have seen is important for distinguishing different speech sounds, cannot be determined by looking at the face. For example, the words 'bat' and 'pat' look identical to the lip-reader. The main difference between them is that vibration of the vocal cords starts at about the same time as the lips start to move apart in the word 'bat', but occurs after a certain time delay in the word 'pat'. Providing information about voicing, via electrical stimulation, makes it possible for the lip-reader to distinguish the sounds, and hence produces marked

Speech Coding 175

Figure 8.6: Block Diagram of Speech Processor of EPI Group.

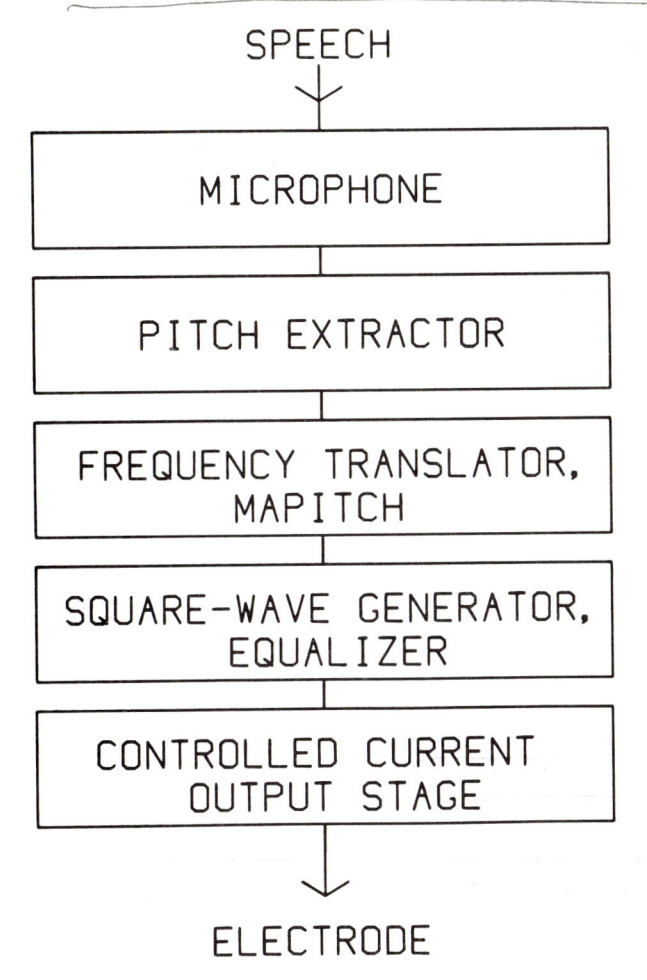

```
              SPEECH
                ↓
         ┌──────────────┐
         │  MICROPHONE  │
         └──────────────┘
                │
         ┌──────────────────┐
         │ PITCH EXTRACTOR  │
         └──────────────────┘
                │
         ┌─────────────────────────┐
         │ FREQUENCY TRANSLATOR,   │
         │       MAPITCH           │
         └─────────────────────────┘
                │
         ┌─────────────────────────┐
         │ SQUARE-WAVE GENERATOR,  │
         │       EQUALIZER         │
         └─────────────────────────┘
                │
         ┌─────────────────────────┐
         │  CONTROLLED CURRENT     │
         │     OUTPUT STAGE        │
         └─────────────────────────┘
                ↓
             ELECTRODE
```

improvements in the accuracy of lip-reading.

The intonation patterns associated with variations in voice fundamental frequency are also invisible to the lip-reader. The provision of information about voice frequency, via electrical stimulation, can produce marked improvements in the speed of lip-reading connected discourse (Moore *et al.*, 1984a, b). Hence we have concentrated on the provision of voicing information, and on its presentation in a form which is as clear as possible for the electrically stimulated patient. It is worth noting that some of the coding schemes described in the previous two sections do not effectively convey voicing information, and in those that do convey voicing this has been almost an accident of the design rather than a deliberate design strategy.

A block diagram of our speech processor is given in Figure 8.6. The first stage in our speech processor is a device which extracts the fundamental frequency of

176   *Speech Coding*

Figure 8.7: Results of a Connected-discourse Tracking Task. See text for explanation.

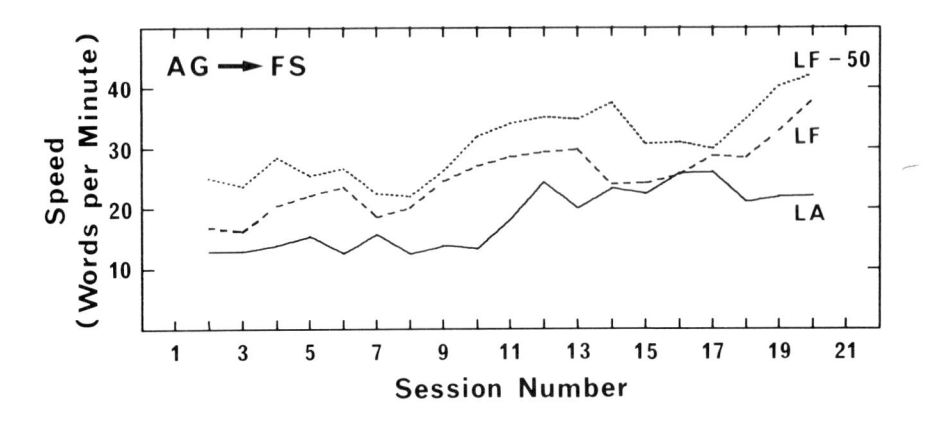

voiced speech sounds — a so-called 'pitch-extractor' (Howard and Fourcin, 1983). This device gives out a single pulse for each period of vocal cord vibration. For male voices these pulses are transformed to squarewaves of the same rate, and these squarewaves are delivered to the electrode via a constant-current stimulator. Squarewaves are used since, as described earlier, they give a maximum dynamic range between threshold and discomfort. The amplitude of the squarewaves (i.e. the peak to peak current) is increased with increasing frequency, so as to keep the stimulation close to the most comfortable level (Moore *et al.*, 1984a; see also Figure 8.2). For male voices the fundamental frequency rarely exceeds 300 Hz, so that the stimulation always falls in the frequency range where the patients are able to detect changes in frequency, and hear them as changes in pitch (see the section on Basic Psychophysics of Electrical Stimulation). Hence there is an intrinsic match between the stimulus and the perceptual abilities of the patients. For the voices of women and children, however, the fundamental frequency often exceeds 300 Hz, thus falling outside the range where discrimination is good. To deal with this our speech processor includes an option called MAPITCH, which allows the fundamental frequency range of the speaker's voice to be mapped into the range optimum for the patient. At present it is operated by a three-position switch. In position A (male), the fundamental frequency is unaltered. In position B (female), 50 Hz is subtracted from the fundamental frequency. In position C (child), 80 Hz is subtracted from the fundamental frequency.

An example of the usefulness of the MAPITCH facility is given in Figure 8.7. It shows the results of a connected-discourse tracking task, in which the patient is required to repeat back everything said by the talker, in this case a woman with a fairly high-pitched voice. Performance is assessed as speed of lip-reading in words per minute, measured over a five minute session, and plotted as a function of session number. The solid curve shows performance with lip-reading alone (LA).

Speech Coding

The dashed curve shows that performance is improved somewhat by the addition of an electrical signal synchronised to the fundamental frequency of the speaker's voice (condition LF). However, performance improves still more when MAPITCH is used to subtract 50 Hz from the fundamental frequency of the speaker's voice (dotted line, labelled LF-50). Relative to lip-reading alone, the mean improvement using unshifted fundamental frequency was 36.5 per cent, and the improvement using MAPITCH was 65.4 per cent.

It should be emphasised that the transformation of speech patterns in this way is readily possible once the patterns have been extracted from the speech. However it is not possible in schemes which use direct analogue transformations of the speech waveform. A further advantage of the pattern-extraction approach is that the hardware performing the 'pitch extraction' can operate successfully even in the presence of moderate levels of background noise. The signal delivered to the patient is noise free. In this way the electronic circuitry can replace some of the analysing capacity which is missing in the electrically stimulated ear, and the range of conditions under which the device can be used is considerably extended.

The EPI group has concentrated on single-channel stimulation applied externally to the cochlea. This approach is conservative, minimising the degree of surgical intervention required, and minimising the possiblity of damage to the cochlea. It is probably capable of providing significant benefit for the majority of candidates for a cochlear implant. However, in some cases it does seem possible to convey more information using a multiple-electrode array within the cochlea. The Australian group (Clark, Tong and Dowell, 1983; Tong et al., 1983) has adopted a pattern-extraction approach, like that of the EPI group, but using an array of ten or more electrodes placed within the cochlea. Like the EPI group, the fundamental frequency of the speaker's voice is conveyed by the rate of stimulation (in the form of biphasic current pulses) applied to a single electrode. Only one electrode is excited at a time. The position of the dominant mid-frequency peak in the sound spectrum (corresponding roughly to the second formant of speech sounds) determines which electrode will be stimulated. More details are given in Chapter 11. Initial results indicate that multiple-channel stimulation may give better speech understanding than single-channel stimulation in a particular individual, although it is not yet clear whether understanding of everyday speech without lip-reading will be possible (Clark et al., 1983).

General Conclusions

We have seen that many different schemes for speech processing and coding have been devised. Some of these schemes are based on sound theoretical ideas, while others have a more empirical flavour. In any case, the results are not always in accord with theoretical expectations, and individual differences between patients are striking. It seems likely that no single scheme will turn out to be the 'best'; rather, different schemes will suit different patients. A major difficulty lies in deciding what form of implant will be most suitable for any particular patient.

Speech Coding

In the meantime, we should realise that research on speech coding is actively proceeding, and that the devices presently available do not represent the limits of what can be achieved.

Acknowledgements

The EPI group is based at the Department of Phonetics and Linguistics, University College London; Guy's Hospital London; and the Department of Experimental Psychology, University of Cambridge. The work of the EPI group has been supported primarily by the Medical Research Council of the United Kingdom. I am grateful to Stuart Rosen and Adrian Fourcin for their comments on an earlier version of this chapter.

References

Banfai, P., Hortmann, G., Karczag, A., Kubik, S. and Wustrow, F. (1984) in W.D. Keidel and P. Finkenzeller (eds.), *Cochlear Implants in Clinical Use*, Karger, Basel

Burian, K., Eisenwort, B., Hochmair, E.S. and Hochmair-Desoyer, I.J. (1984) in W.D. Keidel and P. Finkenzeller (eds.), *Cochlear Implants in Clinical Use*, Karger, Basel

Chouard, C.H,. Fugain, C., Meyer, B., Lacombe, H. and Jegu, D. (1984) in W.D. Keidel and P. Finkenzeller (eds.), *Cochlear Implants in Clinical Use*, Karger, Basel

Clark, G.M., Tong, Y.C. and Dowell, R.C. (1983) in C.W. Parkins and S.W. Anderson (eds.), *Cochlear Prostheses — An International Symposium, Ann. NY Acad. Sci.*, 405

Delgutte, B. (1982) in R. Carlson and B. Granstrom (eds.), *The Representation of Speech in the Peripheral Auditory System*, Elsevier, Amsterdam

Douek, E.E., Fourcin, A.J., Moore, B.C.J. and Clarke, G.P. (1977) *Proc. R. Soc. Med.*, 70, 379–83

Eddington, D.K. (1980) *J. Acoust. Soc. Am.*, 68, 885–91

Edgerton, B.J., House, W.F., Brimacombe, J.A. and Eisenberg, L.S. (1984) in W.D. Keidel and P. Finkenzeller (eds.), *Cochlear Implants in Clinical Use*, Karger, Basel

Flanagan, J.C. (1972) *Speech Analysis*, Springer-Verlag, Berlin

Fourcin, A.J. (1979) in H.A. Beagley (ed.), *Auditory Investigation: the Scientific and Technological Basis*, Clarendon, Oxford

——, Douek, E.E., Moore, B.C.J., Rosen, S., Walliker, J.R., Howard, D.M., Abberton, E. and Frampton, S.L. (1983) in C.W. Parkins and S.W. Anderson (eds.), *Cochlear Prostheses — An International Symposium, Ann. NY Acad. Sci.*, 405

——, Rosen, S.M., Moore, B.C.J., Douek, E.E., Clarke, G.P., Dodson, H. and Bannister, L.H. (1979) *Br. J. Audiol.*, 13, 85–107

Hochmair, E.S. and Hochmair-Desoyer, I.J. (1983) in C.W. Parkins and S.W. Anderson (eds.), *Cochlear Prostheses — An International Symposium, Ann. NY Acad. Sci.*, 405

Hochmair-Desoyer, E.J., Hochmair, E.S. and Burian, K. (1980) *Arch. Otolaryngol.*, 229, 81–98

Hochmair-Desoyer, I.J., Hochmair, E.S. and Stiglbrunner, H.K. (1984) in R.A. Schindler (ed.), *10th Anniversary Conference on Cochlear Implants — An International Symposium*, Raven Press, New York

House, W.F. (1976) *Ann. Otol. Rhinol. Laryngol.*, 85, Suppl. 27

Howard, D.M. and Fourcin, A.J. (1983) *Electron. Lett.*, 19, 776–7

Merzenich, M.M. (1983) in C.W. Parkins and S.W. Anderson (eds.), *Cochlear Prostheses — An International Symposium, Ann. NY Acad. Sci.*, 405

——, Rebscher, S.J., Loeb, G.E., Byers, C.L. and Schindler, R.A. (1984) in W.D. Keidel and P. Finkenzeller (eds.), *Cochlear Implants in Clinical Use*, Karger, Basel

Moore, B.C.J. (1982) *An Introduction to the Psychology of Hearing*, 2nd edn, Academic Press, London

——, Douek, E.E., Fourcin, A.J., Rosen, S.M., Walliker, J.R., Howard, D.M., Abberton, E. and Frampton, S. (1984a) in W.D. Keidel and P. Finkenzeller (eds.), *Cochlear Implants in Clinical Use*, Karger, Basel

——, Fourcin, A.J., Rosen, S., Walliker, J.R., Howard, D.M., Abberton, E., Douek, E.E. and Frampton, S. (1984b) in R.A. Schindler (ed.), *10th Anniversary Conference on Cochlear Implants — An International Symposium*, Raven Press, New York

——, Glasberg, B.R. and Shailer, M.J. (1984) *J. Acoust. Soc. Am.*, 75, 550–61

Sachs, M.B., Young, E.D. and Miller, M.I. (1983) in C.W. Parkins and S. Anderson (eds.), *Cochlear Prostheses — An International Symposium, Ann. NY Acad. Sci.*, 405

Shannon, R.V. (1983) *Hearing Res.*, 11, 157–89

Stevens, K.N. (1983) in C.W. Parkins and S. Anderson (eds.), *Cochlear Prostheses — An International Symposium, Ann. NY Acad. Sci.*, 405

Stevens, K.N. and Blumstein, S.E. (1981) in P.D. Eimas and J.L. Miller (eds.), *Perspectives on the Study of Speech*, Laurence Erlbaum, New Jersey

Tong, Y.C., Blamey, P.J., Dowell, R.C. and Clark, G.M. (1983) *J. Acoust. Soc. Am.*, 74, 73–80

White, M.W. (1983) in C.W. Parkins and S.W. Anderson (eds.), *Cochlear Prostheses — An International Symposium, Ann. NY Acad. Sci.*, 405

9 THE RESULTS FROM VARIOUS VIEWPOINTS

John Ballantyne

Introduction

Most of the information currently available about the results of cochlear implantation has been derived from intracochlear stimulation with single electrodes of adults whose deafness has been acquired after the development of normal speech and language.

In October 1977 it was my privilege to visit from Britain, on behalf of the Department of Health and Social Security, three centres in California which were involved in cochlear implant programmes: with me were Professor E.F. Evans, of the Department of Communication and Neuroscience in the University of Keele, and Mr Andrew Morrison, another otologist from the London Hospital. Our report to the Department was published in the following year (Ballantyne *et al.*, 1978) and it is interesting to look at the results as we then interpreted them and to compare them with subsequent developments.

The three centres were in Los Angeles, San Francisco and Stanford. At that time, 22 patients had been implanted with single-channel electrodes in Los Angeles, seven patients had received bipolar single-channel implants in San Francisco, and three had been implanted with multichannel systems in Stanford. We met five of the patients in Los Angeles, two in San Francisco and one in Stanford; and we concluded that cochlear implants had brought demonstrable benefits to a number of totally deaf adults.

Psychological Effect

Perhaps the most consistent benefit claimed for the implant was the release from total auditory abandonment. As one patient said: 'It's the feeling of not being isolated'; and another commented that it had taken her 'out of total silence'. Furthermore, all the patients who were satisfied with their implants were convinced that the sensation which they experienced was one of 'real sound'.

Identification of Environmental Sounds

There was a greater awareness of some important environmental sounds, including such warning sounds as bells and traffic noise, and with practice it was possible to identify them, and to recognise familiar voices.

Effect on Lip-Reading

When activated, the implant may act as an aid to lip-reading, with an improvement in speech scores and a reduction in the tension and effort involved in it. One of the patients seen in San Francisco claimed that, with the implant, there had been a marked improvement in his lip-reading ability (which was very poor without the implant), especially in his ability to distinguish /b/, /t/ and /p/.

Effect on Patients' Speech

In many cases there is an improvement in the intonation, articulation and volume control of the implanted subject's speech: in three of the five patients seen in Los Angeles, these were noticeably better than one expects to hear usually in totally deaf adults, and in two of them intonation and articulation were excellent.

Effect on Tinnitus

A diminution of, or relief from, tinnitus occurred in some cases and two of the patients whom we saw in Los Angeles had in fact lost their tinnitus entirely, both of them (interestingly) about 1.5 months after the surgery.

Effect on Speech Discrimination

Although electrical stimulation has produced sensations of 'real sound' in several subjects, none of the sounds experienced with such stimulation has ever been exactly the same as those experienced by the subjects before they became deaf.

Furthermore, no single-channel device alone has conveyed adequate discrimination of speech sounds; nor can it be expected to do so. Whether or not multi-channel devices will be able to transmit such information, remains to be seen. This is discussed later.

Despite the obvious shortcomings of single-channel devices, they have enabled many patients to detect some of the prosodic features of speech, such as duration, rhythm and intonation.

Bilger and his colleagues in Pittsburgh (Bilger *et al.*, 1977) carried out intensive tests on 13 patients who had been implanted in Los Angeles and San Francisco, and their conclusions were much the same as our own.

Subsequent independent visits to two of the Californian centres and to others led us to revise our earlier report, and we sent an updated report to the Department of Health in 1982 (Ballantyne *et al.*, 1982). Two rather striking observations followed visits to Los Angeles, by Professor Evans in November 1979 and Mr Morrison in February 1981.

In the first of these, the discriminative ability of a sample of postlingually deaf users of cochlear implants had been examined, and the scores obtained with the implants had been compared with the scores obtained by the same subjects with hearing aids: after several months of training, the scores obtained with the implants were significantly better than those obtained with hearing aids.

The second observation was that, among patients being stimulated regularly with the implants, 80 per cent of those with tinnitus obtained significant relief from this symptom.

It should be emphasised that the results of implantation reported up to that point had been obtained from a limited number of centres in California, mainly with single-channel stimulation, and that essentially they were subjective.

However, many other centres in various parts of the world have become involved with electrical stimulation of the cochlea, and many new approaches (e.g.

multichannel stimulation and extracochlear stimulation) have been used. Furthermore, much more sophisticated information about the results of electrical stimulation of the cochlea has now been obtained from audiological, clinical and histological studies, both in experimental animals and in man.

Audiological Results of Electrical Stimulation

Effects on Responses to Electrically Generated Tones

Engelmann *et al.* (1981) in Oklahoma City assessed the responses of nine implanted patients to stimulation by narrow band noise, through hearing aids and through single-channel intracochlear implants.

The threshold responses to pure tone air conduction audiometry were recorded and analysed. The mean threshold in the frequency range between 500 Hz and 3,000 Hz was 114 dB (Figure 9.1). Pulsed narrow bands of noise, centred at octave and mid-octave intervals from 250–8,000 Hz, were used as test signals for monitoring the free-field thresholds during the testing of hearing aids *before surgery* (in seven of the nine patients) and of the cochlear implants (in all the patients) *after* completion of a programme of *rehabilitation*.

When tested with hearing aids, two of the seven patients obtained no response at all at levels (in the free field) which placed the aid's maximum power output into saturation. (The mean thresholds are shown by the open circles.) When the cochlear implants were used (solid circles), all the patients were able to detect the narrow band noise signals at all the frequencies tested.

In comparing the threshold response obtained during the use of the cochlear implants with those obtained by the use of the hearing aids, the sensitivity with the implants averaged 15.7 dB better than with the hearing aids, only one patient showing a poorer threshold response with the implant than with a hearing aid.

In a report (Hough *et al.*, 1982) on 16 patients implanted in the same department, these results were essentially confirmed.

Effects on Discrimination of Complex Sounds

The same investigators (Engelmann *et al.*, 1981) have studied the responses of eight patients to environmental sounds and to speech sounds, comparing the results obtained with hearing aids and with cochlear implants.

These subjects consisted of three of the first four recipients of implants (Group I) — the test not being available before surgery for the fourth patient — and five others (Group II).

Environmental Sounds. The sounds used in these tests were those devised by the Hearing Rehabilitation Research Center (HRRC) in Los Angeles. These consist of several lists, each containing five environmental sounds: for example, mooing of cow; thunder; vacuum cleaner; person whistling; hammering. The subject is asked to listen to a recorded sound and to select the correct one from the list.

The mean scores (Figure 9.2) achieved by the use of a cochlear implant (76.7

Figure 9.1: Mean Thresholds for Implanted Ear.

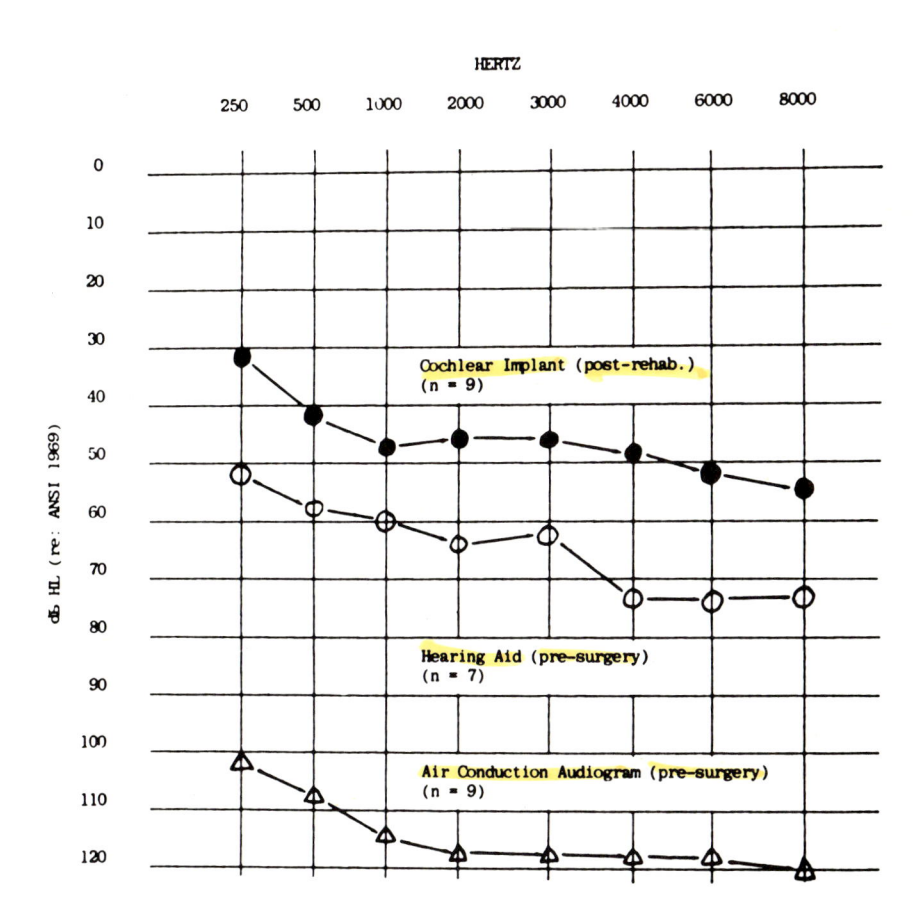

Source: Courtesy Dr J.V.D. Hough and the editor of *The Laryngoscope*.

per cent in Group I and 67 per cent in Group II) were significantly better than those obtained by the use of a hearing aid (45.6 per cent and 14 per cent respectively, in Groups I and II).

In their later study (Hough *et al.*, 1982), it was shown that subjects' responses to environmental sounds continued to improve up to six months after surgery, with an average improvement of 35 per cent rehabilitation.

Speech Sounds. The five patients in Group II implanted in Oklahoma (Englemann *et al.*, 1981) were tested for word recognition and stress recognition. The test used was the MTS Test (M = monosyllables; T = trochees, e.g. chicken, doctor; S = spondees, e.g. baseball, toothpaste).

184   *The Results*

Figure 9.2: Mean Scores from HRRC Environmental Sounds Test for Inner Ear.

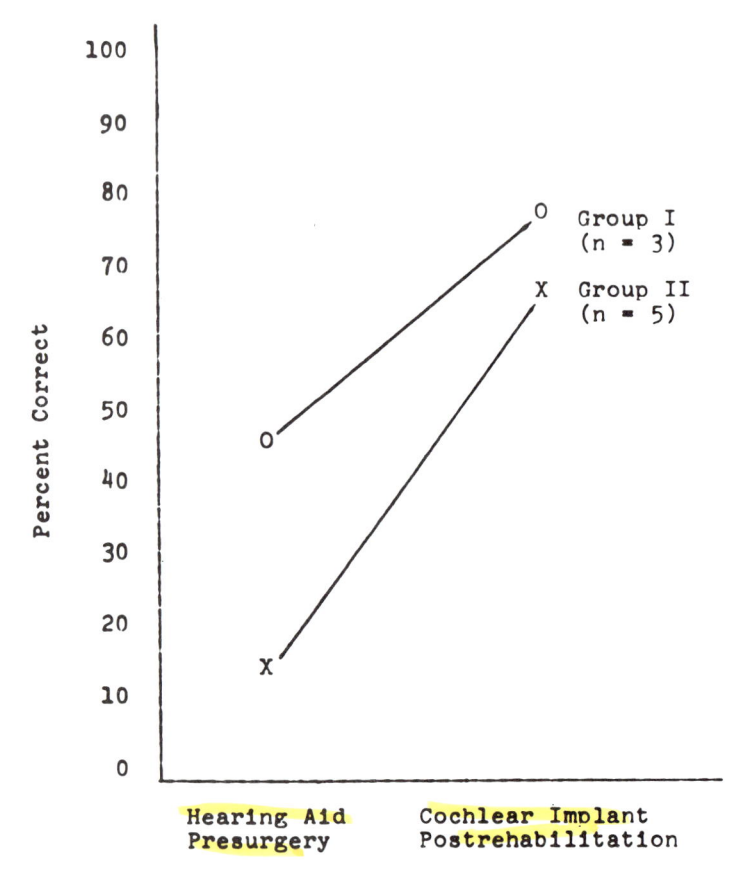

```
100
 90
 80                          O    Group I
 70                               (n = 3)
                             X    Group II
 60                               (n = 5)
 50
    O
 40
 30
 20
    X
 10
  0
      Hearing Aid    Cochlear Implant
      Presurgery     Postrehabilitation
```

Percent Correct

Source: Courtesy Dr J.V.D. Hough and the editor of *The Laryngoscope*.

The patient is allowed to look at the list of words and he is asked to respond after each word has been presented. Two separate scores are made: one for understanding words correctly; one for recognising the correct stress pattern (Hough *et al.*, 1982).

The responses of these five patients are shown in Figure 9.3, which shows that their performance, both for word recognition and for stress recognition, was significantly better with the cochlear implant *after rehabilitation* than with a hearing aid *before surgery*. The mean scores with the implant (of 43.3 per cent for word recognition and 83.3 per cent for stress recognition) were much better than the mean scores with a hearing aid (of 10 per cent for word recognition and 30.8 per cent for stress recognition).

Stress recognition continues to improve even a year after surgery, and this improvement permits a greater recognition of the thought content of words when

The Results 185

Figure 9.3: Mean Scores from Monosyllable, Trochee, Spondee (MTS) Test for Implanted Ear.

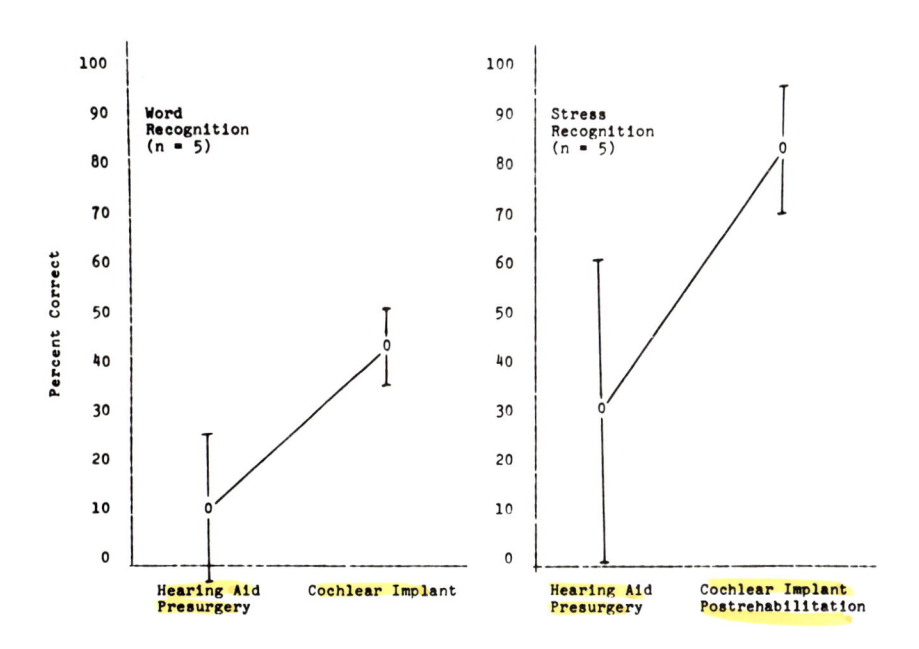

Source: Courtesy Dr J.V.D. Hough and the editor of *The Laryngoscope*.

applied to the augmentation of lip-reading skills.

It should be emphasised again that, in all these audiological tests, the responses of implanted patients after a programme of rehabilitation are being compared with those obtained by the same patients with hearing aids, but without the same intensive training.

Effects on Lip-Reading

Improvement in lip-reading ability is one of the major gains to be obtained by combining visual cues with the limited sound cues so far provided by electrical stimulation of the cochlea. Indeed, many recipients have regarded this as the main benefit of an implant.

The Oklahoma group (Hough *et al.*, 1982) have reported an impressive gain of 35 per cent in conversational cues, after several months of rehabilitation, from the use of electrical stimulation combined with lip-reading.

It is interesting that, when lip-reading skills were tested after only one week of active stimulation, most of the patients found the new sound cues to be a distraction to their lip-reading, and the scores actually declined in some. It is of further interest that, after a period of rehabilitation, these patients obtained much higher scores *even without the use of the stimulator* (Englemann et al., 1981).

It may be that some of the lip-reading skills acquired through bi-sensory learning are retained, even after the acoustic cues have been eliminated; but this observation also leads one to question to what extent the improvement was due to the stimulation and to what extent to the programme of rehabilitation; and also to ask whether hearing aids might have produced similar benefits after equally intensive training.

Effects on Subjects' Own Speech

Most of the subjects who have been implanted to date with intracochlear devices have been postlingually deafened adults with reasonable qualities of voice and speech. However, several have exhibited harshness of vocal quality and difficulty with controlling the loudness of their voice; others have had abnormalities of inflection and articulation.

These have been largely eliminated by training, but they tend to recur unless the stimulator is activated regularly.

Effects of Using a Cochlear Implant and a Hearing Aid Simultaneously

Of the first 27 patients implanted by the Oklahoma group (Hough et al., 1982), two had worn hearing aids before receiving the implant device and both had received some benefit from them, at least in their awareness of environmental sounds.

Although neither of these subjects showed, in the ear in which they wore the aid, any response to audiometric pure tones at less than 100 dB or to speech at maximum loudness, they both continued to wear it even after they had been implanted in the other ear, which was totally unresponsive to an aid; and although they both preferred the implant to the hearing aid, they both enjoyed using the two instruments simultaneously. This observation could lead to a future extension of indications for an implant.

Histological Changes After Implantation

Several studies have been undertaken to assess the histological changes in the cochlea and auditory nerve of animals following acute and chronic implantation and stimulation; and the temporal bones of one human being who had been implanted bilaterally have also been examined.

Animal Studies

The Coleman Laboratory in San Francisco has carried out extensive studies on implanted cochleas in cats and, even within a few weeks following implantation, they have invariably shown extensive or complete loss of hair cells (and of some supporting cells) in that part of the organ of Corti which was in direct contact with the implant. Less extensive loss of hair cells was observed in other turns of the cochlea (Ballantyne et al., 1978).

In the region of the cochlea containing the implant, there was also some loss of ganglion cells, and in those cases in which the implant had penetrated the cochlear partition, there was extensive neuronal degeneration in the region of penetration.

In longer-term studies, however, it was found that the majority of cochlear nerve fibres and ganglion cells survived for eight months, with survival of some ganglion cells for as long as 2.5 years; the complement of ganglion cells was relatively unimpaired in unimplanted regions. No evidence was found of perilymphatic fistulae, or of acute or chronic labyrinthitis.

Although more recent experiments at the Coleman Laboratory have shown that bone formation can occur with long-term electrical stimulation of intracochlear implants, they have also shown that osteogenesis and further nerve damage occur only with currents which are two–three times the maximum required for practicable operation of the implants. Furthermore, they have demonstrated that the nerve loss is related to damage caused by the insertion and presence of the electrodes rather than to their stimulation.

Several studies in cats (Clark et al., 1975; Clark, 1977; Michelson, 1971; Schindler and Bjorkroth, 1979; Simmons, 1967) have confirmed that implants can induce the formation of a fibrous capsule around the electrode tip, degeneration of the organ of Corti and osteogenesis.

In monkeys, Sutton et al. (1980) observed encapsulation, loss of structure in the organ of Corti and loss of myelinated nerve fibres in the osseous spiral lamina; they also found degeneration of cells in the spiral ganglion. A comparison of the effects of a moulded electrode (designed to fill the scala tympani of the basal turn) with those of a small-diameter electrode (fitting loosely in the scala tympani) showed that the former produced greater damage than the latter; but both of them created pathological changes in the cochlea.

In a more recent study, Sutton and Miller (1983) reported their observations on the effects of free-fitting multi-electrode scala tympani implants on the survival of ganglion cells; and they found that all the implanted monkeys showed loss of ganglion cells in that segment which corresponded to the basal turn of the cochlea, even when the implants had been in place for only one month, and in one animal whose implant had not been stimulated.

Animals implanted for four months or less had, for the most part, 50 per cent or greater survival of ganglion cells in the basal segment, with but a few degenerating cells in the regions serving the middle and apical turns; more prolonged periods of implantation led to greater local loss of ganglion cells at the level of the implant and, to a lesser extent, apical to this region.

Sutton and Miller also demonstrated that implantation may produce *progressive* degeneration in the cochlea so that, for example, 28 months after implantation few healthy ganglion cells were found. As 'acute' degeneration was still taking place at that time, it is a matter for conjecture whether, in the longer term, all the cells in the spiral ganglion might ultimately disappear.

In one monkey which was implanted bilaterally, one cochlea was stimulated electrically but the other was not; there was little or no difference in the degree of degeneration seen in the two ears. This would tend to confirm the view that it is the physical presence of electrodes in the scala tympani rather than their stimulation which causes the pathological changes.

Human Subject

The one human subject whose temporal bones have been examined was a 63-year-old male whose profound deafness was due to acquired syphilis. At the time of his death, a single induction coil had been present in his right ear for three years, multiple (five) electrodes in his left ear for eight years. The changes found in these ears were reported by Johnsson, House and Linthicum in 1979.

In the right ear, in which a single coil had been inserted into the scala tympani at the basal end of the cochlea, supporting elements and numerous nerve fibres were still present in the apical turn, and the scala tympani was normal in shape and appearance; the electrode appeared to have been tolerated reasonably well. In the left ear, which had five electrodes implanted chronically, there were no nerve fibres in the osseous spiral lamina and there was extensive new bone formation in the scala tympani.

In both cochleas, the implants had strayed from their intended courses and entered the scala media, about 17 mm from the opening in the niche of the round window.

In the right ear, there was a dense layer of fibroblasts, tightly surrounding the implant, and some loose connective tissue in the scala tympani, adjacent to the electrode. The maximal damage had occurred in the upper basal turn and only two tiny 'islands' of the organ of Corti remained, each with its small bundle of nerve fibres, apical to the tip of the implant.

In the left ear, the organ of Corti was completely absent and some hydrops was present. The new bone formation, which surrounded the implant throughout its course in the scala tympani, occluded in the scala completely in the lower half of the basal turn.

It seems likely that the membranous walls of the cochlea were ruptured during the insertion of the implant. However, it must be pointed out that the electrodes were implanted in these patients in the relative infancy of cochlear implantation; and Schindler *et al.* (1977) have shown that, provided that there is no direct penetration of the cochlear partition, only the hair cells degenerate, not the nerve fibres. Furthermore they have shown that, in cats with induced pre-existing pathology, the insertion and stimulation of intracochlear electrodes do not produce any further neural degeneration.

Single-channel Versus Multichannel Implants

Most of what has been written so far relates to various results of single-channel intracochlear implantation, but it is generally accepted that true speech discrimination will never be achieved with this type of implant.

In our first report to the Department of Health (Ballantyne et al., 1978), my colleagues and I stated that: 'While multiple channel stimulation provides the only hope for restoring *unaided* intelligibility of speech, it has proved *so far* to be no more effective than single-channel implants, because of the insufficient number and inappropriate location of channels used, and inadequate inter-electrode isolation'.

However, more optimistic results have now been reported which suggest that subjects implanted with multichannel devices may be able to make use of the tonotopic organisation of the cochlea.

The perception of pitch is critically important to the feasibility of artificial hearing by multichannel stimulation, and if the placement of several electrodes does not enable the subject to determine the pitch of the sounds elicited, there can be little hope that multichannel stimulation will ever restore the perception of intelligible speech.

Eddington and his colleagues in Salt Lake City, Utah, in conjunction with Brackmann in Los Angeles (Eddington et al., 1978), have reported the results of multichannel stimulation of five human volunteers: one had been implanted by Dr William House in Los Angeles in 1969; one had been deaf bilaterally since birth; one had been deaf unilaterally for 15 years; and the remaining two had been implanted more recently.

Pitch is detected by the location of the activated electrode in the cochlea (place pitch) and concurrently by the frequency of stimulation (periodicity pitch). Generally speaking, basal electrodes elicit a higher pitch than apical electrodes; and as the frequency of stimulation is increased from 70 Hz to 800 Hz, so the pitch perceived becomes higher.

Place pitch and periodicity pitch were both observed in all five volunteers studied by Eddington *et al.* (1978), and preliminary experiments in one of these subjects with the recognition of tunes showed that he was able to recognise simple melodies with periodicity pitch cues.

A later study by Eddington (1980) provided evidence that the sensations of pitch produced (in one subject) by the activation of individual electrodes (in a six-electrode system) were consistent with their placement in the cochlea, pitch increasing from the apical to the basal electrode. There was also a trend for the sensation of pitch and the 'just noticeable difference' between pitches to increase, between 80 Hz and 500 Hz, when the rate of repetition of the stimulus was increased.

(The subject was also able to discriminate between 'da' and 'ta' with single-channel stimulation, a distinction which is not possible with lip-reading, and Eddington believed that this was probably based on his ability to distinguish voiced from unvoiced speech sounds.)

Clark and Tong (1982), in Melbourne, studied two patients who had been implanted with ten-electrode arrays. Various psychophysical tests were begun four weeks after the surgery and they continued for several months.

With a laboratory-based speech processor, both patients were able to recognise a certain amount of speech when the processor was activated; and when it was used in conjunction with lip-reading, there was a substantial improvement in their scores compared with those obtained by lip-reading alone.

When spondee words were used, the scores achieved by these patients were considerably better than those reported by Bilger *et al.* (1977) for single-channel implants; and when a twelve-consonant test was applied, the *improvement* in scores obtained by these subjects when they used the speech processor in combination with lip-reading (64 per cent), as compared with lip-reading alone (38 per cent), was much greater than those (45 per cent and 43 per cent, respectively) obtained by Fourcin *et al.* (1979) with single-channel extracochlear stimulation.

Not so optimistic are the predictions of Quentin Summerfield (1983), in Nottingham, who has suggested that the spread of current *between* electrodes severely limits the frequency resolution achieved by a multichannel system. 'In effect', he writes, 'many nerve fibres are stimulated by each electrode, frequency selectivity is largely lost and the implant becomes an elongated single-channel device.' Not that this outcome, he argues, is necessarily a bad thing, for the most effective way to ensure that as many functioning neurons as possible are stimulated (when only a few may be functional) is to use a multi-electrode array distributed over a considerable length of the cochlear partition.

Even more serious, perhaps, is the warning of Sutton and Miller (1983) who, from their histological studies in monkeys, have emphasised that a continuing process of degeneration in the structures of the inner ear could result in a system which would be capable of resolving a complex input only to a very limited degree; and this could become a major consideration in the future of multichannel intracochlear implantation.

Intracochlear versus Extracochlear Stimulation

Most of the teams involved in electrical stimulation of cochlear nerve fibres have used electrodes, either single or multiple, implanted inside the cochlea, most often in the scala tympani. However, a team based in London and Cambridge (Douek *et al.*, 1977) has used a non-invasive stimulation with electrodes outside the cochlea, either at the round window or on the promontory; others have followed suit.

Extracochlear stimulation can claim several advantages over intracochlear stimulation: in particular, neither the structures of the middle ear nor those of the inner ear are disturbed; there is minimal risk of infection; and the process can be reversed. It therefore allows for the application of future improvements without any risk of irreversible damage.

So far only single-channel stimulation has been used with this approach, the signal being designed to match both the lip-reading needs of the subject and his restricted auditory ability.

Information about the intonation of speech sounds is carried largely by the subject's ability to perceive differences in pitch. It has been demonstrated that, in some patients at least, single-channel extracochlear stimulation has evoked genuine sensations of pitch, but changes in stimulating frequency are heard as changes in pitch only for stimulating frequencies below about 400–500 Hz (Rosen et al., 1982).

Some subjects have been able to detect *changes* in pitch, the range of frequencies over which such changes can be heard corresponding with the range of fundamental frequencies of the adult human voice. One of the pieces of information contained in the fundamental frequencies of a speaker's voice is whether a question is being asked or a statement is being made: questions tend to be signalled by a rise in the fundamental frequency over the course of an utterance; statements tend to be signalled by falls.

One particular patient was very successful at distinguishing rises from falls, and she was also able to recognise simple musical melodies, reporting that the notes sounded 'in tune'.

She and one other subject also had good temporal acuity, measured by presenting either a single click or a number of clicks, and asking the subject to judge whether one or two sounds were present. Since the discrimination of different frequencies of electrical stimulation depends primarily on the ability to discriminate temporal patterns of nerve impulses, it is reasonable to expect that tests of temporal acuity (or the ability to discriminate temporal patterns) will produce results which correlate with those for frequency discrimination; and in those subjects for whom sufficient results are available, the data have borne out this expectation.

In yet another subject, who had some slight residual hearing in one ear (with losses greater than 90 dB between 1 kHz and 8 kHz), that ear was stimulated acoustically through headphones. Her ability to discriminate different sounds in this was very severely limited, and far worse than she obtained with electrical stimulation of the opposite, totally deaf, ear.

Some subjects have been able to distinguish between voiced and voiceless speech sounds, this ability helping the lip-reader to distinguish sounds which look almost identical on the face (such as 'ba' and 'pa'); and sometimes stress patterns in speech have been detected.

Summary and Conclusions

Theoretically, one would expect a greater dynamic range from intracochlear than from extracochlear stimulation, and more useful information from multichannel than from single-channel stimulation; but the results obtained to date by these different modes of stimulation remain inconclusive.

Every group working with implants — notably in the United States, Europe and Australia — has been able to claim some successes, especially in terms of an awareness of environmental sounds and of facilitation of lip-reading skills; and a number of subjects, by whatever mode of stimulation, have been able in the short term to detect changes in pitch and some of the prosodic features of speech: duration, rhythm and intonation. But the understanding of normal consecutive speech is still a long way off, and the long-term results are far from certain.

Although it is known that an individual with but a few surviving cells can still perform useful discriminations, Otte et al. (1978) have expressed concern about the minimum number of cells required for speech perception.

Varying degrees of damage to the cochlea and its nerve fibres have been reported, both from animal experiments and from examination of the temporal bones of one human subject, following intracochlear implantation; and more widespread damage might be expected from multiple than from single electrodes. No such damage has been found, in animal experiments, following the extracochlear placement and stimulation of electrodes.

Responses to electrical stimulation vary so much from one deaf individual to another that it is to be hoped that a device will soon be designed which will permit comparison, in one and the same ear, of intracochlear with extracochlear stimulation, and of single-channel with multichannel stimulation; and that each of these modes will be compared with preoperative responses to hearing aids and vibro-tactile devices, each with the same programme of rehabilitation.

It may seem that, to someone who has nothing, anything — or almost anything — should be better; but it is of the utmost importance that any potential recipient of a 'bionic ear' should have a realistic attitude to what may be expected of it in the current state of the art, and he should be thoroughly conversant with its limitations.

References

Ballantyne, J.C., Evans, E.F. and Morrison, A.W. (1978) *J. Laryngol. Otol. Suppl., 1*, 1-117
——, —— and —— (1982) *J. Laryngol. Otol., 96*, 811-16
Bilger, R.C., Black, F.O., Myers, E.N., Hopkinson, N.T., Vega, A. and Wolf, R.V. (1977) *Ann. Otol. Rhinol. Laryngol., 86* (Suppl. 38), 1-176
Clark, G.M. (1977) *J. Laryngol. Otol., 91*, 185-98
——, Kranz, H.G., Minas, H. and Nathar, J.M. (1975) *J. Laryngol. Otol., 89*, 495-504
—— and Tong, Y.C. (1982) *Arch. Otolaryngol., 108*, 214-17
Douek, E., Fourcin, A.J., Moore, B.C.J. and Clarke, G.P. (1977) *Proc. R. Soc. Med., 70*, 379-83
Eddington, D.K. (1980) *J. Acoust. Soc. Am., 63*, 885-91
Eddington, D.K., Dobelle, W.H., Brackmann, D.E., Mladejovsky, M.G. and Parkin, J.L. (1978) *Ann. Otol. Rhinol. Laryngol., 87* (Suppl. 53), 1-39
Engelmann, L.R., Waterfall, M. Kathleen and Hough, J.V.D. (1981) *Laryngoscope, 91*, 1821-32
Fourcin, A.J., Rosen, S.M., Moore, B.C., Douek, E.E., Clarke, G.P., Dodson, H. and Bannister, L.H. (1979) *Br. J. Audiol., 13*, 85-107
Hough, J.V.D., McGee, M., Richard, G., Waterfall, M. Kathleen, Dormer, K.J., Guthrey, G., Engelmann, L.R. and Shaefer, Arlene B. (1982) *Laryngoscope, 92*, 863-72
Johnsson, L-G., House, W.F. and Linthicum, F.H. (1979) *Laryngoscope, 89*, 759-62
Michelson, R.P. (1971) *Ann. Otol. Rhinol. Laryngol., 80*, 914-19
Otte, J., Schuknecht, H.F. and Kerr, A.G. (1978) *Laryngoscope, 88*, 1231-46
Rosen, S., Fourcin, A.J., Walliker, J.R., Douek, E.E. and Moore, B.C.J. (1982) in J. Raviv (ed.), *Uses of Computers in Aiding the Disabled*, North-Holland Publishing Co., Amsterdam, pp. 167-84

Schindler, R.A. and Bjorkroth, B. (1979) *Laryngoscope, 89*, 752–8
——, Merzenich, M.M., White, M.W. and Bjorkroth, B. (1977) *Arch. Otolaryngol., 103*, 691–9
Simmons, F.B. (1967) *Laryngoscope, 79*, 171–83
Summerfield, A.Q. (1983) in M.E. Lutman and M.P. Haggard (eds.), *Hearing Science and Hearing Disorders*, Academic Press, London, p. 175
Sutton, D. and Miller, J.M. (1983) *Ann. Otol. Rhinol. Laryngol., 92*, 53–8
Sutton, D., Miller, J.M. and Pfingst, B.E. (1980) *Ann. Otol. Rhinol. Laryngol., 89* (Suppl. 66), 11–14

10 REHABILITATION OF THE COCHLEAR-IMPLANT PATIENT

Brigitte Eisenwort, Karin Brauneis, Kurt Burian

Introduction

Hearing impairment like other handicaps cannot be viewed as an isolated deficit, because it is associated with psychosocial restrictions (Richtberg, 1983). Therefore rehabilitation of implant patients serves two purposes. The greater is on improving audiovisual and auditory speech perception, i.e. helping patients to compensate their hearing deficits. The lesser is to relieve the psychosocial restrictions by helping the patient to cope with his hearing handicap in a positive manner and to acquire purposeful and effective communication. Communication training and counselling achieve this second goal.

Our rehabilitation programme focuses on auditory training (see below). We developed a programme of five stages which is modelled on the process of normal auditory speech perception. In communication training (see below) the patients learn to *use* the auditory speech perception acquired in training. Communication strategies are analysed and new ones proposed for ineffective ones.

Counselling sessions offered to cochlear-implant patients before operation are continued afterwards. Their aim is to facilitate the transition from a world of silence to a world of sound.

Target Population

Hearing people live in a world of environmental sounds and noises. Very early in infancy they acquire an acoustic orientation. Nevertheless, speech is the most important acoustic event for them, because speech is our prime way of communicating. Speech is communicative because it is coded to form words and sentences in a language. As speech possesses an emotional function reflected in paralinguistic features like voice quality, rhythm, accent and intonation (unless these are used linguistically) and a semantically significant function, the contact in communication is a double one, namely on an emotional and on a logically abstract level.

Severe hearing impairment causes a communicative breakdown. To understand a message individuals with impaired hearing have to be more attentive than normally hearing people. Although they pay more attention to understanding, they cannot be sure to have understood correctly, because they must concentrate mainly on the segmental structure of speech and on the words. Therefore, they are not flexible enough to follow the underlying ideas. But the uncertainty of understanding also relates to the emotional level. In everyday communication situations patients with impaired hearing often are not sure whether they have grasped the emotional situation. Uncertainty combined with distrust is the affective ground which breeds suspicion. Affects of this kind impair relaxed and appropriate reactions. Besides, such stress tends to enhance the functional impairment which, in turn, makes reactions increasingly inadequate. This may establish a vicious circle (Richtberg, 1983).

Pre- and Postlingual Deafness

The communicative ability and the psychosocial effect caused by hearing impairment are different in cases of prelingual and postlingual deafness. A poverty of language is one of the main problems of prelingual deafness. Typical deficits include voice problems, articulation errors, poor knowledge of morphological and syntactic rules and reduced vocabulary of their mother tongue. Retarded language competence affects cognitive development.

Cognition is based on concepts which, while not concrete in themselves, have as far as this is possible, a concrete basis. This concrete component of concepts, i.e. the acoustic realisation of the word, does not exist for prelingually deaf children. Therefore, the concepts of prelingually deaf are incomplete with regard to content (Lindner, 1981, pp. 143–4). Because prelingually deaf children cannot understand the affective content of speech found in the paralinguistic features, they often have a poorly developed emotional life and are insensitive to the feelings of others (Richtberg, 1980, p. 23). Reduced social competence of the prelingually deaf may also be the result of their life conditions during childhood and youth.

The postlingually deaf do not face all these problems, except for voice and articulation errors which may occur when auditory feedback has long been missing. Their specific problems mainly result from the psychosocial restrictions caused by their hearing loss. Myklebust (1964) claimed that the following factors played important roles in the life of postlingually deaf people:

(1) more stress in daily life;
(2) dependence on family members in everyday needs;
(3) change of social interactions after the hearing loss;
(4) difficulty in maintaining social interactions dating from the time before hearing loss;
(5) isolation.

Other investigations showed similar results. In a study by Richtberg (1980) postlingually deaf people complained of social isolation and of being heavily weighed down by pain and conflicts.

Psychosomatic complaints, e.g. headache, insomnia, sensitivity to weather and nervous diseases of the heart, were found to be most prominent in postlingual deafness. This is explained by a higher cognitive and affective involvement in everyday orientation. As the psycho-automatic excitation level is increased, psychosomatic diseases become prominent. Whereas prelingual deafness was regarded as a more severe handicap in the past than postlingual deafness, it has become increasingly evident that the two handicaps defy comparison. Therefore,

196 *Rehabilitation*

any rehabilitation programme should be geared to the individual problems of the two groups.

Counselling

Counselling Before Surgery

According to Alpiner (1982, pp. 146–7) there are four basic tools of counselling: information, assessment scales and indices, the environment and the counsellor.

In the first interview we only present information. This information relates to (a) the cochlear implant, its components, the possibilities of wearing a speech processor, how to hide the cable, how to change the batteries, etc.; (b) criteria for patient selection, i.e. patients are informed about criteria regarding residual hearing and lip-reading ability, and preoperative electrical stimulation; (c) operation, duration and risks, hospitalisation time; (d) rehabilitation procedures, auditory training, communication training and counselling, follow-up investigations after 3 and 9 months; and (e) results, speech perception, psychological changes. The patients are given an information leaflet, which explains everything they need to know about the cochlear implant. Then the presurgical tests are performed. If found medically suitable for a cochlear implant patients are introduced to the counselling process.

As assessment scales we use the 'Denver Scale of Communication Function' for postlingually deaf patients. Prelingually deaf patients are requested to fill in a questionnaire which is very similar to the 'Denver Scale', but the items are easier to understand. Care should be taken to make the counselling situation as agreeable as possible for the patient. It is important to provide adequate seating, particularly if patients are accompanied by relatives or friends. Patients should face the counsellor and not be made to look into a light source.

The counselling guidelines we use are based on the theory of counselling developed by Rogers (1951, 1961). The main concept underlying client-centred counselling is that human beings are inherently motivated to grow, improve their existence and realise their maximal potential. This process of growing can be encouraged by a friendly atmosphere.

Three factors characterise the role of the counsellor: (1) empathy; (2) acceptance and (3) self-congruence. We believe that adults with hearing impairment, especially those with cochlear implants, will find the plan of action best suited to them, provided that they are supplied with sufficient information and an atmosphere of trust and acceptance.

Presurgical counselling of postlingually deaf aims at (a) coping with the crisis caused by their hearing loss to the point of accepting their handicap; and (b) overcoming their psychosocial restrictions.

(a) Patients should come to the point of accepting their handicap. Ideal implant candidates have coped with their crisis well enough to look actively for possibilities to compensate their handicap (lip-reading, relaxation training, etc.)

and to organise with other hearing-impaired individuals (Schuchardt, 1980, pp. 94–113).

(b) Patients should learn that overcoming their psychosocial restrictions is not dependent on a cochlear implant. Coping with everyday stress situations can be learned by relaxation training. Problems in the family can be solved through family counselling. Isolation can be overcome by client-centred psychotherapy (Rogers, 1961).

Besides counselling, patients are encouraged to meet other implant patients and ask them about their experiences, to attend lip-reading courses, self-experience groups, and undergo psychotherapy etc., as needed.

Depending on the patient's needs three to five counselling sessions are offered. After these patients should have acquired a more realistic outlook, they should have grasped that they will still be handicapped in spite of their cochlear implant and that their implant can at best help them to communicate more easily in everyday life.

Prelingually deaf individuals have much less realistic expectations of the auditory information transmitted by a cochlear implant than those with postlingual deafness. This has a dual explanation:

(1) As they lack acoustic information of any kind, they cannot know what type of acoustic information the cochlear implant will transmit.
(2) Because of their poverty of language which affects cognition, they have difficulties in understanding their counsellor, even if they are given instructions and explanations in writing.

In our experience, prelingually deaf subjects tend to present one of two extreme attitudes. They are either unmotivated for a cochlear implant, because they are well integrated in the deaf community and do not miss acoustic sensations and their parents or hearing relatives want them to be provided with an implant. Or they are highly motivated because, owing to the complete lack of acoustic and linguistic experience, they harbour entirely unrealistic expectations.

Presurgical counselling of the prelingually deaf aims at (1) acquiring realistic expectations of the auditory information transmitted through the cochlear implant; and (2) making patients aware of problems of social integration in both the groups of hearing and deaf subjects, which they may face.

(1) Patients are told that they will be hard of hearing after implantation and resultant problems are discussed.
(2) Patients are made aware of the problems they may face if their speech comprehension is not good enough for integration in the hearing community, but too good for continued acceptance in the deaf group to which they had previously belonged.

We encourage our prelingually deaf to meet other prelingually deaf subjects wearing implants and to talk to them about their experiences. Prelingually deaf patients in general need more time for counselling than the postlingually deaf.

The counsellor should be trained in communication with patients who have a retarded language competence. Before operation patients should have some idea about what they can expect in terms of auditory information through the implant, and they should be aware of problems of social integration.

Counselling During the Postsurgical Period

Using the counselling guidelines of Rogers (1951, 1961) we continue to help our patients after implantation in coping with their specific problems and with the general problems caused by the introduction or reintroduction to the world of sound.

In general, reintroduction to the acoustic environment of postlingually deaf patients seems to be less problematic than the introduction of prelingually deaf. As a consequence, postlingually deaf patients focus on their psychosocial problems during counselling sessions. Isolation, coping with stress and relational problems are topics many of the postlingually deaf want to discuss. Most of the prelingually deaf patients have major problems with the sounds of the acoustic environment, especially in the first week after implantation. Negative reactions to their new auditory ability by their deaf friends, family members, etc. often also are troubling.

Problems shared by both patient groups are those of frustration with prosthetic hearing, especially if expectations were too high; problems resulting from too many tests during rehabilitation; and problems inherent in the interaction with doctors, audiologists, therapists etc. Patients who come from other cities often complain of being separated from their families and friends for six weeks.

While counselling sessions are offered to all of our patients, they can choose themselves whether or not they want to speak about their problems.

Auditory Training

Auditory Speech Perception in the Hearing and Its Consequence for Auditory Training

Prelingually as well as postlingually deaf adults who are provided with a cochlear implant are in a unique situation in that they have to be introduced or reintroduced to the acoustic environment, especially to auditory perception of speech. This implies that the sequence of confrontation with environmental sounds and especially with linguistic structures, their inherent hierarchy of complexity or the speech material chosen to represent these structures is very important.

The Defects of Word Lists. The literature on auditory training and testing of speech perception in implanted patients shows that most research groups used word lists for rehabilitation which were not selected on the basis of special criteria. These open or closed sets had to be learned by heart by the patients and were rated by tests. The percentage of correct answers was published as speech perception results gathered from an open or closed set (Banfai, 1981; Hochmair-Desoyer *et al.*, 1980). If our goal is to make cochlear implant patients use the available auditory information for speech perception in everyday life, we need an auditory training programme based on what we know about normal speech perception.

The Basis of Perception. Speech perception involves interaction of acoustic-driven and knowledge-driven processes (Cooper, 1983). The former are provided by the acoustic signal and the latter by the listener's competence. Both play an important role, because for the acoustic signal precise comprehension is simply impossible unless the listener receives at least some portion of the signal, whereas without linguistic competence the listener has no expectations about what will follow and cannot segment the speech stream into words.

First we will focus on acoustic-driven processes. Decoding of the speech chain proceeds chronologically from extraction of basic features like voice quality and prosodics to extraction of allophones, phonemes, words, sentences and ideas.

Extraction of time pattern, loudness and frequency from the sound stream is a prerequisite of perceiving linguistic information of a higher order. But it also provides a number of cues about characteristics of the speaker's sex, age, personality, etc. These perceptual judgements occur automatically and do not disrupt the listener's processing of the linguistic content.

Suprasegmental features associated with the acoustic cues of duration, intensity and fundamental voice frequency convey clues to higher-order linguistic structures. Variations in voice frequency, duration and intensity influence the listener's perception of stressed words with greater stress perceived on a syllable associated with higher voice frequency, longer duration and greater intensity (Fry, 1955).

Suprasegmental features also provide many cues to the syntactic structure of an utterance (Liebermann, 1967). For example, the boundaries between major clauses are demarcated by segmental lengthening of the final word and a fall-rise pattern of the fundamental frequency (Cooper and Sorensen, 1981). Sometimes optional pausing serves to demarcate boundaries between major clauses or phrase boundaries within clauses. Variations in fundamental voice frequency are used in many languages (e.g. English–German) to interpret a given utterance as a statement (falling frequency on the last word) or a question (rising on the last word) (Cooper, 1983).

Phonemes are basic units in speech production and perception. Although many authors deny today that speech is processed phoneme by phoneme and argue in favour of units of various sizes depending on the requirement of the communication situation (Neisser, 1967), perception of a certain amount of phonemes is, nevertheless, necessary for word understanding.

Considering that the phonemes of speech occur at a rate of 8 to 10 per second and that many languages have phonemic inventories of 40 to 50 members, it seems more plausible that the presence or absence of acoustic features is perceived (Pickett, 1983). Stevens (1983) argues for some acoustic properties, namely the presence of low-frequency periodicity, of noise or aperiodicity, a high or low amplitude of turbulence noise, an abrupt or gradual rise in amplitude, certain gross characteristics of the spectrum sampled near the release of a consonant, and the relative positions for spectral prominences for vowels, that the listener needs to

200 *Rehabilitation*

distinguish between English phonemes.

Perception of words occurs in this way. Words stored in the memory in terms of patterns of these acoustic properties are recognised by the listener at a particular point in time when one of these properties is present in a word. After a particular pattern of acoustic features is detected in the speech wave during an utterance, the listener checks his lexicon and identifies the word which fits best. In this way subsequent words in the sentence are analysed.

The use of knowledge is very important for perception at all linguistic levels. Cooper (1983) differentiates between pure knowledge resident in long-term memory and short-term contextual information, which includes a combination of acoustic-driven and knowledge-driven sources. First short-term contextual information is used and then the listener relies exclusively on pure knowledge.

Segmentation of the sound stream into words and identification of these words require knowledge of a mental lexicon, which allows the listener to distinguish plausible words from non-words, as well as a variety of linguistic and pragmatic rules. The importance of context for word identification can be explained by the fact the listeners make use of higher-order grammatical context, relying on their implicit knowledge of linguistic rules in guiding their recognition of words.

It seems that the influence of knowledge-driven processes becomes more and more important for higher-order linguistic structures. Perception of sentences and texts is impossible without the use of linguistic knowledge.

Although the process of auditory speech perception is not yet fully understood, training of auditory function should be based on what we know about it.

Figure 10.1 shows the speech perception model underlying our auditory training programme. Figure 10.2 shows the consequence of our auditory speech perception model for the hierarchy of difficulty in auditory training.

Auditory Training Programme

The Training Programme developed at this department consists of gradual exercises designed to accustom the cochlear-implant patient to his new acoustic environment on one hand and on the other to improve his speech.

The patients receive beside the auditory training also a speech training:

Target	Auditory Training	Speech Training
I	Accustoming the patient to the new auditory environment	Accustoming the patient to the sound of his own voice
II	Auditory recognition and differentiation of tones and everyday sounds without visual clues.	Control of own voice (volume and pitch)
III	Using auditory information as support for speech-reading, thereby improving general understanding of speech.	Development or improvement of stress, rhythm and intonation in the patient's spontaneous speech.

| IV | Improvement of speech comprehension via auditory input alone (without speech-reading). Recognition of speech in the presence of background noise. | Improvement of the patient's speech through articulation exercises. Teaching the patient to monitor his own speech (articulation and volume) in specific situations: e.g. background noise, distance from listener. |

Figure 10.1: Auditory Speech Perception.

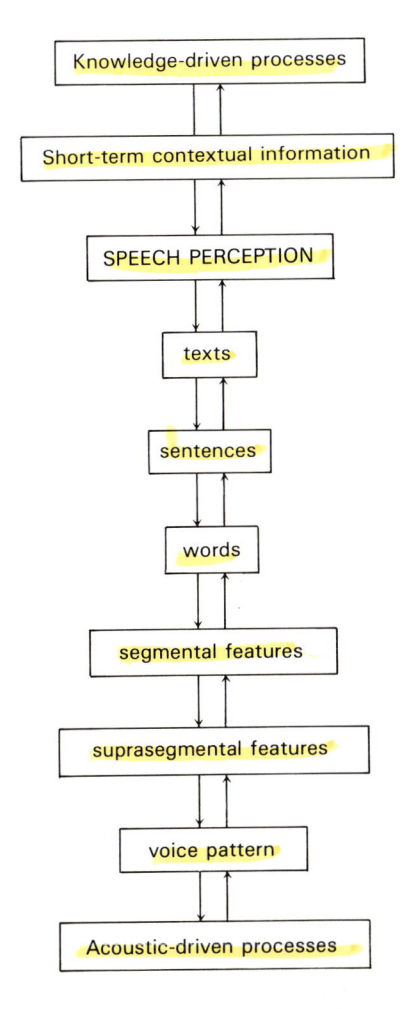

```
        Knowledge-driven processes
                  ↕
       Short-term contextual information
                  ↕
             SPEECH PERCEPTION
                  ↕
                texts
                  ↕
              sentences
                  ↕
                words
                  ↕
           segmental features
                  ↕
         suprasegmental features
                  ↕
             voice pattern
                  ↕
        Acoustic-driven processes
```

Training is commenced immediately after the speech processor has been fitted and adjusted. Training sessions are twice daily over a period of two weeks. Each session lasts 30–60 minutes depending on the patient's concentration span and

202 *Rehabilitation*

Figure 10.2: Stages in Auditory Training.

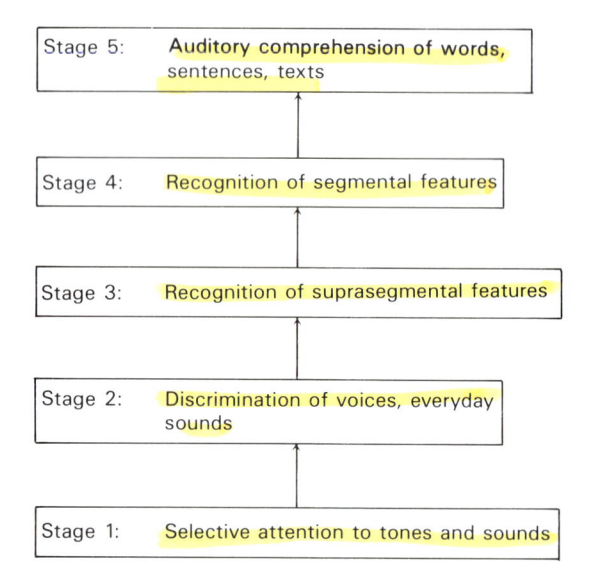

Stage 5:	Auditory comprehension of words, sentences, texts
Stage 4:	Recognition of segmental features
Stage 3:	Recognition of suprasegmental features
Stage 2:	Discrimination of voices, everyday sounds
Stage 1:	Selective attention to tones and sounds

tolerance of acoustic stimuli. After this, training is once a week over at least 18 months. In addition to this the patient gets a home training programme which allows him to do daily exercises.

For those patients for whom it is impossible to attend the weekly training at the clinic, a correspondence course has been developed. But this course requires a trained aid who can work regularly with the patient and also periodic supervision by the therapist.

Each exercise is practised as follows:

(1) Combination of auditory and visual stimuli so that the patient can associate the new auditory impressions with familiar clues.
(2) Repetition of the same exercise with only auditory input in a *quiet* room.
(3) Repetition of the same exercise with only auditory input in the presence of background noise.

The auditory training section is described in Table 10.1.

Immediately after adjustment of the speech processor, three and nine months later an auditory speech test battery (Eisenwort and Benkö, 1983) is used to measure speech perception by lip-reading, electrostimulation alone and lip-reading + electrostimulation, in three linguistic areas, namely (1) recognition of suprasegmental features, (2) recognition of segmental features and (3) auditory-cognitive ability. Besides offering objective evidence of the patient's progress, this also motivates patients for auditory training.

Table 10.1: Auditory Training Programme

I. Selective Attention to Tones and Sounds

Aim	Stimulus	Response
Detection of onset and stop of acoustic stimuli	Tones. Free field pure tone audiometer. 1. BLS[a] 2. ELS[b]	Pt. indicates onset and stop of stimulus by raising his hand.
Recognition of number of units presented	Tones, sounds. Up to 10 presentations, whereby length of stimulus and pauses, as well as frequency and loudness are constantly varied. 1. BLS 2. ELS	Pt. states the number he hears.
Differentiation of temporal aspects	2 tones or sounds which differ in length. Contrast of long/short is gradually reduced. Frequency and loudness are varied. 1. BLS 2. ELS	Pt. states whether the first or second stimulus was the longer/shorter one. Written symbols may also be used. (- . / . -)
Loudness variation	2 tones or sounds which differ in loudness. Contrast of loud/soft is gradually reduced. Frequency and length of stimuli are varied. 1. BLS 2. ELS	Pt. states whether the first or second stimulus was the louder/softer one. Written symbols may also be used. (o O / O o)
Frequency variation	2 tones or sounds which differ in frequency. Contrast of high/low is gradually reduced. Loudness and length of stimuli are varied. 1. BLS 2. ELS	Pt. indicates which stimulus was the higher (or lower) one. (_ - / - _)

Notes: a. Basic Level Sound (BLS): Frequency, volume and duration of stimuli as well as length of pauses are determined by the patient's individual hearing ability. b. Everyday Level Sound (ELS): Everyday level of frequency, volume, duration of stimuli and pauses are used. c. Basic Level Speech (BLSp): The presentation of speech stimuli is very slow, clearly articulated and with marked stress and intonation. d. Everyday Level Speech (ELSp): Speech is of average conversational speech style. Each exercise is commenced at the basic level and then gradually approximated to the everyday level.

Table 10.1 *(contd.)*

Aim	Stimulus	Response
Discrimination of everyday sounds	Real life or taped presentation of everyday sounds with increasing complexity. (a) gross differentiation (clock ticking/door slamming) (b) fine differentiation (clock ticking/telephone ringing) Sound level is adjusted to a loudness comfortable for the patient and then gradually approximated to normal everyday level (either louder or softer).	Pt. has lists of 2 then 3 and more sounds in front of him. He indicates which sound was presented.
Discrimination of voices	Real life or taped presentation of voice samples. (a) male, female voices (b) male, female, children's voices (c) familiar, unfamiliar voices Several speakers of each type should be used to avoid orientation by individual speech characteristics.	Pt. has lists of 2 then 3 and more speakers in front of him. He has to recognise the speaker.
Following speech on the basis of voice patterns	Real life or taped presentation of poems and prose. Care is taken that in live presentation Pt. has no opportunity to speed-read or see jaw movement (pure auditory input). 1. BLSp[c] 2. ELSp[d]	Pt. has text in front of him and points to each word as it is read aloud.

II. Discrimination

III. Suprasegmental Features

Aim	Stimulus	Response

Determination of number of syllables	Words with varying syllable number.
	(a) monosyllables (door, bell, etc.)
	(b) polysyllables
	  1. spondees (sailboat, wastebasket etc.)
	  2. trochees (mother, vinegar)
	Stress pattern should be taken into consideration when selecting the words.
	1. BLSp
	2. ELSp
		Pt. states number of syllables he hears in the presented word.
		No word comprehension is required.

Determination of number of words	Sentences with varying word number, whereby only monosyllabic words are used. 1. BLSp 2. ELSp	Pt. has to state the number of words he hears. No sentence comprehension is required.

Table 10.1 *(contd.)*

Aim	Stimulus	Response
Development of a sense for the length of words	Word pairs consisting of words of varying length. (a) compounds and their parts (window/windowsill), (doorbell/door) (b) words selected according to their length (tin/carpet), (furniture/window) 1. BLSp 2. ELSp	Pt. indicates which word was the longer/shorter one. No word comprehension is required.
Development of a sense for the length of phrases/sentences	Pairs consisting of phrases/sentences of varying length. (Good morning/The weather is fine today.) (How are you?/Hello.) A distinct pause must be made between the two units. 1. BLSp 2. ELSp	Pt. indicates which unit was the shorter one. No comprehension is required.
Recognition of sentence accent	Sentences with variation of the most prominent word. (The *naughty* boy climbed the tree.) (The naughty boy *climbed* the three.) etc. 1. BLSp 2. ELSp	Pt. repeats the most prominent word in the sentence presented. Pt. is familiar with the sentence.
Recognition of word accent	Polysyllabic words with varying word accentual patterns. (enter*tain*) (*del*icate) (*Ja*pan) Exercises are commenced with three-syllable words. 1. BLSp 2. ELSp	Pt. states which syllable has the primary accent.
Recognition of sentence forms	Sentences. (a) pairs (question/statement or statement/question) It's his daughter?/It's his daughter. (b) single (either question or statement) That's enough. 1. BLSp 2. ELSp	Pt. states: (a) Which sentence was the question/statement. (b) Whether the presented sentence was a question or a statement.

Table 10.1 *(contd.)*

IV. Segmental Features

Aim	Stimulus	Response
Recognition of one word of a presented pair (A) syllable number/word length	Word pairs consisting of words which differ in syllable number. (a) compounds and their parts (basket/wastebasket) (b) words selected according to their length (book/market) 1. BLSp 2. ELSp	Pt. has lists of word pairs in front of him and repeats the word he has heard. Pt. is advised to listen carefully and not to forget to concentrate on the word length as an additional help.
Recognition of one word of a presented pair (B) word level accent	Word pairs consisting of words differing in their word-level accent, but not in syllable number. (*apple/demand*) (*beautiful/tomato*) (*yesterday/tomorrow*) 1. BLSp 2. ELSp	Pt. has lists of word pairs in front of him and repeats the word he has heard. Pt. is advised to listen carefully and not to forget to concentrate on the word-level accent as an additional help.
Recognition of one word of a presented pair (C) length of vowels	Word pairs consisting of words differing in the length of one vowel. (*beat/bit*) (*sleep/slip*) (*coat/cot*) 1. BLSp 2. ELSp	Pt. has lists of word pairs in front of him and repeats the word he has heard. Pt. is advised to concentrate on the length of the vowels.
Recognition of word of a presented pair (D) vowels	Word pairs consisting of words differing only in one vowel. (*cup/cap*) (*and/end*) (*thing/thong*) 1. BLSp 2. ELSp	Pt. has lists of word pairs in front of him and repeats the word he has heard. Pt. is advided to concentrated on the vowel sound.
Recognition of one word of a presented pair (E) consonants	Word pairs consisting of words differing only in one consonant. (*peace/peach*) (*tie/shy*) (*pat/bat*) 1. BLSp 2. ELSp	Pt. has lists of word pairs in front of him and repeats the word he has heard. Pt. is advised to concentrate on the consonant sound.

Table 10.1 *(contd.)*

Aim	Stimulus	Response

Recognition of a familiar word in a list of unfamiliar words	List of words.
	Target word is presented several times e.g. cat.
	List: ball
	          door
	          cat
	          tin
	          cat
	1. BSLp
	2. ELSp
		Pt. indicates after each presented word, whether it was the target (familiar) word or not.

Recognition of a familiar sentence in a list of unfamiliar sentences	List of sentences.
	Target sentence is presented several times e.g. The dog barks.
	List: The bird sings.
	          The dog barks.
	          The horse jumps.
	          The dog barks.
	1. BSLp
	2. ELSp
		Pt. indicates after each presented sentence, whether it was the target one or not.

Comprehension of numbers
(a) **closed lists**
(b) **open lists**
	Numbers
	(a) closed list:
	     list of 5, 10, 15 or more numbers
	(b) open list:
	     any number between 1 and 1000
	1. BLSp
	2. ELSp
		Pt. repeats the number
		(a) with the help of a list of the numbers
		(b) Pt. has no written support.

V. Auditory Comprehension

Table 10.1 *(contd.)*

Aim	Stimulus	Response
Comprehension of phrases (a) closed lists (b) open lists	Common phrases (a) closed list: list of 5, 10, 15 or more phrases (b) open list: all the phrases learned to date at random 1. BLSp 2. ELSp	Pt. repeats the phrases (a) with the help of a list of the phrases (b) Pt. has no written support.
Comprehension of words (a) closed lists (b) open lists	Words in concept groups (a) closed list: list of 5, 10, 15 or more words (b) open list: all the words learned to date at random 1. BLSp 2. ELSp	Pt. repeats word (a) with the help of the word list (b) Pt. has no written support.
Comprehension of sentences (a) closed lists (b) open lists	Sentences in concept groups (a) closed list: list of 5, 10, 15 or more sentences (b) open list: all the sentences learned to date at random 1. BLSp 2. ELSp	Pt. repeats sentence (a) with the help of the sentence list (b) Pt. has no written support.
Comprehension of text A	Story, supported by appropriate pictures is read aloud to Pt.	Pt. has to answer questions about the story.
Comprehension of text B	Story is read aloud to Pt. who only has title as support.	Pt. has to answer questions about the story.
Comparison of visual and auditory stimuli	Text, presented orally to the Pt.	Pt. with text in front of him has to recognise differences between oral presentation and written text.
Everyday interactions	Practice of everyday situations (e.g. shopping, restaurant, meeting people) with preliminary discussion and review of the vocabulary and questions to be expected.	

Communication Training

Regan (1977) claims:

> Regardless of the whys and hows of audiologic site-of-lesion assessment, we are confronted with a communicative breakdown, the causative factors of which encompass the entire communicative event, not merely the hearing sensitivity curve of the patient (cited from Alpiner, 1982: Ch. 1).

Effective communication strategies can help to compensate a deficit in speech perception.

But as a matter of fact many hearing-impaired individuals acquired ineffective communication strategies which prevent them from communicating satisfactorily. Some typical ineffective communication strategies of hearing-impaired individuals are:

(1) To concentrate only on visual or only on auditory information;
(2) To be unrelaxed during audiovisual communication;
(3) To miss non-linguistic cues as an orientational aid;
(4) To be unable (a) to create good optical and acoustic conditions for audiovisual speech perception and (b) to educate the communication partner because of lacking self-confidence and acceptance of the handicap;
(5) To overtax the attention of others by speaking the whole time rather than listening.

The programme for communication training is outlined in Table 10.2.

Table 10.2: Communication Training

Aim	Material	Method
1. Relaxation during communication situation	written instructions role play stories	1. training of relaxation in group or individual sessions
2. Use of non-linguistic cues	role play	1. training of use of mimics and gestures 2. training of use of situational cues
3. Combination of visual and auditory information	stories articles role play	1. modality: (a) lip-reading (b) electrostimulation (c) lip-reading + electrostimulation 2. hierarchy of difficulty: variation of acoustic and optic conditions from good to bad.
4. Acquisition of ability to create good optic and acoustic conditions for audiovisual speech perception and to educate the communication partner	counselling role play	1. learning to cope with lack of self-confidence 2. learning to create good conditions for audiovisual speech perception in role play
5. Balance of speaking and listening in communication situation	counselling role play	1. cause for overtaxing communitions partner is identified 2. confrontation with overtaxing communication partner in role play 3. new strategies are proposed

Conclusion

The rehabilitation programme teaches the cochlear implant patient to achieve maximum use of his hearing prosthesis in everyday life. The aims are to reduce the psychological restrictions caused by the severe preoperative hearing deficit and to introduce the patient to his new acoustic environment. In our experience only a complete rehabilitation procedure can enable the patient to take his place in the hearing world.

References

Alpiner, J.G. (1982) *Handbook of Adult Rehabilitative Audiology*, Williams and Wilkins, Company, Baltimore

Banfai, P., Hortmann, G., Wustrow, F., Kubik, S. and Zeisberg, B. (1981) Meßdaten und psychoakustische Auswertung mit 8-Kanal-Hörprothese. *HNO, 29*, 22-6

Cooper, W. (1983) The perception of fluent speech, in C.W. Parkins and S.W. Anderson (eds.), *Proceedings of Cochlear Prostheses: An International Symposium, Ann. NY Acad. Sci., 405*, 48-63

—— and Sorenson, J.M. (1981) *Fundamental Frequency in Sentence Production*, Springer, New York

Eisenwort, B. and Benkö, E. (1983) Kommunikative Kompetenz bei Hörgeschädigten. Ansätze zu einem Trainings- und Testprogram für Cochlearimplantat-Träger und Hörgeräte-Träger. *Folia phoniatrice, 35*, 273-85

Fry, B.D. (1955) Duration and intensity as physical correlates of linguistic stress. *J. Acoust. Soc. Am., 27*, 765-8

Hochmair-Desoyer, I.J., Hochmair, E.S., Fischer, R. and Burian, K. (1980) Cochlear prostheses in use: recent psychophysical data and speech comprehension results. *Arch. Otorhinolaryngol., 229*, 81-98

Liebermann, P. (1967) Intonation and syntactic processing of speech, in W. Wathen-Dunn (ed.), *Models for the Perception of Speech and Visual Form*, MIT Press, Cambridge, MA

Lindner, G. (1981) *Grundlagen der Pädagogischen Audiologie*, VEB Verlag Volk und Gesundheit, Berlin

Myklebust, H.R (1964) *The Psychology of Deafness*, Grune and Stratton, London

Neisser, V. (1967) *Cognitive Psychology*, Appleton-Century-Crofts, New York

Pickett, J.M. (1983) Theoretical considerations in testing speech perception through electroauditory stimulation, in C.W. Parkins and S.W. Anderson (eds.), *Proceedings of Cochlear Prostheses: An International Symposium, Ann. NY Acad. Sci., 405*, 425-34

Regan, D.E. (1977) Problem reduction approach to aural rehabilitation. *Audiol. Hear. Educ., 3*, 6-7, 48

Richtberg, W. (1980) *Hörbehinderung als psychosoziales Leiden*, Forschungsbericht, Frankfurt/Main, Gesundheitsforschung 32

—— (1983) Psychosoziale Behinderung bei Hörgeschädigten, in Bölling-Bechinger, and May (eds.), *Psychologische Hilfen für Hörgeschädigte*, Julius Gross Verlag, Heidelberg, pp. 14-34

Rogers, C. (1951) *Client Centred Counselling*, Houghton Mifflin, Boston

—— (1961) *On Becoming a Person*, Houghton Mifflin, Boston

Schuchardt, E. (1980) *Weiterbildung als Krisenverarbeitung*, Vol. 2, Westermann, Braunschweig

Stevens, K.N. (1983) Acoustic properties used for the identification of speech sounds, in C.W. Parkins and S.W. Anderson (eds.), *Proceedings of Cochlear Prostheses: An International Symposium, Ann. NY Acad. Sci., 405*, 2-17

11 THE ENGINEERING OF FUTURE COCHLEAR IMPLANTS

Graeme M. Clark and Yit C. Tong

Introduction

Speech is a complex acoustic signal, and information is transmitted to the brain at a rapid rate. For example during a conversation ten phonemes are uttered per second. Furthermore, these complex speech sounds are coded into patterns of neural discharges that enable the subject to understand speech. In order, therefore, to bring speech signals directly to residual auditory nerve fibres, considerable processing of the speech signal is required before the central nervous system will recognise and comprehend it. The magnitude of the task can be further appreciated when one considers that there are an average of 31,400 nerve fibres in the human auditory nerve and a large proportion of these convey information to the brain about the speech frequencies. Research studies are showing, however, that the perception of ongoing speech with cochlear implants may be achieved with speech processing strategies which can be achieved by current electronic technology.

The components of the prosthesis that need to be considered are illustrated in Figure 11.1. The speech signals need to be picked up by the patient's microphone and relayed to his/her speech processor. This will mean extracting speech signals from a noisy environment if a patient is going to obtain maximum use from the device both at home and at work. Within the processor the speech signals then need to be transformed from an acoustic to electronic code that will excite auditory neurones, and provide patterns of neural discharges that are perceived by the brain as ongoing speech. This information must be transmitted accurately to the implanted device for decoding into electrical stimuli. An implanted receiver-stimulator is essential for multichannel stimulation, and provides different stimuli for each of the electrodes, under instruction from the external speech processor. As nerve fibres require currents to excite them, power will also be needed. The electronics for the receiver-stimulator should be reliable, and not fail after use over many years. They should also be designed so that the stimulus parameters can be varied to enable different speech processing strategies to be evaluated. It is easier to provide a patient with an alternative speech processor that can be worn, than it is surgically to remove the receiver-stimulator and replace it with a more up-to-date model.

The implanted receiver-stimulator and electrode array must be biocompatible, and not lead to long-term adverse effects. The method of signal transmission through the skin should not cause tissue damage, and the receiver-stimulator and electrode array should be manufactured from materials that are non-toxic. The electronics for the receiver-stimulator should be sealed within a container so that corrosive body fluids cannot enter and cause a device failure. Special care must be given to the sealing of the points where electrical wires enter or leave the implanted

Figure 11.1: Diagram of a Cochlear Prosthesis which Includes: Microphone, Speech Processor, Transmitter-coil, Receiver-coil, Receiver-stimulator and Electrode Array.

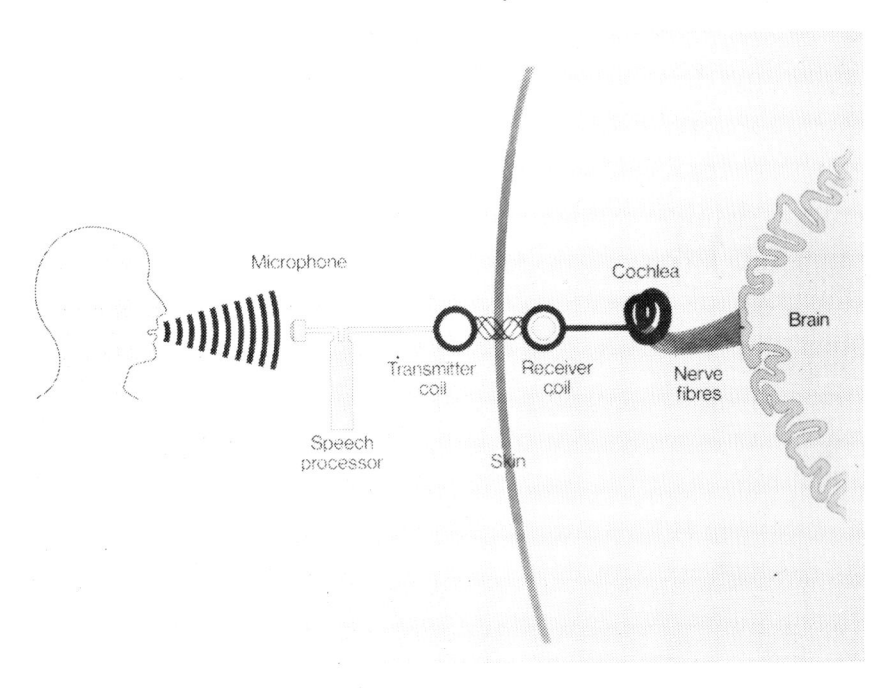

package. It is also desirable to design the device with a connector so that the receiver-stimulator can be removed and replaced without disturbing the implanted electrode array if an electrode failure occurs. The prosthesis must be robust so that it will not be damaged by an impact such as a blow to the skull. It should also be engineered so that repeated small body movements do not lead to metal fatigue and fracture, particularly at the point where the electrode array leaves the receiver-stimulator unit.

Finally, cochlear prostheses should be engineered so that they are cosmetically and socially acceptable as well as cost effective. The implant should be as small as possible. This is particularly important when it is for use in children. The wearable speech-processor needs to be compact and light and comfortable to wear.

The power consumption should be a minimum for a long battery life. There should be few controls on the processor and these need to be easy to manipulate for the elderly and handicapped. The electronics for the speech processor should be enclosed so they cannot be tampered with, and the leads robust so that they will not break with repeated fixing and pulling. The system for transmitting power and signals to the implanted device should be easy to apply and remove, and be cosmetically acceptable.

Speech Processor

In the design of speech processors for cochlear implants, it is important to consider the physical characteristics of the acoustic signal, the linguistic units related to these characteristics, the biophysical, physiological and psychological principles governing the processing of acoustic and electric signals by the auditory system, and the constraints imposed by such considerations as power consumption, size and cost. With reference to the later sections of this chapter, it is also important to consider the limited repertoire of electric signals that can be generated at the electrode tips.

Speech Sounds: Simplified Descriptions

Acoustic speech sounds can be broadly classified into two categories: voiced and voiceless sounds. Voiced speech sounds include all the vowels and some of the consonants, and are produced with a sequence of periodic air pulses created by forcing air from the lung through the vibrating vocal cords. The frequency of this periodic vibration is called the fundamental frequency of voiced speech sounds. The remaining consonants are voiceless, and are produced with a random turbulence of air created by forcing air from the lung through a narrow constriction in the mouth. The sequence of periodic air pulses or random turbulence is modified by the spatial configuration of the speech producing organs (tongue, lips, teeth, palate, etc.) to form individual speech sounds. Vowels and consonants (both voiced and voiceless) are produced by relatively static configurations and are characterised acoustically by three to four dominant frequency components called formant frequencies. The transitions from vowel to consonant and from consonant to vowel in an utterance are accompanied by transitions of these frequency components known as formant frequency transitions. So far we have only described speech sounds in terms of their (fundamental and formant) frequency components. Another very important speech parameter is the intensity, or alternatively the amplitude, of the speech sound. The variation of the amplitude during an utterance is called the amplitude envelope.

Three Important Speech Parameters. The presence and absence of voicing, the fundamental frequency, the formant frequencies and their transitions, and the amplitude envelope described as simplified acoustic characterisation of speech sounds in the last paragraph have also been found in psychological experiments to be essential information for the recognition of speech sounds.

Information about these speech parameters should therefore be presented to cochlear-implant patients. To illustrate the way in which these acoustic parameters can be converted into electric parameters in speech processors for implant patients, let us consider the strategies in the following subsection.

Strategies

Amplitude. Firstly, an implanted electrode can be driven at a fixed frequency (or pulse rate if pulsatile stimulation is used) with the electric current modulated by the amplitude envelope of the ongoing speech. This simple strategy provides the patient with the information about not only the boundaries of occurrence of gross speech events such as syllables, words, phrases and sentences, but also the 'stress' words or syllables where extra vocal effort was applied. In addition, the amplitude envelope also provides information about the occurrence of certain speech sounds (such as p, b, t, d, k, g) and concatenation of speech sounds. For this strategy to be effective, the electrode must be capable of activating residual nerve fibres in the patient, and higher current levels should activate a larger population of fibres. Moreover, the patient's brain must be capable of interpreting this variation in active fibre population as a change in loudness.

Fundamental Voicing Frequency. In addition to the amplitude envelope, information about the fundamental frequency and the presence or absence of voicing can be presented by modulating the frequency (or pulse rate) of the current delivered to the electrode. For example, in the case of voiced sounds, the stimulus rate can be made proportional to the acoustic fundamental frequency, while in the case of voiceless sounds a random electric stimulus pattern can be used. It has been shown that the fundamental frequency (coded as stimulus rate for cochlear implant patients) provides linguistic information about the stress and intonation of the speech message, and voiced/voiceless distinction is one of the important factors for the successful recognition of a large number of speech sounds. For this strategy to work in practice, different stimulus patterns delivered to the implanted electrode must be capable of generating different neural discharge patterns. Furthermore, the patient's brain must be capable of interpreting these different neural discharge patterns as the occurrence of periodic or random speech signals, and in the case of a periodic signal, the variation in periodicity must be interpreted as a change in the pitch (stress and intonation) of speech.

Formant Frequencies. Our final strategy presents formant frequency (and transition) information to patients by switching the active electrode from one place to another according to the formant frequencies of the speech sound. This provides the patient with the information necessary for the identification of most of the speech sounds. The requirements for this strategy are that current delivered to different electrode positions must be capable of activating different groups of the residual nerve fibres, and the brain must be capable of perceiving the sensation so produced as sounds of different timbres.

These three strategies are selected as examples because, for patients who became deaf after the acquisition of language, the operational requirements are, by and large, fulfilled (Tong *et al.*, 1979, 1980b, 1981, 1982, 1983a, b). There are, of course, exceptions to the rule. In particular, the mapping of formant frequency to electrode position described in the last paragraph is less effective for multiple-channel cochlear implant patients with residual auditory nerve fibres sparsely distributed in the cochlea. For these patients and for patients who received single-channel cochlear implants, a speech processor based on amplitude and fundamental frequency information can be designed. In addition, for patients who were born deaf, it is not known whether or not these requirements are fulfilled, and so further research with these patients is necessary.

It should be noted that many other strategies and requirements may be suggested on the basis of biophysical, physiological and psychological considerations (Burian *et al.*, 1979; Clark *et al.*, 1978; Eddington *et al.*, 1978; Fourcin *et al.*, 1979; House, 1976; Merzenich *et al.*, 1979; Pialoux *et al.*, 1979; Simmons *et al.*, 1979) and scientific procedures can be used to test the validity of these hypotheses. Some of the research studies currently carried out in the world are summarised in the other chapters in this volume.

In the next subsection, we shall describe, some of the tactics involved in the implementation of the three chosen strategies. (In this chapter, strategy refers to the choice of electric parameters to encode information about acoustic parameters while tactics refers to the means employed in the implementation of a strategy.)

Tactics

Figure 11.2 shows a block diagram of an implementation of the strategies described in the last subsection. The signal is picked up by a microphone, and passed through an automatic gain control amplifier. The amplified signal is then directed along three parallel paths for the extraction of the three parameters: amplitude envelopes, fundamental frequency and formant frequency. Note that only one formant frequency measurement is depicted in this block diagram: further blocks for formant frequencies can be added if required. The output of the amplitude envelope detector is converted into stimulus current level, the estimated fundamental frequency to stimulus pulse rate, and formant frequency to electrode position. These three parameters are fed into the microprocessor and output generator which generates the radio frequency signal to be transmitted to the implanted receiver-stimulator.

With the exception of the microphone, the component blocks in Figure 11.2 can be constructed using digital or analogue circuitry or a combination. The instantaneous values of the signals in a digital system are described by (or quantitated to) a finite set of numbers, and the processing of the signals involves the mathematical manipulation of these numbers by adders, multipliers and other digital circuits. The numbers are represented by the presence or absence of electric pulses. In an analogue system, continuous variations of the instantaneous values of the signals are allowed. In contrast to digital signals, continuous variation for analogue signals implies, in mathematical terms, that an infinite set of numbers is required for the specification of these signals. To perform the mathematical manipulation of the signals in analogue processing, the continuous signals are fed through and modified by various physical devices such as transistors, resistors and capacitors. The form and degree of modification are dependent on the characteristics of the physical device.

Digital processing offers several advantages over analogue processing. Firstly, because of the lack of passive components, digital circuits can be integrated into a small silicon chip using large-scale-integration technology. Secondly, digital processing is more stable and repeatable. This is because the amplitude of the electric

Figure 11.2: A Block Diagram of a Speech Processor.

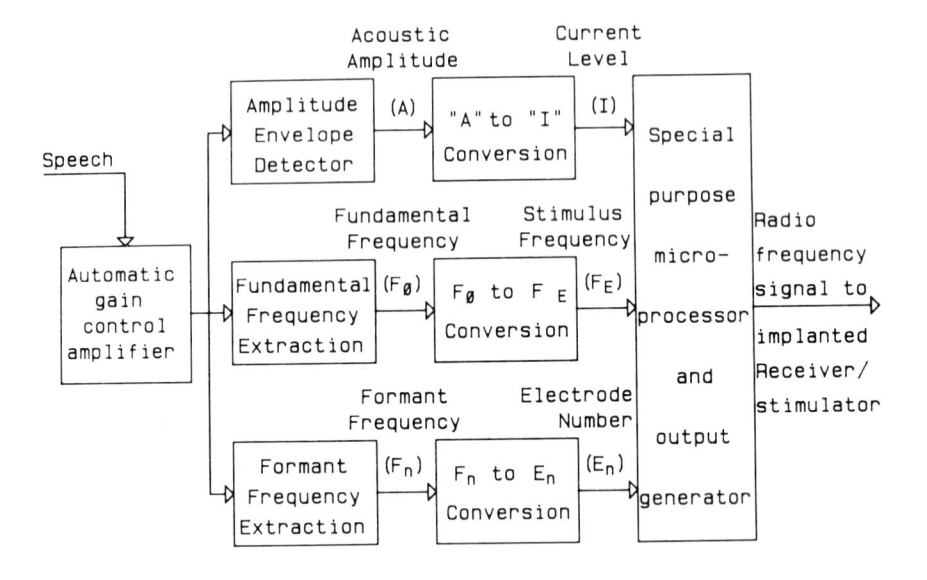

pulses representing the numbers in a digital system can be badly distorted without affecting the precision of the numerical operation. By contrast, any distortion of the continuous signals in an analogue system directly affects the precision of the mathematical manipulation. The major disadvantage of digital processing, however, is that, with existing semiconductor technologies, the power consumption for implementation of some of the electronic subsystems described in this section significantly exceeds that for analogue implementation. As a result of the stringent power requirements for a wearable unit, both digital and analogue techniques were used in the realisation of the speech processor depicted in Figure 11.2.

Construction of the Speech Processor. The microphone converts acoustic speech sounds into electric signals to be processed.

The Microphone. For cochlear implant patients, it is important that a directional microphone should be used. A directional microphone enhances sound signals coming from the front and reduces those coming from other directions. As a result, if the microphone is pointed towards the sound source, the speech signal in the noisy environment will be enhanced. Another consideration for microphone selection is that it should be small to enable ease of carrying and for cosmetic reasons. Furthermore, the site where the microphone is placed on the patient must be carefully chosen because of variations in microphone frequency response characteristics at different locations.

The First Amplifier. The automatic gain control amplifier reduces the range of amplitude values of the speech sounds to be processed by the device. It keeps the peaks of the output amplitude at a level which is acceptable for subsequent processing and comfortable to the patient while the input amplitude varies over a wide range. The amount of dynamic range reduction and the time delay over which this reduction is achieved for ongoing speech are factors which must be carefully controlled to ensure a minimum amount of distortion of the speech signals.

Amplitude Detection. The analogue amplitude envelope detector consists of a full wave rectifier followed by a lowpass filter. Electric current has been found in psychophysical experiments to be related to acoustic amplitude by a power function, and the index of the power function can be determined by psychophysical means. It should be noted that the power coefficient may vary from electrode to electrode depending on the size and location of the electrodes and on the density of residual auditory nerve fibres in the cochlea. Directed by the microprocessor (Figure 11.2) the acoustic amplitude is sampled by an analogue-to-digital converter. The digitised acoustic amplitude is converted into a number representing the current level by referring to a table prepared according to the already mentioned power function. This table is stored in a block of digital memory controlled by the microprocessor.

Fundamental Voicing Frequency. Fundamental frequency can be measured in an analogue system by passing the outputs of the automatic gain control amplifier sequentially through a rectifier, a low pass filter, a zero crossings counter, and a frequency to voltage converter. A voltage proportional to the fundamental frequency is produced at the output of the frequency to voltage converter. This voltage is used to determine the rate of stimulation during voiced speech. For unvoiced speech, the stimuli are random and produce something which sounds like noise.

Formant Frequencies. The formant frequency is similarly measured in an analogue system. It is estimated from the output of a formant filter which is designed to cover the frequency range of the formant frequencies in question. The filter output is fed through a zero crossings counter and frequency-to-voltage converter to produce a voltage proportional to the formant frequency. Directed by the microprocessor (Figure 11.2) this voltage is sampled by an analogue-to-digital converter, and the electrode number read from a table in the digital memory. The correspondence between formant frequency and electrode number can be determined in psychophysical studies, or derived on the basis of the spacing between the electrodes in the cochlea and known physiological principles.

The Signals Combined. The three signal parameters corresponding to the three branches of the block diagram are continuously fed to the microprocessor and output section in real time. The microprocessor controls the instances at which the electric parameter values are sampled, and configures the radio frequency signal to be transmitted to the implanted receiver-stimulator.

218 *Engineering of Future Cochlear Implants*

Figure 11.3: Photograph of Speech Processor, Manufactured by Nucleus Ltd, Lane Cove, Australia.

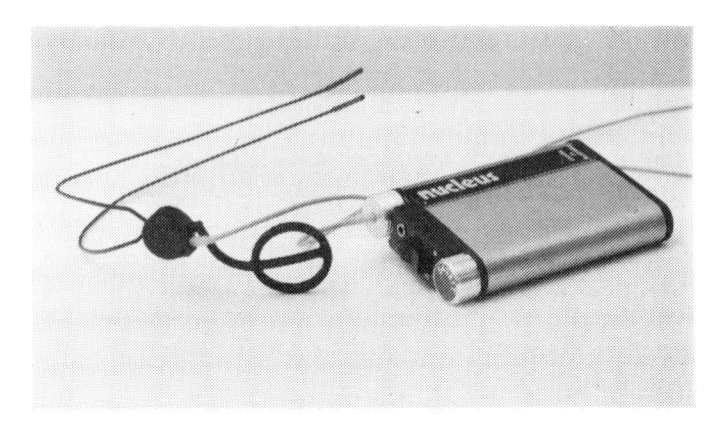

Standard Integrated Circuits. The speech processor as shown in Figure 11.2 can be implanted using standard integrated circuits. The size of the speech processor can be reduced by using hybrid circuits in which the integrated circuit chips are mounted directly onto a ceramic interconnecting substrate. A further reduction in size (and in power) may be achieved by the semi-conductor fabrication of specially designed integrated circuit chips which perform some of the major functions depicted in Figure 11.2, and combining these with standard integrated circuits as a hybrid. Such a mixed implementation was employed by Nucleus Limited Australia in the speech processor shown in Figure 11.3. In the engineering of future speech processors, it is envisaged that most of the major functional blocks in Figure 11.2 will be implemented on a single silicon chip with low power technology such as CMOS.

There are other ways of constructing speech processors of course but it is worth noting that optimum (or even satisfactory) engineering solutions can only be achieved after considerable research and development. More sophisticated algorithms and circuits may be used in the measurement of the speech parameters depicted in the block diagram in Figure 11.2. The functional relationships between speech and electric parameters may be better specified with further psychological and physiological research. The adequacy of different algorithms, circuits and functional relationships can be assessed by physical measurements and psychological evaluation using speech materials. Finally, the choice of the strategies is also influenced by the availability of adequate tactics. After all, as engineers would agree, conceptions based on scientific principles can be turned into good engineering solutions only if they can be constructed within the constraints imposed by the design objectives.

Transmission of Speech Data and Power to the Implanted Receiver-Stimulator

Speech information transformed into electric signals needs to be transmitted to electrodes to excite the residual auditory nerves. Electric power must also be provided.

The speech data can be transmitted to the stimulating electrodes by a direct electrical link, or indirectly through intact skin. Electromagnetism, light or ultrasound energy may be used as the carrier for the signal. Power is best transmitted by a link which passes physically through the skin to the implanted device, or indirectly by electromagnetic inductive coupling.

It is important that the method of transmitting the coded speech signal to the electrodes be 'transparent', allowing the independent and continuous variation of stimulus parameters and be tolerant of changes in the coil position. The method adopted should also be harmless in the short and long term.

The most 'transparent' transmission link is one with electrode wires passing directly through the skin. In this case there should also be a socket to receive the plug from the speech processor. This type of link, however, is not very satisfactory for a number of reasons. Infection is prone to occur when foreign material passes through the skin. It may spread along the electrode wire or develop in a sinus around its point of entry. For example, infection was reported in the 21 patients implanted by Pialoux *et al.* (1979, pp. 185–9) and the Teflon plug needed to be removed. On the other hand, animal experimental studies on percutaneous plugs (Merzenich *et al.*, 1981) and through the skin wire cables (Rebscher *et al.*, 1982) have shown the incidence of infection after short-term implantation to be acceptably low. Nevertheless, as infection is an ever-present risk connections should be placed at some distance from the cochlea, and this can be surgically inconvenient. Another major problem with percutaneous connectors is fracturing of the electrode wires by bumping, fingering and other body movements that cannot always be predicted from animal experiments. Finally, the plug is not aesthetically pleasing to all patients.

In view of the problems with a percutaneous system a number of links have been developed which transmit energy through the intact skin. These include sending data and power electromagnetically on a single channel (Dobelle *et al.*, 1974, pp. 81–6); power by electromagnetic induction and data transtympanically using a pulse modulated optical signal (White, 1974, pp. 199–207); power by electromagnetic induction and data with an ultrasonic link (Gheewala *et al.*, 1975, pp. 472–9) and both power and data by electromagnetic induction at two separate carrier frequencies (Forster, 1978).

Electromagnetic Induction

This is the most efficient and reliable method of transmitting signals. It is based on the principle illustrated in Figure 11.4 that a magnetic flux produced by passing a current through a coil (external) will induce a current in a second coil (internal). This method has been used for both power and data in the device shown

220   *Engineering of Future Cochlear Implants*

Figure 11.4: Diagram of External Transmitter Coil with Electromagnetic Energy Passing Through the Skin to Induce a Current in the Receiver Coil.

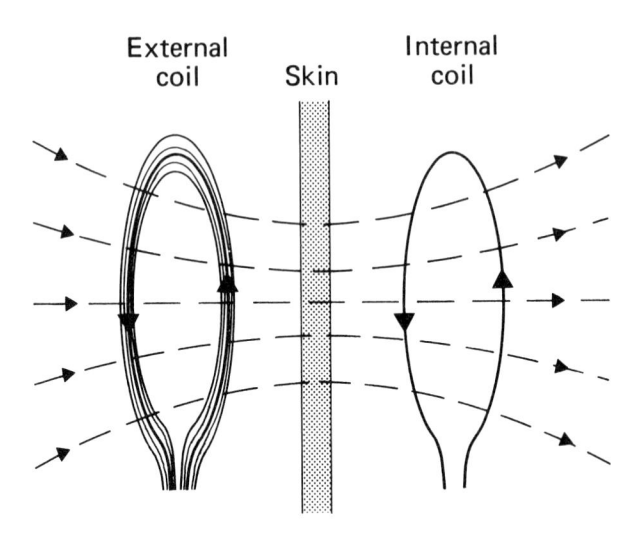

Figure 11.5: Photograph of a Multichannel Receiver-Stimulator and Electrode Array, Manufactured by Nucleus Ltd, Lane Cove, Australia.

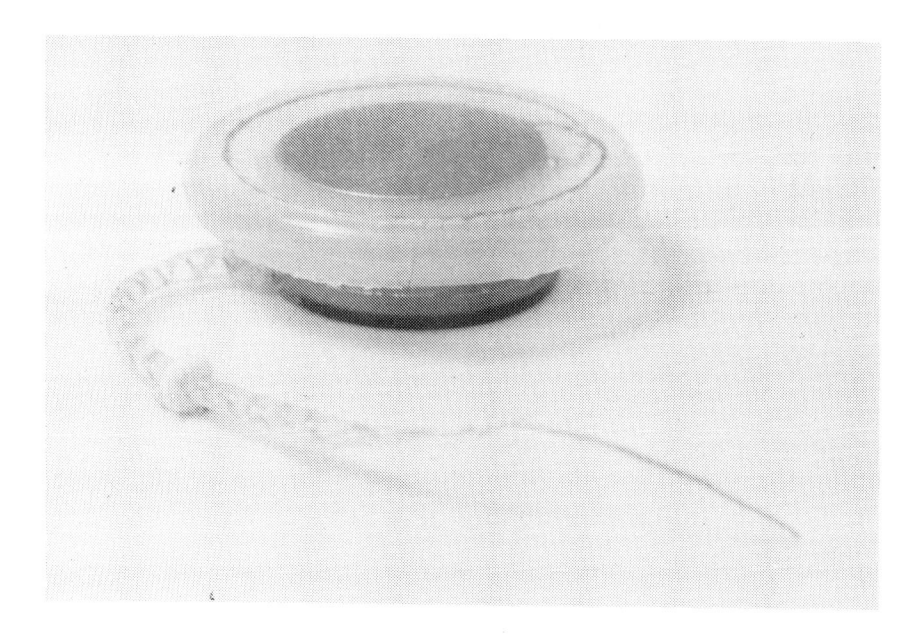

Engineering of Future Cochlear Implants 221

in Figure 11.5.

Adequate power must be transferred from the external to internal coils over a distance that will vary depending on the thickness of patient's skin and underlying tissues. It is desirable that some lateral misalignment be possible between the two coils. Even if magnets in the centre of both coils are used to help the patients bring the external coil into the correct position, precise coaxial alignment will be difficult, and the coil may be displaced. There should be adequate power transfer over a distance of up to 10 mm when the coils are coaxial, with some degree of misalignment possible at shorter distances.

A high frequency carrier wave is used, and this is modulated by the coded speech signal. A high frequency modulated wave is desirable as it permits a small aerial to be used, and a large amount of speech data to be transmitted efficiently. Examples of a carrier wave modulated by varying either its amplitude or frequency are illustrated in Figure 11.6.

Figure 11.6: A Diagram of Amplitude and Frequency Modulated Carrier Waves.

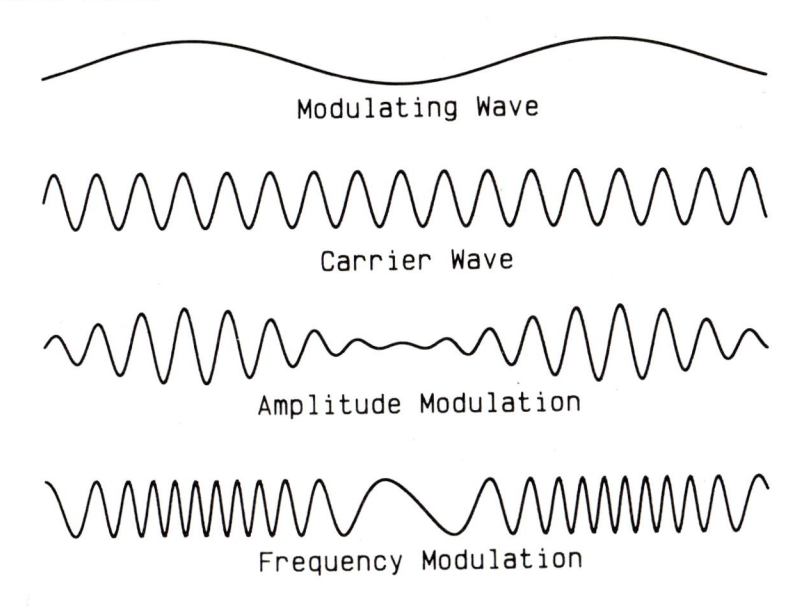

Modulating Wave

Carrier Wave

Amplitude Modulation

Frequency Modulation

Radio-frequency carrier waves may cause long-term adverse effects on the body tissues. This could take place from the absorption of energy by ions, or dipole-induced vibrations in protein molecules (Johnson and Guy, 1972, pp. 692–718). The energy absorbed by tissues increases with the carrier frequency and safety levels are being established (Tyler, 1975, pp. 1–545). It is therefore important to keep the carrier frequency as low as possible, and the energy absorbed within the safety limit.

Implantable Receiver-Stimulator Design

Design Principles

When implants were first made it was considered that there should be almost complete flexibility with the stimuli so that a patient's percepts for different current levels, pulse widths, pulse rates and so on could be determined. For this reason there was an initial emphasis on percutaneous plugs, and receiver-stimulators that could best achieve this goal. Now that more is known about the range of percepts possible, a receiver-stimulator can be designed to provide the appropriate stimuli without having to be quite so flexible.

The first consideration is whether constant current or constant voltage stimulation should be employed. The interface impedance between electrode and tissue may change, in which case the current flowing through the nerve will vary. This may be avoided by constant current stimulation.

The electric stimuli produced by the receiver-stimulator should be charge balanced biphasic pulses to minimise corrosion of electrodes, and the production of toxic products at the electrode-tissue interface, and neural and other tissue damage.

The number of stimulus channels to be incorporated in the receiver-stimulator is also a matter of importance. This has been under discussion for some time. On theoretical grounds it was proposed by Evans (1975) that there should be a minimum of 10 channels, and Clark *et al.* (1977, pp. 935–45) recommended 15 or more. Since then multiple-channel devices have been implanted with the number of channels varying from 4 to 12 (Hochmair-Desoyer *et al.*, 1981, pp. 107–19). More recently a 21-channel device was implanted in ten patients (Clark *et al.*, 1984a) and the psychophysical results (Dowell *et al.*, in press) have shown that most of these patients were able to perceive pitch difference for all 21 channels. These 21 channels have been used in the speech processor and given encouraging results.

The next question to resolve is whether to use either bipolar stimulation alone or have the facility of also using an intracochlear common-ground stimulus mode. Monopolar stimulation, however, has no place in multichannel stimulation as the spread of current is too great. With bipolar stimulation all the stimulus current flows from one electrode to another. Common-ground stimulation, however, occurs between an active electrode and a ground made up of all the other electrodes connected together (Figure 11.7).

The bipolar mode has the advantage of providing a more localised stimulus (Merzenich *et al.*, 1981). One method of achieving this and maintaining low threshold currents is a moulded array with small electrodes placed so they will be close to auditory neurons in the osseous spiral lamina. This array has been designed with a central rib to prevent axial rotation during insertion (Rebscher *et al.*, 1982). If misplacement of electrodes occurs, however, high threshold currents will be required, and metal corrosion and tissue damage are possible. On the other hand, the banded electrode (Clark *et al.*, 1979, pp. 107–9) has certain advantages as the electrodes are circumferential and is therefore more tolerant of misplacement during insertion. It is also easier to fabricate.

Figure 11.7: Diagram Showing Bipolar, Bipolar Plus One, Common-Ground and Monopolar Stimulus Modes.

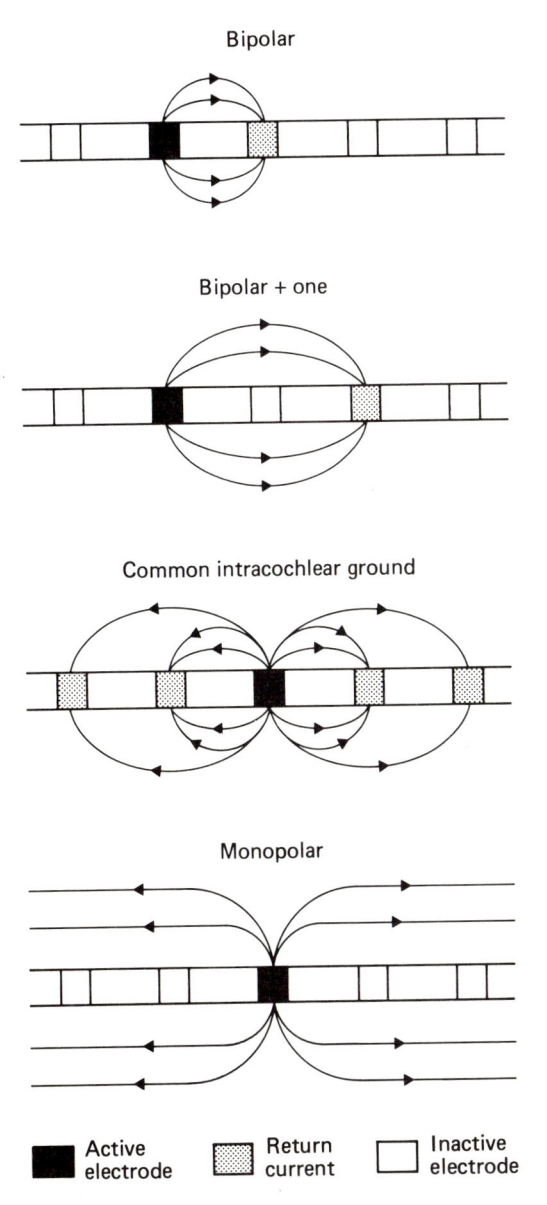

Bipolar

Bipolar + one

Common intracochlear ground

Monopolar

■ Active electrode   ▨ Return current   ☐ Inactive electrode

The minimum current level required depends on the lowest threshold level, and this will vary with the type of electrode array. The maximum current depends on the highest threshold as well as the greatest discomfort level expected. Furthermore if some of the electrodes are not placed close to the auditory nerve fibres, or are subsequently displaced by fibrous tissue and bone, greater stimulus levels will be required. Although it is desirable to have current levels vary continuously, this is probably not necessary as patients cannot perceive variations less than 0.7 per cent (Hochmair-Desoyer *et al.*, 1983), and furthermore intensity changes are not as important in speech perception as frequency cues.

Charge densities should not be used that are damaging to the spiral ganglion cells. With the banded electrode our animal studies have shown that continuous stimulation at charge densities of 18–32 $\mu C/cm^2$ geom./phase will not lead to damage of spiral ganglion cells (Shepherd *et al.*, 1983). It has also been shown that charge densities of 20–40 $\mu C/cm^2$ geom./phase are within biologically safe limits (Leake-Jones *et al.*, 1981, pp. 6–8).

It may be necessary to change the pulse width as variations in this parameter can be used as an alternative to current level to produce changes in loudness. We have shown that it is possible to trade off current level for pulse width and maintain equal loudness. With the device shown in Figure 11.5 the pulse width can be varied from 20 μs to 400 μs per phase in steps of 0.4 μs.

As the perception of pitch is important so also is the facility to vary the rate of stimulation. The upper limit on the perception of variations in the rate of stimulation has been shown to be about 400–800 pulses/s in humans (Simmons, 1966, pp. 2–76), and 200–800 pulses/s in animal experimental studies (Clark, 1969, pp. 124–36; Clark *et al.*, 1973, pp. 190–200). There is therefore no necessity to provide stimulus rates in excess of 1000 pulses/s. Although there are very real limits on the perception of variations in pulse rate, the effects of changes in this parameter on speech perception have not been fully explored, and the fine time structure of electric pulses delivered to the electrodes may be important. For this reason there is still a need to have adequate control of stimulus timing especially between channels.

Design Realisation

In the realisation of the receiver-stimulator design an important decision is whether to use analogue or digital circuitry or a combination of both. Analogue circuits are those where continuously varying physical parameters such as voltages can be altered or combined. With analogue circuitry the instantaneous amplitude of speech could be converted into a voltage proportional to the amplitude. The voltage could be transmitted indirectly to the receiver-stimulator where the induced voltage (or current) be used to excite nerve fibres near electrodes.

With analogue circuits variations in the speech amplitude could lead to similar variations in the voltages produced across the electrodes. If a number of electrodes were to be stimulated, however, it is more attractive to use digital circuitry. First, it is straightforward to combine (multiplex) the control information for each electrode into a single signal, and to recover this information in the stimulator. A single transmission path can then be used for a multichannel implant. Secondly, digitally controlled current sources deliver well-defined stimuli, and the speech processor can be precisely adjusted to suit individual patients. Finally, integrated circuit silicon chip technology is currently more readily available for digital designs, and can therefore be more conveniently used with cochlear prostheses.

With a receiver-stimulator that is predominantly digital in design, speech data are transmitted through the skin as a coded signal. This code specifies the electrode to be stimulated, the mode (bipolar with various electrode spacings, common ground), the rate, the current amplitude and the pulse width.

The circuits must implement the instructions from the speech processor and the digital information finally converted into an electrode voltage or current for neural stimulation.

Power Transmission. Power is best transferred by inductive coupling. This power transfer should be efficient to spare the batteries. This will be a concern of future cochlear prosthesis designs as batteries have become the largest component in wearable speech processors, and there will be a steady pressure from patients to make the device comparable in size to present hearing aids. Therefore attention needs to be given to the design of the power generating circuitry, the transmitter and receiver coupling elements, and the receiver-stimulator power conversion circuitry (Forster, 1978).

Integrated circuit technology used will affect power consumption. As CMOS gate arrays for silicon chips are readily available, cheaper than the equivalent full custom integrated circuits and of low power consumption, they are preferred.

Other considerations are that the receiver-stimulator circuit be isolated from the receiving coil so that the coil will not act as an extracochlear electrode should there be an electrical current path to the surrounding tissues. This is important as medical grade encapsulating materials like Silastic should not be relied upon to prevent these current paths or the possibility of corrosion. Finally the electrode circuitry should be designed so that accidental exposure to a stray electromagnetic field will not damage electronic components or cause unwanted stimulation.

Packaging the Receiver-stimulator

The receiver-stimulator electronics need to be packaged in an hermetically sealed container impervious to body fluids. The standards required need to be high as body fluids and enzymes permeate along minute pathways or seek cracks creating points of entry.

Once a reliable procedure has been found the technique needs to be validated by helium leak testing. Helium is used as it can be detected in very small concentrations, and has a very fast diffusion rate.

A great deal has been learnt from pacemaker technology about sealing electronic units, and this can be applied to cochlear implants. For example, epoxy resins were originally used, but led to later electronic failures. Kovar containers with glass feed-throughs and sealed by soldering have been used in space programmes. They were also used for packaging our first multichannel implants. Although these containers were satisfactory for space flights the body is a more hostile environment. It is quite likely to erode the glass insulation around the wires entering and leaving the package, or surface tension forces may enlarge small cracks in the glass so they become fluid entry paths. Furthermore with time the metals in the solder can migrate or produce corrosion from an electrolytic reaction and thus lead to weaknesses in the seal.

The most realiable packaging material is titanium which has now been used for many years in heart pacemakers. It is an inert metal and the seal can be made by welding the edges of the two halves of the containers together. In this way the seal is made of the same material as the container so no electrochemical reaction can be set up, and cause corrosion.

However, the use of titanium or other metal presents two problems. Firstly, there needs to be an effective seal and adequate insulation, at the points where the wires enter or leave the package. Glass is not really effective for long-term use in the body, and ceramics are to be preferred. Ceramics have been found reliable in heart pacemakers, and can form a good bond with metal. In the device shown in Figure 11.5 special ceramic feed-throughs have developed (Patrick *et al.*, 1984). Unfortunately the receiving coil cannot be placed inside the package, as electromagnetic energy cannot be transmitted through the metal. The coil can, however, be placed around the titanium capsule as illustrated in Figure 11.5 without actually increasing its thickness.

Although titanium is at present the most reliable method of packaging receiver-stimulator electronics, implants in the future will need to be made smaller for children, and ceramics may be of use. Although methods of sealing are not at the moment as reliable as those used for titanium packages, ceramics have the advantage that a coil can be placed inside the package. White (1974) has also emphasised the difficulties of achieving a good seal around the electrode feed-throughs in ceramic packages, especially when glass is used.

The receiver-stimulator may need a connector so that it can be replaced if there is an electronic failure. It should be added, however, that with heart pacemakers the least likely failure is an electronic one, and the same situation will most probably occur with cochlear implants. Failures are more likely with the electrodes or the connectors themselves.

Connectors therefore may not be essential in the future, especially as reinsertions may be possible with minimal damage to cochlear tissues and auditory neurones.

If a connector is used pressure between contact points needs to be maintained for many years, and the same metals be used to avoid corrosion. Furthermore, the connector should be designed so that body fluids cannot enter and cause current leaks between the electrodes. The device shown in Figure 11.5 has an improved connector which uses an intermediary pad locked into place between the package and electrode assembly pad (Patrick *et al.*, 1984). The pad has been designed to reduce the possibility of loss of compression and electrode contact over time.

A simple connection and disconnection procedure is essential. The surgical theatre is not the place for complicated mechanical equipment and manoeuvres with consequent breaks in sterility.

The implantable receiver-stimulator should be mechanically robust. Our first series of three implants in 1978 and 1979 showed that the area most vulnerable to repeated small body movements was the point where the electrode array emerged from the package. Any movements transmitted from rubbing the skin or adjusting the transmitter coil will result in maximum bending at this junctional area. Consequently, designs should incorporate stress relief of the electrode wires emerging from the receiver-stimulator so that metal fatigue and fractures of electrode wires will not develop months or years after implantation. This has been achieved by spiralling the electrode wires. It is also recommended (Clark *et al.*, 1984b) during implantation that this bundle of electrode wires be placed in a groove under the mastoid cortex.

The receiver-stimulator should be designed for ease of surgical placement and cosmetic acceptability. Surgical experience as a result of implanting our first prototype in 1978, which was rectangular in shape, and a series of six implants in 1982 using the device shown in Figure 11.5 confirmed the view that a round device is to be preferred. The bed can be made very neatly with a milling burr (Clark *et al.*, 1984b). A round shape is also desirable for other reasons. It conforms best to a circular receiver coil, and has no sharp angles where stress concentration can occur and sealing become inadequate.

Our anatomical and surgical studies showed that the maximum depth a bed could be drilled in the mastoid and occipital bones was 6 mm, but 3–4 mm was more usual. The maximum height superficial to the bone that is cosmetically acceptable is about 5–6 mm. Acceptability could be improved by rounding off the edges. It was also our experience that the maximum diameter of the device in adults was about 35–40 mm. In the package shown in Figure 11.5, stability was helped by making the implant mushroom-shaped. The titanium capsule and connector having a diameter of 20 mm made the stalk, while the receiving coil with a diameter of approximately 30 mm helped make up the cap. Engineering receiver-stimulators in the future will need to reduce these dimensions to make them more acceptable for children.

References

Burian, K., Hochmair, E., Hochmair-Desoyer, I. and Lessel, M.R. (1979) *Acta Oto. Laryngol.*, 87, 190–5
Byers, C.L., Leale-Jones, P.A., Rebscher, S.J. and Merzenich, M.M. (1982) *Progress Report*. NIH Contract No. 1-NS-0-2337
Clark, G.M. (1969) *Expl. Neurol.*, 24, 124–36
——, Black, R.C., Dewhurst, D.J., Forster, I.C., Patrick, J.F. and Tong, Y.C. (1977) *Med. Prog. Technol.*, 5, 127–40
——, ——, Forster, I.C., Patrick, J.F. and Tong, Y.C. (1978) *J. Acoust. Soc. Am.*, 63, 631–3
——, Dowell, R.C., Pyman, B.C., Brown, A.M., Webb, R.L., Tong, Y.C., Bailey, Q.R. and Seligman, P.M. (1984a) *Aust. N.Z. J. Surg.*, 54, 519–26
——, Kranz, K.G. and Minas, H. (1973) *Expl. Neurol.*, 41, 190–200
——, Patrick, J.F. and Bailey, Q. (1979) *J. Laryngol. Otol.*, 93, 107–9
——, Pyman, B.C., Webb, R.L., Bailey, Q.R. and Shepherd, R.K. (1984b) *Ann. Otol. Rhinol. Laryngol.*, 93, 204–7
——, Tong, Y.C., Black, R.C., Forster, I.C., Patrick, J.F. and Dewhurst, D.J. (1977) *J. Laryngol. Otol.*, 91, 935–45
Dobelle, W.H., Fordemnalt, J.N., Hanson, J.W., Hill, D.R., Huber, R.J., Mladejovsky, M.G. and Smith, K.R (1974) *Electronics*, 47, 81–6

Dowell, R.C., Tong, Y.C., Blamey, P.J. and Clark, G.M. (in press) *Proc. 10th Anniversary Cochlear Implant Conf.*, San Francisco

Eddington, D.K., Dobelle, W.H., Brackmann, D.E., Mladejovsky, M.G. and Parkin, J.L. (1978) *Ann. Otol.* (Suppl. 53), *87*, 5–39

Evans, E.F. (1975) *Proc. 2nd Br. Conf. Audiol*

Forster, I.C. (1978) The Bioengineering Development of a Hearing Prosthesis for the Profoundly Deaf. PhD Thesis, University of Melbourne

Fourcin, A.J., Rosen, S.M., Moore, B.C.J., Douek, E.E., Clarke, G.P., Dodson, H. and Baunister, L.H. (1979) *Br. J. Audiol., 13*, 85–107

Gheewala, I.R., Melen, R.D. and White, R.L. (1975) *IEEE J. Solid State Circuits, 6*, 472–9

Hochmair-Desoyer, I.J., Hochmair, E.S., Burian, K. and Fisher, R.E. (1981) *Med. Prog. Technol., 8*, 107–19

Hochmair-Desoyer, I.J., Hochmair, E.S., Burian, K. and Stiglbrunner, H.K. (1983) *Ann. N.Y. Acad. Sci., 405*, 295–306

House, W.F. (1976) *Ann. Otol.* (Suppl. 27), *85*, 1–93

——— and Urban, J. (1973) *Arch. Otolaryngol., 82*, 504–17

Johnson, C.C. and Guy, A.W. (1972) *Proc. IEEE, 60*, 692–718

Leake-Jones, P.A., Walsh, S.M. and Merzenich, M.M. (1981) *Ann. Otol. Rhinol. Laryngol., 82*, 90, 6–8

Merzenich, M.M., White, M., Vivion, M.C., Leake-Jones, P.A. and Walsh, S. (1979) *Acta Otolaryngol., 87*, 196–202

———, White, M.W., Shannon, R.V., Gray, R.F., Byers, C.L., Rebscher, S.J. and Casey, D.E. (1981) *Seventh Quarterly Progress Report*. NIH contract No 1-NS-0-2337

Patrick, J.F., Crosby, P.A., Kuzma, J.A., Money, D.K., Ridler, J. and Seligman, P.M. (1984) in R.A. Schindler (ed.), *Proc. 10th Anniversary Cochlear Implant Conf.*, San Francisco, Raven Press, New York

Pialoux, P., Chouard, C.H., Meyer, B. and Fugain, C. (1979) *Acta Otolaryngol., 87*, 185–9

Proc. Symp. Artificial Auditory Stimulation, 29 Sept.–2 Oct. 1981. Erlangen, West Germany

Rebscher, S.J., Byers, C.L., Leake-Jones, P.A., Aird, D.W., Gardi, J.N. and Gray, R.F. (1982) *Eighth Quarterly Progress Report*, NIH Contract No. NS-0-2357

Shepherd, R.K., Clark, G.M. and Black, R.C. (1983) *Acta Otolaryngol.* Suppl. 399, 19–31

Simmons, F.B. (1966) *Arch. Otolaryngol., 84*, 2–76

———, Matthews, R.G., Walker, M.G. and White, R.L. (1979) *Acta Otolaryngol., 87*, 170–5

Tong, Y.C., Black, R.C., Clark, G.H., Forster, I.C., Millar, J.B., O'Loughlin, B.J. and Patrick, J.F. (1979) *J. Laryngol. Otol., 93*, 679–95

———, Blamey, P.J., Dowell, R.C. and Clark, G.M. (1983b) *J. Acoust. Soc. Am., 74*, 73–80

———, Clark, G.M., Blamey, P.J., Busby, P.A. and Dowell, R.C. (1982) *J. Acoust. Soc. Am., 71*, 153–60

———, ———, Dowell, R.C., Martin, L.F.A., Seligman, P.M. and Patrick, J.F. (1981) *Acta Otolaryngol., 92*, 193–8

———, Dowell, R.C., Blamey, P.J. and Clark, G.M. (1983a) *Science, 219*, 993–4

———, Millar, J.B., Clark, G.M., Martin, L.F., Busby, P.A. and Patrick, J.F. (1980b) *J. Laryngol. Otol., 94*, 1241–56

Tyler, P.E. (ed.) (1975) Biologic Effects of Nonionizing Radiation. *Ann. N.Y. Acad. Soc., 277*, 1–545

White, R.L. (1974) Integrated circuits and multiple electrode arrays, in M.M. Merzenich, R.A. Schindler and F.A. Sooy (eds.), *Electrical Stimulation of the Acoustic Nerve in Man*, Velo-Bind, San Francisco, pp. 199–207

GLOSSARY

Apical turn: Most inaccessible part of the cochlea responsive to low frequency sounds.

Atticotomy: Surgical approach to the cavity of the middle ear which contains the heads of the malleus and incus.

Auditory brainstem responses: Very small electrical potentials which may be measured in response to acoustic or electrical stimulation of the ear. Five waves are recognised as the impulse passes upwards, each peak associated with synapses in brainstem nuclei.

Automatic gain control (AGC): When allied to an amplifier automatically controls the gain in response to signal amplitude. A useful technique where soft sounds need amplification and loud ones do not. Loudness discomfort is a leading cause of distress to the deaf. Compression circuits actually reduce the signal strength to avoid discomfort when input is high.

Basal turn: First turn of the cochlea housing the neural elements responsive to high frequencies. This part of the cochlea is easily reached through the round window.

Biphasic pulses: The use of a steady or alternating current of fixed polarity may result in electrolysis and gas production at the electrode tissue interface. Pulses of opposite polarity, one phase positive and one phase negative minimise this problem.

Bipolar electrodes: Two wires terminating within the tissues close to each other such that an electrical current may pass from one to the other traversing a small volume of tissue. Spread of excitation within adjacent neurones is therefore limited.

Biocompatible: Material used within body tissues known to produce minimal adverse effects.

BSER: Brainstem evoked responses, see Auditory brainstem responses.

Cholesteatoma: Also called keratoma this is a collection of dead skin scales which accumulate in the middle ear and mastoid. Often infected and the source of offensive ear drainage the keratin mass has the power of eroding bone and causing complications such as deafness, facial paralysis and brain abcesses. The treatment is radical surgery which leaves an open ear cavity.

Cochlear partition: The bony spiral passage of the cochlea is divided into two compartments or levels by a structure called the cochlear partition. This partition contains the sensory apparatus of hearing called the organ of Corti.

Conductive deafness: Hearing loss due to mechanical obstruction to the passage of sound vibrations across the outer or middle ears. A fracture of the incus, for example, results in discontinuity of the ossicular chain. Surgical repair is often successful in conductive deafness and a hearing aid gives a very good result. Even when deafness is bilateral the subject can still hear and moderate his or her voice as it is well conducted through the bone of the skull.

Decibel: Unit of sound pressure. 0 dB is the limit of normal hearing, a conversational voice is about 50 dB and heavy machinery about 90 dB. Injury to ears occurs at sustained sound pressure levels above 90 dB.

Dynamic range: An audiograph may be marked with the maximum comfortable loudness levels at various frequencies. The part of the chart which lies between threshold and discomfort presents the dynamic range at that frequency. This range may be determined for both electrical and acoustic stimulation.

Electrode: The termination of a wire within the tissues. Often used to indicate a bundle of insulated wires passing into the cochlea.

Electrophonic hearing: Place skin disk electrodes near the ear and deliver the electrical analogue of speech at a suitable amplitude (an audio signal) and speech will be perceived. The skin-electrode interface acts as a small loudspeaker and the effect is absent in a deaf ear.

Extracochlear stimulation: Electrical stimulation by an electrode placed as near the cochlea as possible, usually in the round window niche or on the promontory.

Facial recess: Hollow in the wall of the middle ear cavity next to the descending portion of the facial nerve. The recess may be entered from the mastoid side by drilling.

Formants of speech: Sound energy in speech is not evenly distributed across the frequency spectrum. Peaks of energy occur in up to four narrow pitch bands and make each sound unique. The first is the low frequency laryngeal band and the second, third and fourth bands originate in the resonance of the pharynx, nose and mouth. They are called the first, second and third formants.

Ganglion cells: The 32,000 or so cochlear nerve fibres connecting each ear to the brain have their cell bodies in the centre of the spiral core of the cochlea. This concentration of cell bodies is called the spiral ganglion.

Hard wired: see Percutaneous connector.

Indifferent electrode: The ground or earth electrode required to complete a circuit. Often this is buried in the temporalis muscle.

Intracochlear stimulation: Electrical stimulation by an electrode or electrodes within the bony cochlea, usually passed through the round window into the scala tympani.

Inductive link: Two wire coils in close proximity, one inducing a current in the other. A signal may thus be passed through the skin to an implanted device from a surface antenna coil, without the need of cables through holes in the skin.

Labyrinthitis: Inflammation of the passages within the organ of hearing or balance is usually due to viral or bacterial proliferation in the spaces and results in loss of function. New bone may be laid down and obliterate the bony passages.

Mastoidectomy: Surgical approach to the middle ear by removing all or part of the party wall between middle ear and mastoid air cell spaces. Performed through an incision behind the ear, it is a common operation for cholesteatoma (see above).

Middle turn: Part of the cochlea responsive to middle sound frequencies.

Modiolus: Axial bony spiral of the cochlea hollowed out to accommodate the cell bodies of the cochlea nerve (the spiral ganglion).

Monpolar electrode: A wire terminating near or in the tissues of the cochlea which when electrically active passes a current through a wide volume of tissue to a remote, indifferent or ground electrode. This is usually located in the Eustachian tube or the temporalis muscle. Spread of excitation in surrounding neurones is controlled by current size.

Multichannel: Device in which several signals may be simultaneously delivered to two or more sites within the cochlea.

Neuroprosthesis: A device to stimulate or inhibit nerve impulses by manipulation of electrical current applied to nervous tissue. A cochlear implant is an example.

Organ of Corti: The hair cells, supporting cells and the connecting fibres of the auditory nerve are collected together in a strip running from base to apex of the cochlea, bathed in the fluid of the middle compartment. This is the place where mechanical movement is changed into nerve impulses and is called Corti's organ.

Osteoneogenesis: New bone formation.

Osseous lamina: Spiral shelf of bone in the cochlea which supports the membrane on which the organ of Corti rests. Contains terminal fibres of the auditory nerve.

Percutaneous connector: Wires or a plug passing out through the skin. Hard wired is a less precise term for the same arrangement. Good for electrical access to the electrode but prone to infection and only used for short periods.

Perilymph: Fluid filling the bony passages of the cochlea and semicircular canals. Fluid within the inner membraneous passages is called endolymph.

Place-pitch: The organisation of the cochlea into regions each most sensitive to a specific sound frequency. The travelling wave has its peak amplitude in the basal turn for high pitches and in the apical turn for low pitches.

Postlingually deaf: Severe or total loss of hearing after the acquisition of a spoken language, these are the people most likely to benefit from a cochlear implant. The first four years of childhood are crucial.

Prelingually deaf: Severe or total loss of hearing at a very young age. Most deaf people who prefer to communicate by sign language were deafened before or at birth. If part of the brain is set aside as a reference library for syntax, grammar and vocabulary of a spoken language this remains unfilled. The same features of a signed language are probably located in association with the visual cortex rather than the acoustic cortex of the brain. Cochlear implants are theoretically of no benefit to the prelingually deafened adult; those that have been fitted with implants tend not to use them.

Promontory: The bulge in the wall of the middle ear opposite the tympanic membrane. The promontory is grooved by the sensory nerves of the middle ear, indented by the round and oval windows, and partly encases the basal turn of the cochlea.

Radical cavity: The space left when surgery to remove middle ear and mastoid disease has been performed. This space is accessible through the ear canal which is generally made wide for this purpose.

Scala tympani: A tapering passage 36 mm long within the bony cochlea, beginning at the round window and ending at the cochlear apex. This is the most common site for an intracochlear electrode.

Sensory-neural deafness: Deafness due to loss of sensory hair cells and cochlear nerve fibres. It is characterised by loudness discomfort and loss of discrimination.

Speech processor: An amplifier, usually worn on the body, delivering an electrical analogue of speech to the implanted electrode. Elements of the speech signal, thought to be most readily passed to the brain through the implant, may be selected and the range of loudness is strictly controlled.

Speech reading: Lip-reading enhanced by a lively appreciation of the speaker's position, posture and gestures, all of which are social signals or clues to the content or significance of speech.

Swage: Die or former for shaping metal parts by hammering or pressure.

Thresholds: The limits of perception, in this case for sound.

Tinnitus: Sounds perceived to originate in the ears or head when in a quiet place. The sufferer hears a sound like escaping steam or a radio out of tune and this may be so loud as to prevent sleep or drown conversation. In the worst case the sounds are continuous, life long, unrelieved by conventional treatment and lead to suicidal despair. In less serious cases the sounds may be ignored or masked by a suitable sound or the use of a hearing aid to relieve the associated deafness. Electrical stimulation of the cochlea sometimes relieves tinnitus.

Travelling waves: Von Bekesy saw that sound waves entering the cochlea by movement of the stapes produce a displacement of the basilar membrane which travels like a wave up to the apex. The envelope of the wave has a static maximum point for any given frequency.

Tono-topic: see Place-pitch.

Vibro tactile: Sensation of sound in the very low pitches which may be perceived not only by the ear but also by the fingers. Pitch discrimination of a very limited sort is possible; this help is all that some deaf people get from high power hearing aids.

Vestibular tests: Tests of function of the balancing organ.

INDEX

Ageing 58, 128
Allergy to materials 79
Anaesthesia 141
Audiometry (pure tone) 130
Audiometry (special) 129
Auditory nerve physiology 46-8
Australia 15, 17
Austria 15, 17

Ballantyne J.C. 10, 13, 18
Bacterial labyrinthitis 127
Banfai P. 19
Biomaterials 77
Biostim 109
Bipolar stimulation 223

California, University of 22
Caloric responses 136
Canal route 141
Carbon 88
Carcinogenesis of foreign bodies 79
Carrier wave 221
Ceramics 86
Cerebrospinal Fluid (CSF) leaks 152
Charge densities 224
Clark G. 15, 17, 113, Chapter 11
Children 128, 161
Chouard C.H. 14, 19, 111
Circuits
    digital 215
    integrated 218
Cochlear mechanics 27-32
Cochlear transduction 32-9
Common ground stimulation mode 223
Complications of surgery 152
Congenital deafness — ganglion cell
    survival 128
Consent to surgery 138
Consonants, voiced and unvoiced 174
Copenhagen 116
Corrosion 89
Current, effects of 58
Current densities 90

Dacron 83
Damage by electrodes 62
Davis H. 39
Deafness
    congenital 128
    total 130
    syphilitic 127
    traumatic 127
    vascular 127
Degeneration of neurones 52

Design of implants 74
Digital Circuits 215
Djourno 1, 2; *see also* **Eyries**
Douek E.E. 16, 118

Eddington D.K. 110
Electrode 11
    bipolar 6, 7
    hard wire gold 4
    modiolar 4, 5, 8
    monopolar 6
    pseudobipolar 6
    stainless steel 4
Electrode insertion 146
Electrode types 11, 97, 103, 108-20
Electrolysis 66, 156
Electrophonic hearing 1, 4
Encapsulation 91
Environmental sounds 180
Epoxy 91
Evoked responses (ERA) 131
Expectations, questionnaire for 138
External Pattern Input Group (EPI) 18,
    176
Extracochlear devices 118
Extracochlear stimulation 190
Eyries 1, 2; *see also* **Djourno**

Facial recess route 148
Failure, insulation 154
Failure of electronic components 157
First International Conference on Electrical
    Stimulation 9-10
Fisch V. 16, 19
France 14, 19
Frequency
    formant 214
    fundamental 214
    transformation, use of 176
    voicing 174

Ganglion cell survival 55, 125

Hair cells
    anatomy 32-7
    inner 39-41
    outer 41-3
    physiology 37-49
Hearing aid, implant used with 186
Histological changes 186
Hochmair E.S. 111
Hochmair-Desoyer I.J. 15, 17
House W.F. 2, 7, 12, 108
House Ear Institute 13, 28

234 Index

Implant used with hearing aid 186
Inductive link 220
Infection 80
Inflammatory reaction to implants 78
Injuries to implants 154
Instruments 143
Insulation failures 155
Integrated circuits 218

Kemp D.T. 42
Kiang N.Y.S. 8

Labyrinthitis (bacterial and viral) 127
Leak testing 93
Leaks, Cebrospinal Fluid (CSF) 152
Lip-reading, improvements in 175, 180, 185
Los Angeles Group 7, 22

Menieres Disease 127
Merzenich M.M. 7, 22
Metals for implantation 88, 90
Michelson R.P. 5, 7, 12, 22
Microphone 216
Minimum Auditory Capability (MAC) Test 131
Modiolar electrodes 151
Monopolar stimulation 223
Multichannel 189

Nerve fibre counts 70
Nucleus Ltd (Australia) 113, Chapter 11, 212

Olivocochlear bundle 41
Otitis externa 127
Otosclerosis 127
Ototoxic deafness 54, 127

Packaging the receiver stimulator 225
Parylene 85
Patient selection 10–11
Percutaneous cable 103
Pitch extraction 174
Pittsburgh Group 10
Polyester 83
Polyethylene 82
Polymers 80, 81
Polymethylmethacrylate 85
Polyurethane 84
Post mortem of temporal bones 61
Posterior tympanotomy approach 148
Postoperative care 149
Power consumption 212
Power transmission 225
Project Ear Foundation 18
Psychological assessment 137
Pure tone audiometry 130

Questionnaire for expectations 138
Questionnaire for selection 125

Radiological examination 133, 160
Receivers 107
Receiver-stimulator 222
Rehabilitation, effects of 184
Round window anatomy 60

San Francisco Group 9, 10, 12, 22
Schlinder R.A. 9
Sealing implants 91, 211, 226
Selection, questionnaire for 125
Sellick P.M. 29
Silicones 83
Simmons F.B. 4, 8, 9, 12, 21, 114
Single channel 189
Sounds
  environmental 180
  voiced and unvoiced 213
Speech
  discrimination 181
  processors 170, 174, 213
  production, effects on 186
  signal, amplitude of 213
Spoendlin H. 9
Stanford Group 10, 12, 21, 114
Sterilisation 154
Stimulation
  bipolar 223
  extracochlear 190
  monopolar 223
Stimulation mode, common-ground 223
Stress fractures 227
Surgery, complications of 152
Surgical approaches 12
Switzerland 16, 19
Syphilitic deafness 127

Teflon 82
Tinnitus and suppression of 136, 153, 181
Torpedo fish 1
Total deafness 130
Transmission links 11–12, 219
Traumatic deafness 127
Travelling wave 27–32
Tuning curves 41–7

University of California San Francisco (UCSF) 22
  cochlear implant system 96
University College Hospital London 18
University of Utah 13, 22–3
University of Washington 13, 23
Urban J. 7

Vascular deafness 127

Vestibular nerve 56, 64
Viral labyrinthitis 127
Voice, production and pathology 139
Voiced and unvoiced sounds, consonants 174, 213

Voicing frequency 174
Volta A. 1
Von Bekesy G. 27

West Germany 19